RETHINKING
AIDS PREVENTION

RETHINKING AIDS PREVENTION

Learning from Successes in Developing Countries

Edward C. Green

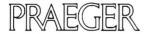

Westport, Connecticut
London

Library of Congress Cataloging-in-Publication Data

Green, Edward C. (Edward Crocker), 1944–
    Rethinking AIDS prevention : learning from successes in developing countries / Edward C.
Green
      p.   cm.
    Includes bibliographical references and index.
    ISBN 0–86569–316–1 (alk. paper)
    1. AIDS (Disease)—Prevention.   2. AIDS (Disease)—Developing countries—Prevention.   3.
AIDS (Disease)—International cooperation.   I. Title.
RA643.8.G74 2003
616.97'9205—dc22   2003059691

British Library Cataloguing in Publication Data is available.

Library of Congress Catalog Card Number: 2003059691
ISBN: 0–86569–316–1

First published in 2003

Praeger Publishers, 88 Post Road West, Westport, CT 06881
An imprint of Greenwood Publishing Group, Inc.
www.praeger.com

Printed in the United States of America

The paper used in this book complies with the
Permanent Paper Standard issued by the National
Information Standards Organization (Z39.48–1984).

10 9 8 7 6 5 4 3

Every reasonable effort has been made to trace the owners of copyright materials in this book, but
in some instances this has proven impossible. The author and publisher will be glad to receive
information leading to more complete acknowledgments in subsequent printings of the book and
in the meantime extend their apologies for any omissions.

Contents

Preface

Books and articles about global AIDS, particularly if they focus on Africa, are usually of the doom and gloom variety. They typically provide updated statistics on the soaring number of people infected and indirectly affected by HIV, as well as the cumulative numbers of AIDS deaths. We are reminded that the situation is catastrophic and whatever the amount of money has been available to address the problem, it is only a tiny fraction of what is needed. We are assured that there are great hidden epidemics in countries like Indonesia and the Philippines, where official HIV infection rates remain very low. We are warned that in Africa, where infection rates are already the highest anywhere, they are actually higher than we think because sentinel surveillance of HIV infection rates is greatly underestimating actual rates.

Another, far less-common genre of global AIDS literature urges us not to give up on the problem because there are two or three rays of hope in the less-developed parts of the world. Thailand and Uganda are often mentioned, as are condoms. The present book resembles the latter genre in that I believe there is, indeed, hope. I focus a great deal on countries that have achieved at least a measure of success. But their success stories are not unfolding the way most of us anticipated.

Acknowledgments

Thanks for support are due to Harvard University's Takemi fellowship in International Health program, the Harvard Center for Population and Development Studies, and USAID. All but one of my information-gathering trips to Uganda were under USAID funding. USAID also supported some of the research that went into this book under its ABC Study, a joint initiative that involved the Office of HIV/AIDS and the Office of Family Planning. The literature review that underlies some of the sections on faith-based organizations was supported by USAID under the Synergy project. Of course, the views expressed are mine alone. I also wish to thank a number of individuals for intellectual and moral support. Listing them should not be taken as evidence that all necessarily agree with my views or conclusions, for which I am solely responsible. They are listed here in alphabetical order: Saiffudin Ahmed, Milton Amayan, Stephanie Baldock, Tom Barton, Tony Bennett, H. Russell Bernard, Ruth Bessinger, Jim Coates, Jim Chin, Paul DeLay, Amitai Etzioni, Nomi Fuchs, Daniel Halperin, Norman Hearst, Penn Hendwerker, Alan Hill, Jan Hogle, William W. Howells, Doug Kirby, Emmanuel Kusemererwa, Daniel Low-Beer, Ray Martin, Tom Merrick, Marc Mitchell, Henry Mosley, Elaine Murphy, Vinand Nantulya, Yaa Oppong, Anne Peterson, Michael Reich, Rev. Sam Ruteikara, Rand Stoneburner, Jim Shelton, Jeff Spieler, and Martin Ssempa. I am happy to report that when I began to come forward with the evidence in this book, there were enough open- and fairminded officials at both USAID and the World Bank to keep me going.

I also wish to sincerely thank Greenwood Publishing for instantly recognizing the significance of my original book proposal, and for being such pleasant people to work with throughout this undertaking.

Abbreviations and Acronyms

ABC	Abstain, Be Faithful, or Use Condoms
ACP	AIDS Control Program
AIC	AIDS Information Centre (Uganda)
AIDS	Acquired Immune Deficiency Syndrome
AMREF	African Medical and Research Foundation
ANC	Antenatal Clinics
APCP	AIDS Prevention and Control Project (Uganda)
ARV	Antiretroviral
BCC	Behavior Change Communications
BSS	Behavioral Sentinel Surveillance
CBD	Community-based Distribution
CBO	Community-based Organization
CDC	Centers for Disease Control
CHUSA	Church Human Services AIDS Prevention and Care (Uganda)
CRS	Catholic Relief Services
CSW	Commercial Sex Worker
DHS	Demographic and Health Surveys
EPMS	Extra- and Premarital Sex
FBI	Faith-based Intiative
FBO	Faith-based Organization
FDA	Food and Drug Administration
FHI	Family Health International

FSW   Female Sex Worker
GFATM   Global Fund to Fight AIDS, Tuberculosis, and Malaria
GPA   Global Program on AIDS
HAART   Highly Active Antiretroviral Therapy
HEART   Helping Each Other Act Responsibly Together
HIV   Human Immunodeficiency Virus
IDU   Injecting Drug Use
IEC   Information, Education, Communication
IMAU   Islamic Medical Association of Uganda
KABP   Knowledge, Attitudes, Behaviors, Practices
LAC   Latin America/Caribbean (region)
MAP   Multicountry HIV/AIDS Program
MSM   Men Who Have Sex with Men
NGO   Nongovernmental Organization
NIH   National Institutes of Health
NRC   National Research Council
PBC   Primary Behavior Change
PDA   Population and Community Development Association
PLWHA   Person Living with HIV/AIDS
PVO   Private, Voluntary Organization
RBIs   Religious-based Initiatives
SBC   Sexual Behavior Change
SHEP   School Health Education Program (Uganda)
STD   Sexually Transmitted Disease
STI   Sexually Transmitted Infection
TASO   The AIDS Support Organization (Uganda)
THETA   Traditional and Modern Health Practioners Together
           against AIDS (Uganda)
UNAIDS   Joint United Nations Program on HIV/AIDS
UNFPA   United Nations Population Fund
UNGASS   United Nations General Assembly Special Session
UNICEF   United Nations Children's Fund
USAID   U.S. Agency for International Development
VCT   Voluntary Counseling and Testing
WHO   World Health Organization
WLI   World Learning Inc.

INTRODUCTION

Why Do We Need to Rethink AIDS Prevention?

When I started this book in 2001, there were plans afoot to develop a U.N. war chest of $7–10 billion per year to address the AIDS crisis, along with tuberculosis and malaria. This was sometimes referred to as a kind of relief Marshall Plan which was urgently required to save lives. By early 2002, the Global Fund had been established. The first meeting of the board of the Global Fund to Fight AIDS, Tuberculosis, and Malaria (GFATM) took place in Geneva on January 28–29, 2002. It was appearing as if the Global Fund would become the largest donor for international AIDS programs. The World Bank was also adding an additional $500 million to its Multi-Country HIV/AIDS Program (MAP) for Africa.

Then in January 2003, President Bush announced a U.S. initiative of spending $15 billion over five years. It appeared that the United States would control most of this money bilaterally, which is to say it would go through American government agencies. Thus, U.S. AIDS policy promises to become even more important in the future than it has been in the past. But whoever spends the funds, we are seeing the greatest mobilization of resources ever directed toward a health problem.

Where will these billions go? Will they be put to good use? Or will most money continue to go to drugs and drug companies, consultants, and condoms? Could billions of dollars be put to better use in AIDS prevention?

From both the scientific literature and public discourse about global AIDS, including discussions about the new Global Fund, the impression is certainly given that experts know how to prevent AIDS. AIDS prevention organizations in the private sector, whether for profit or not-for-profit, speak confidently about "proven interventions," which refer to condoms (female, as well as male, nowadays) and treatment of sexually transmitted infections (STIs). The first applications for grants under the Global Fund sometimes used titles such as Cambodia's "Partnership for Going to Scale with Proven Interventions for HIV/AIDS, TB, and Malaria" (this received about $16 million).

Carael and Holmes (2001), in their introduction to a special issue of *AIDS*, note that many in the AIDS field believe that, two decades into the global pandemic, we understand the epidemiology of the disease and what the appropriate interventions should be—it is only a matter of raising adequate funds and scaling up the known interventions. Yet these authors suggest that better understanding of HIV dynamics might lead us to refocus on new and more appropriate interventions. This understanding ought to come from research directed at the central questions of why HIV infection rates vary so greatly in different parts of the world, and how epidemics of 30 percent of the adult populations of some African cities can be *sustained* "despite the impact of AIDS-related mortality depleting the most vulnerable segments of the populations" (Carael & Holmes, 2001, p. S1).

Yet as two observers admit bluntly in the following:

It is simply untrue that we know what works in HIV control. There have been few controlled trials with HIV infection as an outcome and the distribution of sex acts within partnerships and the associated risks have rarely been measured. It is more accurate to say that we know what might work and as our understanding of transmission improves then we can be more confident in our prescriptions. (Garnett & Rottingen, 2001, p. 641)

Reflecting the latter view, a senior USAID official in Washington also stated candidly in a recent presentation that HIV/AIDS is an imperfectly understood phenomenon, meaning that we do not really know what accounts for wide variation in HIV infection rates, nor do we really know what the critical interventions and key program elements should be to address the pandemic.

Still, we know or ought to know quite a bit. The main objective of this book is to bring greater connectivity between information now available about global AIDS prevention and how we spend billions of dollars in AIDS programs. It would not be too far from the truth to say that how we currently spend AIDS prevention funds worldwide is based to a large extent on what we think we knew about AIDS in America in the mid-1980s.

FOCUS OF THIS BOOK

This book focuses on heterosexual transmission of HIV in less-developed countries, which accounts for most of the AIDS in the world.

The greatest focus, in fact, will be on the part of the world with the highest HIV infection rates, sub-Saharan Africa.[1] This region accounts for 70 percent of the world's HIV infections. There is only one African country with an indisputable and significant decline in national HIV prevalence—Uganda. There are two other possible success stories: Senegal, where HIV prevalence has remained remarkably low and stable; and Zambia, where prevalence has declined among youth. I cover the experience of each of these countries.

I will also be discussing the major virus that causes AIDS—HIV-1. HIV-2 will be differentiated by name when it comes up. The secondary geographic focus will be on the region with the second highest infection rates—the Caribbean. The predominant modes of transmission in both areas are the same, heterosexual vaginal intercourse (see below for characteristics of so-called Pattern II transmission). The focus is also on generalized epidemics and majority (general) populations, rather than on concentrated epidemics and special high-risk groups, such as we find in the epidemics of the United States or Europe. One of the insights that motivated the writing of this book is that the basic model of AIDS prevention adopted virtually everywhere derived in large measure from the first programs designed in the United States for the local epidemic. These programs were developed for high-risk groups. Yet most HIV infections in the world are found in sub-Saharan Africa and the Caribbean, and in majority populations rather than in high-risk groups.

The focus of this book is on sexually transmitted AIDS, which accounts for most transmission. There will be only peripheral discussion about injection drug use, vertical or mother-to-child transmission, and impure blood supplies. The focus is also on AIDS prevention, although there is a short section on care and support of those already HIV infected. In both prevention and care, I hope to show that different approaches are needed in order to have more impact in less-developed countries. Recommendations will be evidence based, which is to say, informed and inspired by empirical findings from biological and behavioral sciences. I believe that current business-as-usual approaches to HIV prevention are driven at least as much by politics, financial or business interests, and entrenched mindsets as by science.

I may be accused of hubris for questioning so much of the received wisdom about AIDS, but I find the courage to raise questions because prevention programs have not been very successful, with a handful of exceptions. Also, there are powerful economic interests and related political forces at work guiding the allocation of billions of dollars. Science, reason, and plain common sense can all become forgotten in the face of such considerations and forces. We who work in AIDS, as in other fields, fall into thinking and operating within certain paradigms which become mindsets, which in turn erect blinders to ideas and evidence that fall outside—or contradict—the prevailing paradigm. Most who work in AIDS, as in any crisis situation I suppose, become so caught up in daily battles that they lack the time and the perspective to think critically about why they are doing what they are doing. Finally, most AIDS professionals know only one part of the world and one pattern of HIV transmission. It is natural to project assumptions and lessons from the area one knows best onto the rest of the world. Yet there are so many highly divergent patterns of HIV transmission that making assumptions about African AIDS based on experience in, say, San Francisco or Bangkok, becomes especially fraught with peril.

METHODS

I consider evidence from available studies, published or in some cases unpublished. The validity and reliability of studies of course vary on the basis of general design (e.g., cross-sectional, cohort studies; community intervention trials; various types of qualitative research, such as focus group discussions or in-depth, key informant interviews), as well as size and representativeness of sample and other factors that determine the quality and overall usefulness of the study. This book is not an extended, formal meta-analysis of data from studies that meet certain predetermined criteria. I reviewed all studies I was able to find within a timeframe of about two years, although I have been accumulating studies about AIDS from the beginning of the pandemic. Some studies are unknown outside of the countries where they were conducted. It helps to be an "insider" who works in international AIDS and has access to unpublished reports, and to reports before they are published. Still, the majority of literature cited is published in peer-reviewed journals and is available to anyone.

I can probably be accused of bias in favor of selecting certain kinds of studies; namely, those that show evidence of the importance of what I call *primary behavior change* (PBC): partner reduction, delay of sexual debut among youth, and abstinence for a specified time period. If I have done this, it is because there are thousands—tens of thousands— of papers that assume or argue that the AIDS prevention interventions heavily favored by the donors are the best, even the only, interventions that ought to be supported. Therefore, I have the task of challenging two decades of research and policy papers in the course of one publication. I am trying to present another view, to show other types of research findings that have rarely been part of the public discourse about AIDS prevention, at least until very recently.

Attribution of causality in the context of a disease like AIDS and change in sexual behavior is difficult under the best of circumstances. In addition to reasons for this inherent in the limitations of various methodologies, it is also the case that people are exposed to multiple messages and other interventions over whatever period of time we are considering. It is usually impossible to isolate the impact of specific factors being investigated. Therefore, at the end of this book, the most we can hope for is something suggestive rather than definitive.

I ask readers to judge the book on the overall weight of evidence presented. Strict methodologists will doubtless find weaknesses in certain studies and perhaps in my interpretation. Some will believe that studies that have not undergone peer review should not even be discussed in this or any book. But adoption of that criterion would force exclusion of rich resources, such as, the Demographic and Health Survey (DHS), which are funded by USAID and are highly influential in decisions made by USAID, UNAIDS, and other major donors. The same can be said of behavioral surveys conducted every two years by the Uganda Ministry of Health. There is also a publication bias in favor of excluding studies with "negative results," even though this evidence may be important. Even if there are some studies that have insufficient sample sizes or are otherwise weak, I hope readers will not take this as a reason to reject the rest of the evidence assembled here. All I hope for by the end of this book is to have convinced readers that there ought to be a broader range of behavioral options promoted in AIDS prevention programs than at present, and that there ought to be more targeting of interventions on the basis of age, gender, group, and other important differentiating criteria. As simple and reasonable as these propositions may appear, accepting them has profound implications in how we spend billions of dollars in AIDS programs. And it is never easy to change how billions are spent.

An economics professor is credited with having said that it is better to be vaguely right than precisely wrong. I hope that I am at least this way.

PERSONAL NOTE

I have found from personal experience that those who raise any sort of question about condom effectiveness or who suggest that reducing the number of sexual partners might help reduce HIV transmission may be accused of being part of the religious right wing, someone beyond the pale of scientific discourse. Therefore, I find it necessary to state up front my liberal, contraceptive, and AIDS credentials.

Starting with contraceptive credentials, I spent three years working for a global contraceptive social marketing project (SOMARC), with special responsibilities for the Dominican Republic, which has one of the best social marketing programs in the world. I have also worked as a consultant for the Pathfinder Fund and for Population Action International (formerly, the Population Crisis Committee) in a project I designed to promote condoms in Nigeria. I have published in the periodical *Studies in Family Planning*. My father was the first ambassador for population affairs at the State Department and was on the board of family planning organizations such as Population Action International. I myself served on the board of the World Population Society for five years. I believe in the need for contraception. But I have come to believe from mounting evidence that AIDS prevention must involve more than contraceptives and drugs.

I have also worked extensively in all parts of Africa, in HIV/AIDS and in other areas of health research and health care provision. I served as an advisor to the Ministries of Health in Swaziland (1981–1983) and Mozambique (1994–1995). I have done a great deal of research on indigenous or traditional health beliefs and behavior, and on indigenous health practitioners. I wrote a book, called *AIDS and STDs in Africa* (Green 1994), based on my research findings and my program experience in several African countries.

As an anthropologist, it is glaringly clear to me that AIDS prevention programs designed by Western experts have been to a large extent incompatible with the cultures of Africa and other resource-poor parts of the world. Why have more Africans and other recipients of donor assistance not complained about this? Simply because people in need of funds quickly learn how to play the game. Whatever donors are prepared to fund, that is what people in need will ask for. They will not risk angering donors by insisting that funds go to interventions that are not in current favor with the donors.

This game reflects badly on donor organizations. It reflects ethnocentrism and technological arrogance. After all, who can know more about how to influence the behavior of Ugandans and Senegalese than Ugandans and Senegalese themselves? In any case, the export of Western models of behavior change has not had much impact on the ultimate measure—national HIV prevalence. Meanwhile, AIDS prevention and behavior change responses that have been to a large extent indigenous seem to have had significant impact on national HIV prevalence. This book summarizes the evidence for this bold statement and makes a plea for evidence-based AIDS prevention, as distinct from consensus-based prevention. In presenting this evidence, I have no moral agenda regarding human sexuality. My only agenda is to give credit to the indigenous prevention approaches that evidence shows have been most effective in the fight against AIDS.

OVERVIEW OF THESIS

The arguments and hypotheses presented in this book are summarized here for the reader who may wish an overview, or who may wish to read only one or two chapters of special interest.

In discussing global AIDS, it is useful to make a distinction between high-risk, core transmitter groups, such as men who have sex with men (MSM), injecting drug users (IDU), commercial sex workers (CSWs), and the like, and the general or majority populations. The latter term denotes those in a population who do not exhibit special high-risk behaviors for HIV infection, relatively speaking. We speak of *generalized epidemics* when most HIV infections are found in the majority population, that is, mostly outside of special high-risk groups. And we speak of *concentrated epidemics* when most infections are found mostly in defined high-risk groups. This book and the summary comments in this section pertain primarily to generalized epidemics and majority populations.

When people in majority populations of developing countries are asked about sexual behavior in surveys (such as, the DHS, and WHO/GPA or UNAIDS surveys), they usually report that they have changed their behavior as a result of AIDS. When asked how their behavior has changed, the most common answers are as follows: fidelity to one's partner, reduction in the number of sexual partners, delay of sexual debut (among youth), and sexual abstinence for a period. It is useful to refer to these actions as primary behavior change.[2] PBC tends to be reported far more frequently than condom use, in fact between five and ten times more frequently in unprompted, open-ended questions. In Africa, PBC is reported frequently in longitudinal or panel surveys, in evaluations of AIDS prevention campaigns, and, indeed, in every type of survey. Answers of this sort also show up in qualitative research. Yet for some reason, these answers are often overlooked or ignored. Some surveys even bury them in the "other" or "miscellaneous" response category.

PBC seems to be the spontaneous, indigenous, or natural response to concern over, or fear of, HIV infection. It is the behavior change that most people choose for themselves, whether or not it is promoted. However, when PBC is actively promoted, even more of this type of behavioral change seems to result than when it is not, plus we are building upon and enhancing what people are already inclined to do, if not already doing. It makes public health sense to build upon what people already do rather than put all or most of AIDS prevention resources into promoting an alien technology, something that involves monetary costs to the target audience and that needs to be constantly resupplied in vast quantities. At least this makes sense if promotion of PBC can be shown to reduce HIV transmission significantly.

When there are behavioral data from DHS from the same country over a period of time, pertaining to age of sexual debut and proportions of sexually active before marriage, as well as proportions reporting multiple partners, the behavioral trend is almost always in the direction of less risk. Condom use also rises (with some exceptions, such as Malawi). Increases in condom use are often noted in DHS reports, while primary behavior changes are seldom if ever commented upon. This partly explains why fundamental changes in sexual behavior have gone largely unnoticed by so many experts. But the bias against PBC goes far beyond DHS.

PBC programs may be the natural response to AIDS of Third World governments as well as their citizens. My Ugandan colleague, Vinand Nantulya, refers to PBC interventions as endogenous responses to AIDS, while condom-drug interventions are considered exogenous responses. Prevention programs developed before foreign donor-driven projects exerted much influence in Uganda and Senegal had strong components of PBC. It is also instructive to look at Jamaica's program since 1995, which has an unusual degree of independence from donor organization design. Jamaica's prevention programs represent a balance of PBC, condom promotion, and STD treatment. Yet prevention programs that emphasize PBC programs may be diluted or thwarted by well-meaning foreign experts who are sure they have the only proven interventions that will prevent AIDS. Most national AIDS prevention programs put few actual resources into PBC, reflecting what I sometimes call the Washington-Geneva consensus that AIDS programs should not interfere with peoples' sexual behavior.

It can only be good that other behaviors beyond condom use are starting to change, since condom use is irregular and inconsistent in Africa and most other parts of the world. A recent Cochrane review found condoms have an 80 percent rate of effectiveness in averting HIV infection if they are used consistently. The great majority of condom use in Africa and elsewhere is inconsistent, plus only 80 percent effectiveness itself represents a significant risk. A recent study in Uganda shows that inconsistent condom use is significantly associated with an increased risk of certain STDs. "Inconsistent condom use may actually be an 'enabling' process allowing individuals to persist in high risk behaviors with the false sense of security" (Ahmed, Lutalo, Wawer, Serwadda, & Sewankambo, 2001, p. 2171). This may explain why African countries that have the highest condom user rates and the highest numbers of condoms available per male ages 15–49 (Zimbabwe, Botswana) also have the highest rates of HIV infection. In fact, there seems to be a significant and unwanted association between these two condom measures (which are also USAID impact indicators) and HIV infection rates, if we examine countries in Africa for which we have data. This association may not be causal, nevertheless it is not the association expected or desired when we promote condoms in Africa or elsewhere. As the levels of these two condom measures increase, HIV prevalence is expected to decrease.

Condom use is most likely to have national impact in countries where HIV is highly concentrated among CSWs and their clients, such as in

Southeast Asia, especially during the early stages of local epidemics. It is relatively easy to persuade men to use condoms with CSWs, or to have CSWs insist on their use as a condition for sex. If there is widespread, consistent use of condoms among these populations (such as happened in Thailand), it seems possible to choke a local HIV epidemic before there has been a great deal of *bridging* to the majority population (this refers to men infected by CSWs then infecting their wives). Yet even in Southeast Asia, men are unlikely to use condoms with wives and regular partners, especially on a regular basis. By the time prevention programs began in most of Africa and much of the Caribbean, HIV was already in the majority population.[3] As elsewhere, African men (who make condom use decisions) have shown great reluctance to use condoms with spouses or regular partners. Added to this are the problems of supplying condoms on a regular basis, condom quality, correct use, and consistent use.

USAID analysts have estimated that even with all the efforts that go into condom supply and promotion, this currently amounts only to 4.6 condoms per male per year in Africa (Shelton & Johnston, 2001). According to this analysis, condom levels peaked in sub-Saharan Africa in the mid-1990s. This means that as AIDS exploded in southern Africa, reaching the highest levels anywhere, ever, condom provision and possibly condom demand remained stable, or actually declined somewhat.

Does PBC have an impact on HIV infection rates? It appears so. The main behavioral changes that occurred in Uganda in its earlier epidemic phase (1986–1991) were partner reduction, followed by delay of sexual debut as well as increased abstinence practiced at later ages. HIV prevalence peaked nationally in 1991 and incidence peaked in about 1989 (Low-Beer, 2002, p. 1788). Even by 1995, only about 6 percent of all Ugandans were using condoms with some regularity. The national rate of condom use was about 5 percent or less before 1991, when HIV prevalence peaked. These figures suggest that condoms did not play much of a role in at least initial HIV decline there. Evidence has also emerged from Zambia that PBC, more than condom use, seems to have resulted in national-level HIV prevalence decline among urban Zambians and youth.

Given Western AIDS experts' phobias associated with the word "abstinence," let it be stressed that partner reduction was the main behavioral change reported in Uganda. HIV prevalence and behavior are measured in people ages 15–49. Most people in these age groups are married, especially in Uganda, where marriage is relatively young, and therefore sexually active. This is why Uganda's main message, for the majority population, was "zero grazing" or sticking to one partner, not abstinence. Zero-grazing (faithfulness, partner reduction) was also the primary response to prevention efforts and to the epidemic, if a distinction can be made. When Ugandans were (and are) asked what is the main thing they have done to avoid AIDS, sticking to one partner is the first and overwhelming response in all age groups except 15–19, whose first answer is delaying or abstaining. Cross-sectional surveys confirm the rank order of protective strategies.

Analysis of what has occurred in at least three other countries where HIV seroprevalence has at least stabilized or begun to decline—Senegal, Jamaica, and the Dominican Republic—suggests that there have been significant amounts of PBC in these countries, seemingly more than in other countries in their respective regions. In each of these three countries, there has been some substantial promotion of PBC along with the more usual and highly-funded condom promotion (and, in the case of Jamaica, an excellent STD case finding and treatment program). There are sections to follow on Senegal and Jamaica.

It is assumed by many who work in AIDS that delay of sexual debut and abstinence are "luxuries" not available to women in Africa and elsewhere due to poverty in general and to the low status of women in particular (e.g., Diarrah & Rielly, 2002). There is some truth to this. Yet there has been a significant and measurable empowerment of women in Uganda, making it possible for women to not only negotiate condom use better than in the past (empowerment in the context of AIDS is usually measured by a condom standard), but also to refuse unwanted sex (a better standard of real empowerment). There has also been an astonishing rise in women's employment in Uganda since the late 1980s. Empowerment of women may prove to be, if not a *sine qua non* factor in HIV prevalence decline, at least a greatly facilitating factor.

As for poverty, its alleviation certainly ought to help AIDS prevention by creating conditions conducive to PBC. But Uganda, Zambia, and Senegal all demonstrate that AIDS can be prevented even among the poorest countries in the world.

As a general rule, PBC may be the most effective intervention aimed at majority populations, at least in generalized epidemics such as those in sub-Saharan Africa and the Caribbean. Likewise, risk reduction interventions (condom promotion and provision, treating STDs) may be the most effective interventions for high-risk groups when targeting either heterosexual and homosexual transmission, not that PBC in the form of partner reduction should not also be promoted. We should support both risk reduction and risk avoidance in national programs, but with emphasis appropriate to groups targeted. For example, delay of sexual debut should probably be emphasized in primary schools, following the example of Uganda. As reasonable as this might sound, virtually all AIDS prevention funds currently go to risk reduction interventions, to interventions requiring medical products.

Research, such as the UNAIDS Multicentre study and modeling studies (e.g., Auvert & Ferry, 2002; Auvert, Buonamico, Lagarde, & Williams, 2000; Bernstein et al., 1998; Robinson, Mulder, Auvert, & Hayes, 1995), suggests that positive changes in age of debut and partner reduction can have significant impact on reducing HIV infection rates at the population level, even more than consistent condom use by large proportions of general or majority populations, something that has never been achieved. Part of the reason behind the impact of later age of sexual debut is that young females have increased biological vulnerability to HIV infection, especially when their partners are older men, as is the pattern in much of Africa and parts of the Caribbean. It should be noted that behaviors that comprise PBC are synergistically related. Several studies in the United States, the United Kingdom, Europe, Africa, and Asia have found that early age of debut is associated with higher number of lifetime partners, either for men or both genders (White, Cleland, & Carael, 2000). The implication is that promotion of delayed sexual debut also pays off in fewer sexual partners in later life.

It would appear on the basis of these findings and considerations that donor organizations and AIDS prevention programs ought to support programs with more of a balance between the elements of A, B, and C in the so-called ABCs of AIDS prevention (Abstain, Be faithful, or use Condoms if you cannot follow A or B). It can be counterargued that we already have the "official" ABC approach to AIDS prevention in many countries, but the truth is that very few resources go into A and B while many or most go to C, and to another risk reduction intervention, namely D (drugs for treatment of the curable STDs).

There are also few program impact indicators that measure A or B interventions. These indicators can be taken as shorthand measures of program activities. That is, if there are genuine, funded AIDS prevention activities, there will be impact indicators associated with them. USAID's behavioral impact indicators until quite recently were focused only on condoms and STD behaviors. More recently, one question concerning casual sex (noncohabiting, nonmarital partners) and one on age of sexual debut were added. Impact indicators are important because they are the basis for measuring progress toward the goals and objectives of program interventions. If no impact indicators exist, it is safe to conclude that there are no associated programs.

Most recently, the United Nations General Assembly Special Session (UNGASS), drawing on the experience of AIDS experts from UNAIDS and elsewhere, has decided to recommend use of only one official behavior-related program impact indicator, namely, condom use. This can be seen in the UNGASS draft Declaration of Commitment. This declaration provides guidance for both governments and civil society in AIDS prevention and mitigation programs, and given its high-level U.N. sponsorship, it will probably influence the programs supported by the new Global Fund for AIDS, TB, and Malaria. It is especially unfortunate that there will be no impact indicators associated with abstinence or delay (or partner reduction) because UNGASS focuses its global AIDS prevention program on youth. This means that condom use is the only behavior change of interest to UNGASS.

If there is evidence that PBC has been a contributor to HIV infection decline in at least some countries, and it has been widely reported in many countries, why have so few experts recognized this? This is a difficult but important question with no simple answer. The main reason may be historical: When interventions were designed for Africa and other resource-poor areas, the only prevention model available was that based on risk reduction that had been designed in the United States for special high-risk, core transmitter groups. The model seemed to work, although it must be admitted that infection rates are rising again among MSM. Nevertheless, this model was applied to populations where most of those infected were not in special high-risk groups but instead in the majority population. In short, we provided Pattern I (American) solutions for Pattern II (African and Caribbean) populations. We put our resources into an approach that has had limited impact, and this diverted attention and resources from an approach that might have had more impact.

Once the risk reduction model was launched in Africa and the developing world in the mid-1980s, it assumed a life of its own. It became the dominant, if not the only, paradigm of AIDS prevention. The few who questioned it were impatiently reminded that condoms—and later, STD treatment—were the only proven interventions. Few researchers tried to gather evidence that other, essentially unfunded interventions might be working. In fact, few donors were willing to fund unorthodox research that challenged basic assumptions about AIDS prevention (one even heard that such research was dangerous to public health). And when evidence supporting the importance of PBC arose in spite of not being specifically sought, it was largely ignored.

Additional reasons for the bias toward the risk reduction medical model relate to professional orientation, stereotypic thinking about sexual behavior as it is imagined to be in some parts of the world, entrenched business interests and powerful financial motivations to carry on business as usual, issues involving family planning, the early history of AIDS in America, and other factors. It nevertheless seems astonishing that evidence of the importance and impact of PBC has been overlooked for so long.

Who can promote PBC effectively? Again, based on the experience of Uganda and a few other countries, two groups stand out: religious groups and schools. The former, faith-based organizations (FBOs), have exactly the interest, motivation and moral authority, not to mention the resources and outreach capability, to promote PBC, or what they may prefer to call premarital chastity and marital fidelity. And schools—many of which are run by FBOs in resource-poor countries— have captive audiences of youth. It seems especially important to reach them before they become sexually active, as Uganda did and does. When we can get over the issues of whether to mention condoms in school-based AIDS education, an issue that unfortunately often keeps AIDS education out of the schools, AIDS preventive education can have great impact on the sexual behavior of youth. Uganda and Jamaica are two countries that have done this quite well. In fact, even these countries have had their problems in school-based programs, but this only suggests that even when done imperfectly, AIDS education in schools at various levels seems to have a high payoff.

People differ in various ways including how they may be willing to change. A single preventive approach to something as complex as human sexual behavior will never appeal to all people, let alone influence their behavior. Some people will continue to have multiple partners; therefore, the only preventive options may be those classifiable as risk reduction, namely, condom use and seeking appropriate treatment for STDs.[4] Yet we know that many men and a large proportion of women simply do not use condoms no matter how much education and social marketing they have been exposed to. Looking at Shelton and Johnston's (2001) condom supply data, demand for condoms seems to have already peaked in Africa in the mid-1990s. This peaking seems to have occurred at well below the levels at which they can make much difference. There need to be other preventive options for condom nonusers. We now know that many men and women respond to the abstinence (or delay) and fidelity (or partner reduction) messages, and it seems that promotion of these options can influence behavior in those directions. It certainly makes public health sense to reach both types of people and to provide the maximum range of prevention options. The current approach of promoting the maximum number of condoms to everyone, everywhere, has not paid off, particularly in Africa, where it counts, in national HIV prevalence decline. A different approach to condom promotion is needed, one that targets particular groups, situations, and behaviors.

The foregoing has broad implications for approaches to AIDS prevention and mitigation efforts. If we begin with the explicit or unconscious premise that people cannot or will not change their sexual behavior, then some sort of risk reduction is the only solution (condoms, treating STDs, clean needles in the case of injecting drug users). But if significant numbers in any population show willingness to change sexual behavior fundamentally, then we need to discover how this came about, and how we can reinforce and encourage more of the same. As noted, there is evidence from all over Africa and other parts of the world with significant national rates of HIV infection (defined roughly as over 1% of the adult population) that people are already changing their sexual behavior, even if it is not in the way most of us anticipated. In Africa, we find the most evidence for primary behavior change in Uganda, where infection rates have fallen by about two-thirds from once very high rates. And we find the most evidence of both relatively low-risk sexual behavior to begin with, and then change toward even lower-risk behavior, in Africa's other main AIDS success story, Senegal.

The evidence from Uganda is particularly compelling since it shows that if we want to achieve PBC, we can use a variety of existing and low-cost channels and mechanisms, such as peer education and sensitizing local leaders. These interventions are low cost in part because PBC promotion does not require distributing or selling any commodities (condoms, drugs, test kits) or treating STDs or any other diseases. It does not require medical or other facilities. This gets us away from the facility-based thinking that prevails among donor organizations. The outline of so many AIDS and related health interventions is dominated by exhortations to improve services, create more demand for services, and teach people the dire consequences of not using services. Some kind of "bricks and mortar" health facility is foremost in mind behind such planning. Yes, we still need to treat STDs, distribute condoms, and take care of other things in health facilities. But AIDS is a behavioral as well as a medical set of issues; therefore, AIDS prevention has much to do with promoting certain behaviors.

The region of Uganda with the lowest HIV seroprevalence (Karamoja) also happens to have the lowest recorded levels of condom use (about 3%). Yet seroprevalence in this region has declined significantly, people know about AIDS, and people have changed or maintained their sexual behavior. People there seem to have learned about AIDS and the need to change behavior mostly from interpersonal, nonfacility-based IEC. In fact, DHS studies have established that this is how most Ugandans learned about AIDS and how to prevent it. It is just that in Karamoja, there were virtually no other interventions (e.g., condom social marketing, voluntary counseling and testing, widespread treatment of STDs) that can be credited with causing or influencing prevalence decline. Nearly the same can be said about Moyo district, which has also had about a 50 percent decline in HIV prevalence, more than any country outside of Uganda.

The evidence from Uganda, and especially from Karamoja and Moyo, suggest that simple, low-cost interventions can greatly reduce HIV infection rates. Yet this realization has yet to catch on among AIDS experts. We have been blinded by an ideology of risk reduction, an approach that relies on medical solutions. We have been conditioned to think that medical commodities (condoms, pills, injections) must be delivered through medical facilities of some sort. We have also been blinded by ethnocentrism, as well as by pride, if not hubris, about which more is written later.

In addition to the central theme of this book, primary behavior change, there are other AIDS-related topics. These include not only the issue that has captured a great deal of current attention, antiretro- viral drugs and the issue of poverty, but also the possibility of new, essentially untried measures of prevention (i.e., involvement of underutilized community-based resources, such as traditional heal- ers). The male circumcision factor is such a potent factor determining HIV infection levels, especially in heterosexually driven epidemics, that it is essential to have some understanding of it to fully compre- hend the relative impact of age of sexual debut and levels of casual sex in different countries. This in fact was a conclusion—far from antici- pated at the outset—of the recent UNAIDS Multicentre study (Auvert, Buvé, Ferry, et al., 2001).[5] However, I decided not to write a section on this complex topic in this book since I would not do the topic justice. A compelling and quickly expanding body of scientific literature exists on the topic of male circumcision and AIDS.

I can say with assurance from the outset that critics will attack the foregoing on the grounds that there is not enough evidence to reach the conclusions I reach, however tentatively and however much they are framed as hypotheses for more rigorous testing. Fine, I agree we need far more research. Yet unless there is more of a consensus than there is at present about the importance of PBC, research pertaining to it is not likely to be supported.[6] I have already noticed that evidence of PBC has a hard time surviving the peer review process in medical journals.

I also predict that critics will charge that I have been selective in the evidence I discuss. My defense is that to challenge a well-entrenched paradigm, one needs to assemble a great deal of contrary evidence. There are thousands of articles, conference papers, and reports that support the reigning paradigm. The viewpoint I am submitting for consideration is seldom read or heard. In fact, one could make the case that it is excluded from public discourse precisely because it chal- lenges the paradigm.

In the early 1990s I argued for treatment of standard, curable STDs in addition to condom promotion as an effective intervention for re- ducing HIV transmission, especially in Africa where it was clear we needed an intervention in addition to condoms. There is an interest- ing lesson about paradigm modification in this intervention. A single study (Grosskurth et al., 1995) conducted in Mwanza, Tanzania, changed the thinking of the major donors, after which significant resources began to be devoted to STD (soon to be renamed STI) control programs. I think the AIDS establishment was quick to adopt the STD treatment intervention because it had all the favorable earmarks: It is a medical solution, one that involves exporting Western technology to populations thought to be deficient in this technology; it is a risk reduction solution; it to a great extent avoids behavior and changing behavior; and it is fairly expensive. Money for this intervention continues to flow even though there have been two other clinical trials in East Africa that basically challenge the findings of the Mwanza study.

Near the end of writing this book, there were signs that the paradigm might be shifting, whereas there were almost no such signs when I began writing. President Bush has recently committed $15 billion for a new global AIDS initiative, with the funding tied to programs—such as those promoting PBC—that will meet the approval of social conservatives. It is only natural that donor organizations will follow the money.

But even before this new funding became available, a few people at USAID (notably, Daniel Halperin) were beginning to think along the lines laid down in this book. I was asked to present my ideas about Uganda to a USAID audience in February 2002. Two colleagues presented similar ideas and conclusions (Nantulya at the same time, Stoneburner a few weeks later). To everyone's surprise, an overflow crowd showed up to listen. These presentations led to USAID funding an ABC study in response to a proposal I wrote with Nantulya's inputs. But the event that may go down in AIDS prevention history was a conference arranged by Kate Crawford, Daniel Halperin, and others at USAID. It was called the "ABC" Experts Technical Meeting and was held in Washington, D.C. on September 17, 2002. Halperin and Kate Crawford and other colleagues brought in key AIDS prevention people from around the world, perhaps favoring those who were or might prove to be open minded about the A and B parts of the equation. I played a minor role because my views were already well known and considered very controversial. Members of FBOs, such as Catholic Relief Services, were there as were top researchers from UNAIDS.

By the end of the one-day conference, there seemed to be consensus that the A and B parts of the ABCs of prevention were important. More attention and resources were therefore needed. It helped enormously to have USAID's new Director of the Office of HIV/AIDS Connie Carrino give her blessing to the conference (her predecessor, Paul DeLay, was supportive earlier). It seemed as if there were many AIDS professionals who had been thinking about A and B interventions but were afraid to say much in public lest they be thought of as Bush administration partisans, or worse, agents of the religious right. Once it became legitimate to discuss abstinence and fidelity as serious public health issues, and USAID seemed to be blessing the endeavor, a tipping point might have been achieved and people almost tripped over one another to identify themselves with the new way of thinking.

It may be useful for the historical record to outline the timelines of my discoveries and efforts to bring the ABC approach and evidence of primary behavior change to the attention of the AIDS establishment and the public.

ABC TIMELINES

1993. My first trip to Uganda. I see a very different type of prevention program there, as well as preliminary evidence of behavioral changes not anticipated by global experts: partner reduction and delay of sexual debut.

1998. My third trip to Uganda, for World Bank. I see convincing evidence of PBC.

1998. I conduct behavioral research in Dominican Republic and find evidence of partner reduction as a strategy to avoid HIV infection. Journals do not want to publish our results.

1998. I begin speaking out. I try to interest people in the ABC approach, but I am met with great resistance and hostility. Yet there is strong interest from the faith-based community and a handful of colleagues in international health.

2000. I become aware of research by Stoneburner and Low-Beer, whose findings on Uganda are very compatible with my own.

2001. I receive a contract to write a book about ABC and PBC.

2001. I am awarded a Takemi Fellowship by Harvard University School of Public Health, thereby providing support and a helpful environment for writing the book.

2001. My fourth trip to Uganda. I find that outside donor organizations have been diluting the ABC approach by promoting the preferred Western model of AIDS prevention. Evidence emerges of a slight trend toward riskier sexual behavior among Ugandans.

2002. Evidence emerges of a slight rise in national HIV prevalence, the first rise in a decade.

2002 (February 2). I am invited to USAID headquarters to present findings about Uganda and behavioral change. I am joined by my new colleague Vinand Nantulya, a Ugandan researcher and physician. The meeting is taped by the Voice of America and broadcast later on African TV.

2002. USAID publishes "What Happened in Uganda?" based on findings by Green, Nantulya, Stoneburner, and Stover.

2002. I submit an unsolicited proposal to USAID to conduct research in Uganda and Tanzania, with Nantulya. USAID funds similar proposal, but suggests focus on six countries.

2002. Various articles begin to appear in newspapers and national magazines about ABC.

2002 (September 17). USAID convenes "ABC" Experts Technical Meeting in Washington, D.C. A report is later published and circulated. More experts seem to begin to accept the ABC approach, as well as the evidence of PBC.

2002 (December). My fifth trip to Uganda, this time as part of a delegation with the deputy secretary of the Department of Health and Human Services, and representatives from the Centers for Disease Control, Alan Guttmacher Foundation, USAID, and the philanthropic sector.

2002 (December). Nantulya assumes a very senior position at the Global Fund for AIDS, Tuberculosis, and Malaria. He disseminates ABC evidence there and gains allies.

2002 (December 24). USAID officially adopts an ABC policy. A cable developed by the USAID administrator and signed by Colin Powell is sent to all USAID missions announcing the new ABC policy.

2003 (January). Announcement of President Bush's AIDS Initiative. President pledges $10 billion in new AIDS money, bringing the U.S. total to $15 billion over next five years.

2003 (March 1). I publish op-ed piece in *New York Times* about Uganda's ABC approach.

2003 (March 20). I testify before Congress about ABC, and brief Senate and House staff, as well as the White House. I try to ensure that the ABC model be recognized in U.S. legislation as an official policy.

2003. New congressional legislation governing the allocation of $15 billion of AIDS funds adopts the language of ABC and the lessons from Uganda.

Yet there is still great resistance to doing AIDS prevention differently. Many or most who work in AIDS persist in thinking of the ABC approach as a conservative plot rather than a proven public health intervention. At this writing, it is not clear what will happen with AIDS prevention in the future.

A note on the ABC abbreviation is in order. Some have criticized use of ABC on various grounds, such as it's too simple. But simplicity can be good. Also in its favor, ABC is immediately understood by the rank and file in Africa and other resource-poor areas of the world. It also signals that there is interest in the contributing role of three interventions and behavior changes, including condoms. It implicitly separates discourse from abstinence-only positions. This linkage helps those committed to condoms accept the A and B options. ABC also implies equivalence among the elements, although their rank order reflects the priority in which arguably they ought to be considered. ABC also implies a balanced approach, a menu of options instead of only one or two. It further implies getting down to basics, to fundamentals, and to simplicity, as in AIDS prevention need not be rocket science. Prevention can be as simple as ABC.

The genius of ABC is that it focuses attention on what individuals themselves can do to change (or maintain) behavior, and thereby avoid or reduce risk of infection. Meanwhile governments and NGOs can and should engage in what some have called A through Z, that is, D for Drugs or Destigmatizing AIDS, E for Equal opportunity or Empowerment of women, and so on.

NOTES

1. Unless otherwise qualified, "Africa" refers to sub-Saharan Africa.

2. The term "behavior change" is widely used by those who work in AIDS. It is often measured only as condom use, so there must be caution when encountering this term. It can have both a more restricted meaning (condom use) or a broader one, perhaps encompassing ABC. Behavior change in the narrow sense is likely to be confused with PBC, so it should be remembered that PBC has a distinctive meaning and that the term is new and not yet in general circulation.

3. Senegal seems to be an exception. It launched a vigorous prevention program before there was significant HIV infection levels in the majority population.

4. I will use STD, rather than the term now favored by Western donor agencies, STI. This is in part because I deal with a fair amount of historical information in this book, and STI is a recent term.

5. The Multicentre Study on Factors Determining the Differential Spread of HIV in Four African Cities (Carael & Holmes, 2001) is referred to here and elsewhere as the Multicentre study.

6. As this book goes to print, this seems to be changing, with USAID's support of the ABC study, which examines the role of PBC along with condom use in impacting HIV infection rates, as well as USAID's convening a conference on September 17, 2002, to discuss these matters in an open, objective manner.

2

Epidemiology

AIDS prevention ought to follow the distinctive epidemiological patterns found in various populations and regions of the world. Prevention also ought to follow what is known about culture of populations of interest, especially if we take culture as a broadly inclusive term that includes behavioral patterns, society, economy, polity, beliefs, values, and the like. Yet there is a deep gulf between epidemiology and culture on the one hand and AIDS prevention strategies and programs on the other. Just considering epidemiology, there are no programs that I am aware of that address risk factors such as heterosexual anal sex or use of vaginal tightening agents, to say nothing of lack of male circumcision. This last factor was found by at least one major multicountry study to be one of the most determining factors in accounting for levels of HIV infection in Africa. It is useful to begin any discussion of AIDS with a review of epidemiology.

EPIDEMIOLOGICAL OVERVIEW

As Figure 2.1 illustrates, there are great differences in the global distribution of HIV. By far the greatest number of cases are found in sub-Saharan Africa, even though areas such as south and east Asia have much greater population concentrations. If we consider prevalence rates of HIV infection, we see that one in ten sexually active adults is infected in sub-Saharan Africa. In parts of southern Africa (South Africa, Botswana, Lesotho, Namibia, Swaziland, Zambia, and Zimbabwe), this rises to one in four, or nearly one in three, the highest rates the world has seen.

Figure 2.1
Adults and Children Estimated to Be Living with HIV/AIDS, End 1999

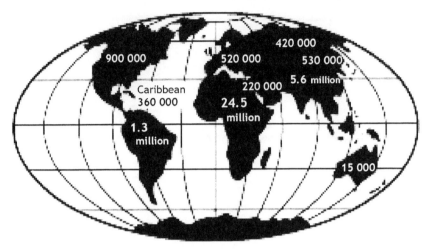

Total = 34.3 million

Source: UNAIDS/MAP 2000.

By contrast, infection rates in Asia are on the order of one in a thousand. In parts of the Caribbean, rates are about one in fifty, making this region second only to sub-Saharan Africa in HIV prevalence rate. All other parts of the world fall between those of Asia and those of the Caribbean, but most are under 1 percent.

Earlier in the epidemic, there was a convenient, shorthand way of referring to different transmission patterns. This shorthand language has been abandoned in recent years, in part because it was believed that differences between transmission patterns would diminish and there would only be one predominant pattern in the world. Yet these patterns have persisted to a large extent. It would make the task of discussing global AIDS and the development of high-impact prevention strategies much easier if we revive the prematurely abandoned typology of HIV transmission patterns. See Table 2.1.

Patterns I, II, and III were developed by the WHO Global Programme on AIDS and widely used for several years. Weniger and Brown (1996) and others proposed a fourth pattern for Southeast Asia just as use of any patterns were going out of style. In Pattern IV, a relatively high proportion of the male population (as high as 70–80% in Thailand in the early 1990s) were having sexual contact with a relatively small proportion of the female population, usually identifiable as direct or indi-

Table 2.1
Formerly Used HIV Transmission Patterns Designation

Pattern by Region	Character
Pattern 1 **Industrialized** **Countries**	• Male/male transmission—IV drug abusers • Male/female infection ratios—10:1-15:1 • Perinatal transmission—rare
Pattern II **Sub-Saharan Africa** **and the Caribbean**	• Male/female transmission • Male/female infection ratio ~1:1 • Perinatal transmission common
Pattern III **Eastern Europe, North** **Africa, Middle East**	Few cases— • Often imported by travelers of those infected by foreigners • Or infection from blood supplies
Pattern IV **Asia**	• Transmission from FSWs to male clients • Male/female infection ratios ~4:1 in early stage, then move toward 2:1

Note: FWS = female sex worker.

rect CSWs. A characteristic of the Asian pattern is maintenance of virginity until marriage and marital fidelity afterward. The pattern of many men with few women is reflected in male–female infection rates in Asia. In early stages, these tend to be 5:1, 4:1, and 3:1, then move toward 2:1 in later stages. In the Philippines, only 17–20 percent of men were visiting CSWs in the mid-1990s (Chin, Bennett, & Mills, 1998), therefore we see at once that there are exceptions to the Asian pattern proposed by Weniger and Brown. But in fact, the elements of Pattern IV seem to hold up quite well for both mainland and Southeast Asia.

Heterosexual epidemics in Southeast Asia usually start when a significant proportion of CSWs (however defined) become HIV infected, so that they constitute a core group, "that subset of the population in which the infection is present and that sustains sex partner exchange rates greater than the critical threshold" (Jones & Wasserheit, 1991, pp. 65–66). A bridge to the majority population then develops, for example, infected male clients of CSWs then infect their wives. Depending on the size of the proportion of men who have contact with the first core group, traffic on the bridge moves either quickly or slowly, so to speak. Infection rates among women in the general population begin to rise, as shown in antenatal clinic surveillance. If infection rates decline among CSWs and their clients, as happened in Thailand, infection rates become more balanced among men and women. Finally, infected mothers in the majority population pass on the infection perinatally, and the number of pediatric cases begins to rise. At least such is the model of Pattern IV.

Given the efficiency of HIV transmission from direct blood-to-blood contact and from anal intercourse, there may be relatively high numbers of IDUs and MSMs early in the development of a general HIV/AIDS epidemic, but these groups are usually quickly overtaken in numbers by heterosexually transmitted cases, at least in countries where males are not circumcised. Epidemiological data suggest that male circumcision provides a significant degree of protection against STD and HIV infection, especially in developing countries with predominantly heterosexual transmission of HIV (Bailey, Plummer, & Moses, 2002; Halperin & Bailey, 1999; Bailey, Neema, & Othieno, 1999; Moses, Bailey, & Ronald, 1998; Moses et al., 1994; Bongaarts, Reining, Way, & Conant, 1989). Since about 1995 there have been occasional calls to add male circumcision to the mix of AIDS preventive interventions, but this has not happened, although at least two clinical trials are underway at this writing, involving voluntary circumcision in Africa.

A paper (written originally in 1995) by Mills, Bennett, and by Chin, Bennett, and Mills (1998) helps explain much of the variation in Asian HIV infection rates (also see Bennett & Mills, 1996). The factors proposed include the following:

1. Levels of STDs in high-risk populations
2. Level of CSW customer turnover (e.g., high in Thai cities, low in the Philippines)
3. Level of male circumcision
4. Extent of bridging between commercial and noncommercial sexual networks (perhaps this should be broadened to read "between core groups and the majority population")

This model, based on Pattern IV epidemiologic factors, predicted in 1995 that not all Asian countries will have HIV prevalence rates as high as Thailand, Cambodia, or Burma. Some AIDS program service providers or advocates don't want to hear this, fearing that HIV/AIDS prevention funds might be diverted away from countries that seem to have low infection rates, like the Philippines and Indonesia. They ask, What if the prediction is wrong? What if current infection rates are much higher than they seem, only there has been poor surveillance? And yet HIV infections have continued to be concentrated among a few high-risk groups in these countries; AIDS has not exploded and it is not likely that it will.

It is interesting to speculate why these shorthand descriptors of global patterns of transmission were dropped from public discourse. My guess is that political pressure was brought to bear on public health professionals. The argument might have been, Let's not single out particular risk groups. That will stigmatize them—blame the victims—and make the general public feel that they are not at risk. So let's make the message more like, We are all at risk of AIDS. This has a nice, egalitarian ring: We are all in this thing together. This message would have been well received by the public health community, including those in ministries of health in developing countries, because it promised to impose no epidemiological restrictions on funds requested. For example, Indonesia, as the fourth largest country in the world, could extrapolate from African epidemiologic data and predict millions of HIV cases by the year 2000. Indonesia could then ask for funding commensurate with such a predicted catastrophe. This would be harder to do if we were still thinking about Pattern I and IV differences, and harder still if we read and understood epidemiological findings about male circumcision.

Since there is a need to distinguish different epidemiologic patterns, new language has inevitably crept back into usage among those working in international AIDS. We now speak of low, concentrated, and generalized epidemics. Countries like the Philippines are considered low. Countries like the United States or Russia have concentrated epidemics, since most infections remain in high-risk groups, even if the debate continues about whether, or the degree to which, this is changing. The countries of sub-Saharan Africa have generalized epidemics because most infections are found outside of specific high-risk groups.

EPIDEMIOLOGIC FACTORS THAT ACCOUNT FOR HIV TRANSMISSION

Policymakers, researchers, and those writing overviews of the AIDS pandemic are still making observations, such as "Reasons for different infection prevalence rates within sub-Saharan Africa are not yet understood" (Schoepf, 2001, p. 336). This is not really the case. We have learned a lot about the epidemiology of HIV/AIDS that explains much of the difference. I agree that there is more to learn, that we do not know as much as we could, perhaps especially about biological factors. But let us review what we do know, beginning with what we knew in 1994.

To explain the differences between HIV transmission in various parts of the world, Peter Piot (who is now director of UNAIDS) summarized a list of probable variables that influence the spread of HIV through sexual intercourse some years ago (Piot, 1994). These include a range of factors, ranging from HIV-1 subtype variation to presence of other STDs, a well-established factor, to various economic and political factors. The list includes the following:

Virological Parameters

Infectivity and virulence of HIV-1 strains

Level of viremia (and immunodeficiency)

Local Genital Factors

Presence of other STDs

Lack of male circumcision

Use of certain vaginal products (e.g., for "dry sex")

Sexual Behavior

Rate of partner change

Sexual mixing patterns

Type of sexual intercourse (e.g., receptive anal intercourse, sex during menses)

Size of and rate of contact with core groups

Level of condom use

Demographic Variables

Proportion of sexually active age groups to other age groups

Male-to-female ratio in the population

Proportion of urban population to rural population

Migration patterns

Economic and Political Factors

Poverty

War and social conflicts

Status of roads and mobility of population

Performance of the health care system

Response to the epidemic

Some of these factors facilitate transmission in a relatively direct way; these are referred to as proximate determinants of infection. Presence of an ulcerative STD is such a determinant. Some STD experts believe chancroid is such an efficient facilitator of HIV that it may deserve to be in a risk factor class of its own. The UNAIDS Multicenter study found additional evidence that male circumcision and herpes (HSV-2) explain much of the HIV prevalence variation in Africa (Carael & Holmes, 2001).

Other factors operate more indirectly, for example, a high male-to-female ratio in the population (related to migration, presence of roads, urbanization) leads to an increase in casual and commercial sexual activity, which in turn increases rate of partner change, sexual mixing patterns, and the size of and rate of contact with core groups. Likewise, poverty and war engender commercial sex work, homeless adults and street children, poorly educated citizens, irregular food supply and poor nutrition, migration and separated families, and—we might add—higher levels of immunodeficiency. However, this is not to say that poverty and war necessarily associate with HIV infection rates in a clear, simple, unidirectional way.

Like any other infectious diseases, HIV transmission depends on the reproduction rate of infection, that is, the average number of susceptible people infected by an infected person over his or her lifetime. Epidemiological models of transmission suggest that the reproductive rate of an infection is determined by (a) the efficiency of transmission during exposure between susceptible and infectious partners, (b) the risk of exposure of susceptible to infectious person, and (c) the duration of infectiousness (St. Louis & Holmes, 1999). The sexual transmission of HIV can be prevented by blocking the reproduction rate of infection in the following three ways: (1) by avoiding the exposure to risk (through sexual abstinence), (2) by reducing the risk of exposure (through partner faithfulness and reduction in partners), and (3) by blocking the efficiency of transmission risk (through using a barrier method, such as condom).[1] Thus we see the elegance of the ABC approach: There are three ways to block sexual transmission at the level of proximate cause, and there are three corresponding types of behavior that prevent sexual transmission. Incidentally, we almost always speak of behavior change, which assumes that current behaviors are high risk. This is not always so, particularly among female populations.

One important factor in the Piot formulation that is implied in "proportion of sexually active age groups to other age groups" is the phenomenon of age disparity. This refers to the pattern we find notably in Africa and parts of the Caribbean of younger females having older men as sexual partners (sometimes referred to as the "sugar daddy" pattern). This is when older men offer gifts of cash or some form of nonfinancial support to young unmarried women in exchange for sexual favors. The pattern has become sufficiently widespread that it often provokes little or no negative social sanction locally (Gupta & Mahy, 2001). It is of concern for several reasons, one being that young females are more susceptible to HIV infection than are males of the same age, or than they themselves would be at a later age. Some of the evidence for this is indirect. A study in Zambia and Kenya found that HIV prevalence was six times higher in women than in men among sexually active fifteen to nineteen-year-olds, three times that in men among twenty to twenty-four-year-olds, and equal to that in men among twenty-five to forty-nine-year-olds. The researchers conclude the following:

Behavioural factors could not fully explain the discrepancy in HIV prevalence between men and women. Despite the tendency for women to have older partners, young men were at least as likely to encounter an HIV-infected partner as young women. It is likely that the greater susceptibility of women to HIV infection is an important factor both in explaining the male–female discrepancy in HIV prevalence and in driving the epidemic. (Glynn, Carael et al., 2001, p. S51)

Genital trauma can also result from intercourse between adult men and young girls and from the breaking of the hymen (Carael, Buvé, & Awusabo-Asare, 1997). We return to this important issue in the section to follow.

Another relatively little-documented risk factor is the use of vaginal drying or tightening agents (mentioned under Local Genital Factors in Piot's list). Dry sex practices involve use of vaginal drying agents or implants which seem to be increasing HIV transmission through microabrasions or irritation of the vaginal lining. Such practices have been best documented in Zambia, former Zaire, and Zimbabwe, although the practice appears to be found (among African-derived populations only) in Guyana, Suriname, and the Dominican Republic, and perhaps elsewhere in the Caribbean (Halperin, 1999a; Brown, Ayowa, & Brown, 1993).

In 1996, the National Research Council (NRC) of the (U.S.) National Academy of Sciences (Cohen & Trussell, 1996) developed a summary table that is even more useful because for each epidemiologic factor, there is comment on what interventions are required and what the general time frame is for the different interventions (see Table 2.2).

Part of the value of a summary table like this is that it puts into perspective the diversity and multiplicity of factors that ought to be considered. When I hear or read about the justification for particular preventive interventions, I am often struck by how seldom the full range of relevant transmission factors are considered. I would like to see a table like this one (especially with a few improvements) made into a five-foot color poster and pinned to the walls of all who work in AIDS prevention including those who make funding decisions. An especially useful feature of the NRC table is the listing of the changes (and implicitly, interventions) associated with particular transmission factors, as well as the feasibility and probable timetable for achieving desired changes. It reminds those who put all their AIDS prevention energies into calling for structural changes, such as eradicating poverty or civil unrest, that these goals may not be achievable before HIV has run its course with particular populations and peaked or declined on its own. At the same time, it shows that societal (or environmental, or structural) factors, such as improvement of the status of women or job opportunities for women, can be achieved within a medium or not-too-distant timeframe.

Table 2.2
Factors Contributing to Sexual Transmission of HIV

Level & Definition	Examples	Changes required
Individual Factors that directly affect the individual and that the individual has some control in changing.	**Biological** History & presence; Lack of male circumcision; Anal intercourse; Sex during menses; Traumatic sex; Cervical ectopy	Prevention, STD treatment; Avoidance of sex during menses; Prevention of traumatic sex **Achievable—short-term**
	Behavioral Frequent change of sex partners; Multiple sex partners; Unprotected intercourse; Sex with a CSW; Sex with an infected partner; Lack of knowledge of STDs/HIV; Low risk perception	Abstinence; Mutual fidelity; Consistent condom use; Knowledge and skill of STD/HIV prevention **Achievable—short-term**
Societal Factors related to societal norms that encourage high-risk sexual behavior.	High rates of prostitution; Multiple partners by men; Gender discrimination; Poor attitudes toward condom use; Low social status of women; Extended postpartum abstinence	Improvement of the status of women; Job opportunities for women; Promotion of mutual fidelity; Changes I societal attitudes toward condom use **Achievable—short- to medium-term**
Infrastructural Factors that directly or indirectly facilitate the spread of HIV, over which the individual has little/no control.	Poor availability of condoms; Poor STD services; High STD prevalence; Poor communication services	Changes in health infrastructure; Improvement in STD care, behavior-change communication, and condom provision **Achievable—short- to medium-term**
Structural Factors related to developmental issues, over which both the individual and the health system have very little control.	Underdevelopment; Poverty; Rural/Urban migration; Civil unrest; Low female literacy rates; Laws/policies non-supportive of human rights Unemployment	General economic development programs; Enactment of appropriate laws/policies; Income-generating opportunities; Improvement in education of women **Feasible—long-term**

Source: NRC, Cohen & Trussell, 1996, pp. 158–159.

Note: CSW = commercial sex worker.

Missing from the NRC table is clade, or "and virulence of HIV-1 strains" in Piot's terms. This may be appropriate since the role of specific clades is still under study and not yet confirmed as a causal factor. Some investigators have suggested that clade B, which predominates in North America and Europe, is less infective than clade A or C, which predominate in Africa, or clade E, which characterizes Thailand and some other Asian populations (Soto-Ramiriz et al., 1996). However, this idea is far from accepted as a determining—or at least significant— factor, in HIV transmission. It may prove that the amount of concentration of HIV in the genital tract is a more important determinant of transmission (Cohen & Eron, 2002).

There are some additional factors directly or indirectly associated with HIV infection. For example, use of alcohol or mood altering drugs is a well-established risk factor, in that use of these substances leads to impairment of judgment, which in turn may lead to unsafe sexual practices (Carael, Cleland, Deheneffe, Ferry, & Inghams, 1995; Magnani et al., 2002).

An extended period of postpartum sexual taboo—more common in West than East Africa—is listed as a risk factor by the NRC but not Piot. There is some controversy over this. As Glynn and colleagues (2001) note, "Prolonged postpartum sexual abstinence could be a risk factor for HIV in women as it encourages husbands to seek extramarital partners. On the other hand it could be protective because it reduces the number of episodes of sexual intercourse for the wife, and may therefore reduce the risk of transmission if the husband is HIV positive." In fact, these authors studied data from six urban clinics in three African countries and found an association between HIV infection only in Yaounde, which had the longest partpartum abstinence of the three countries. But there were confounding factors and the authors cautioned against generalizing from these preliminary findings (Glynn, Buvé, et al., 2001, p. 1061).

Another factor that favored extramarital sex has been labor migration patterns in southern Africa. Black men from South Africa and from neighboring countries were not allowed to bring wives or children with them to the mines, plantations, and factories that served as magnets for employment in the region. This separation of spouses, often for periods of years, led to a great deal of sexual intercourse and sexual partners outside of marriage, and this may be a factor that helps explain why southern Africa has the highest HIV infection rates in the world.

Also missing from the NRC table is Piot's "level of viremia (and immunodeficiency)." Quinn and his colleagues (Quinn, Gray et al., 2000a; Quinn, Wawer et al., 2000b), among others, have shown that viral load is a major predictor in HIV transmission. This factor has become an essential part of the current popular argument that we somehow find the money required to provide antiretroviral drugs for the HIV-infected of

Africa. Part of the argument is that effective treatment of the HIV-infected will lower levels of viremia (viral loads) and thereby diminish the chances of these people infecting others; thus we ought to achieve some measure of prevention as well as treatment for this intervention.

Other biological factors known to increase the probability of the sexual transmission of HIV are acute primary infection or advanced clinical stage of AIDS in a partner, when viral loads are higher, menstruation (mentioned by Piot), and exposure to HIV-1 as distinct from HIV-2. Anal intercourse facilitates transmission, whether it is among MSM or heterosexuals. Heterosexual anal intercourse is widely practiced in North and Latin America as well as parts of South Asia, Africa, and other regions, yet is seldom addressed in preventive interventions (Halperin, 1999b). Use of oral contraceptives and *Depo-Provera* is associated with greater efficiency of HIV transmission, probably because hormones regulate and stimulate HIV excretion (Cohen & Eron, 2002). In addition, one study in Kenya showed that when compared with women who were using no contraceptive method, users of oral contraceptives were at increased risk for acquisition of chlamydia and vaginal candidiasis, which in turn may facilitate HIV transmission (Baeten, Nyange, Richardson et al., 2001).

Unfortunately, the NRC seems not to have gone far enough in translating recommendations found in its summary table into actions actually recommended in the text of its report. In spite of identifying abstinence and mutual fidelity as changes required in its table, these are not found in the NRC's eleven specific, highlighted recommendations at the end of its chapter on Primary HIV Prevention Strategies (Cohen & Trussell, 1996), where in fact the table is found. The specific recommendations have to do with the need for additional research (fully nine of eleven recommendations), condoms, vaginal microbicides, and promotion of gender equality.

TREATMENT OF TREATABLE STDs

Evidence has been accumulating for years that presence of standard STDs enhance the likelihood of HIV transmission. This is particularly true of the ulcerative STDs, but it is also true of nonulcerative STDs. Findings from the recent UNAIDS Multicentre study (Carael & Holmes, 2001) suggests that genital herpes (HSV-2) is a potent biological factor explaining differences in HIV infection rates between West and Southern and East Africa. It has also been observed that ulcerative STDs are far more prevalent in eastern and southern Africa than in West Africa. Some estimates have been made that attribute a high percentage of HIV infections in men in countries like Kenya and Uganda to genital ulceration (Carael, Buvé, & Awusabo-Asare, 1997).

The idea that treatment of the treatable STDs should be part of HIV/AIDS prevention has been discussed since the mid 1980s. It was the main intervention promoted in a book I wrote about AIDS in Africa (Green, 1994). Major donor funding became available after an influential study in Mwanza, Tanzania, suggested that a strong program of treating standard STDs through syndromic management programs could result in a 40 percent or more reduction in HIV infections (Grosskurth et al., 1995). As can be seen in the section on Jamaica, that country has an especially good STD case finding and treatment program. Many who work in AIDS in Jamaica attribute that country's falling STD rates and stabilized HIV rates to STD treatment. Given the modest change in sexual behavior there, STD treatment might prove to be a major factor in HIV stabilization.

However, two other large-scale, community-based, randomized controlled trials investigated the impact of STD treatment on HIV incidence, both in Uganda. Controversy developed about the efficacy of the STD treatment intervention when the Uganda trials seemed to suggest that neither mass treatment of STDs (in Rakai district) nor improved syndromic management of STDs (in Masaka district) had much effect on HIV incidence (Wawer et al., 1999), even if interventions reduced the prevalence of some STDs.

Based on modeling with "STDSIM microsimulation," the difference in outcomes between Tanzania and Uganda seems to be due to differences in stage of the epidemic, to use the language of Barcelona global AIDS conference presentations in July 2002 (Orroth et al., 2002; White et al., 2002). That is, during the periods of these trials, there was a growing epidemic in Mwanza, Tanzania, while there was a mature epidemic in the two Ugandan sites. For example, HIV prevalence was 4.1 percent and rising in Mwanza, while it was 16 percent and declining in Rakai.

However, use of language such as growing and mature obscures the fact that the major difference in outcomes seemed to be due to sexual behavior, specifically to numbers of sexual partners and age of sexual debut, although with contributions from condom use. By the time the STD treatment began in Uganda, people were no longer having multiple partners, for the most part. Researchers found that 54 percent of men reported two or more sexual partners, compared to 27 percent in Rakai and 20 percent in Masaka (see Table 2.3).

Because of risk-reduction or risk-prevention behavioral changes in Uganda, there were relatively few treatable STDs to treat (only chronic STDs such as herpes). Most current transmission in Uganda seemed to occur between discordant couples; partners were not catching treatable STDs from one another. Thus neither mass treatment nor syn-

Table 2.3
Behavioral and STI Comparisons between STI Treatment Sites in
Tanzania and Uganda

	Mwanza		Rakai		Masaka	
	Male	Female	Male	Female	Male	Female
Sexual debut (median age)	15	15	17	16	18	16
Recent sex partners (%)						
2-4	44	11	26	4	18	3
5+	10	1	1	0	2	0
Condom use (%)	2	0	20	6	28	15
STD prevalence (%)						
CT (15-39y)	2.3	13.0	2.7	3.2	2.2	1.6
NG (15-39y)	2.8	2.3	1.1	1.9	0.9	1.8
Active syphilis (15-54y)	5.6	6.3	2.3	1.4	1.2	0.7
HSV-2 (15-29y)	13.3	47.4	21.0	42.8	16.8	44.2

Source: Orroth et al., 2002.

dromic management made much difference to HIV infection levels, as summarized in the following:

Higher risk behaviour, including younger age of sexual debut, higher numbers of recent partners, and lower frequency of condom use, was apparent in Mwanza compared to Masaka and Rakai. Active syphilis, gonorrhoea, chlamydia and trichomoniasis were all more prevalent in Mwanza, except for chlamydia in males. There was little difference in HSV2 seroprevalence between sites. (Orroth et al., 2002)

This issue is summarized succinctly in the following from the Web page of the USAID–funded Horizens project ("The Mwanza and Rakai Studies: Contradictory Results or Unifying Model?"):

In the early phases of an HIV epidemic, STI control has a high impact by greatly reducing the rate at which HIV is transmitted within groups with high rates of partner change and from these groups to people with fewer partners or only one partner.

Once HIV infection has spread to people with low rates of partner change (as in a mature epidemic) and the prevalence of HIV is high enough, STI control has little or no effect on HIV transmission among those with low rates of partner change (the majority of the population). STI control will still be important for adolescents who may have a relatively high number of lifetime partners and go through a phase of frequent partner change. Thus, early in the epidemic, especially in situations where STI prevalence is high, STI prevention and control can reduce HIV incidence. In countries with a mature HIV epidemic, STI control should focus on adolescents. (Posted by the Population Council at: https://www.popcouncil.org/horizons/newsletter/sidebar.html#mwanza)

If we define "mature epidemic" as one where partner reduction (or reduction in rates of partner change) must by definition have occurred, then we can pass lightly over the highly significant behavioral change we find in Uganda, with little recognition of its importance. But to really learn from the experience of these three studies of the impact of STD treatment, we need to fully appreciate the importance of primary behavior change, and indeed recognize that STD treatment seems not to be needed (because it is not cost-effective, nor even effective) if people instead practice A and B behaviors to a sufficient degree, as 95 percent of Ugandans were reporting by 1995 (see below).

We might also conclude that once HIV infection has spread to people with low rates of partner change (as in a mature epidemic) and the prevalence of HIV is high enough, then condoms may not be of much use either. This should be no surprise, considering that most infections in Uganda are probably now among discordant couples. And condoms are rarely used by married or cohabiting partners.

For our purposes, the effects of PBC are confounded by findings of higher reported condom use in the two Ugandan sites than in Mwanza. Thus it could be argued that the lower rates of treatable STDs were due to condom use rather than PBC. However, I would ask whether user rates of 20 percent and 28 percent (no doubt reflecting primarily inconsistent use) would have much effect on STD aversion (see below), and we know that enough PBC occurred to start bringing down new infection rates before 1991, as will be seen in Chapter 6 on Uganda, at a time when condom user rates appear to have been too low to have had much impact on HIV infection rates. Still, I would be satisfied if the conclusion from these three trials were that later sexual debut, fewer partners, and condoms were all needed. And if so, then let's promote all three, not just the third.

BROAD DIFFERENCES IN CASUAL SEX

Prior to the AIDS epidemic, there were few objective measures of sexual behavior in most countries. Anecdotal evidence was often quoted, but survey data were rare. The WHO/GPA conducted a series of surveys in countries the WHO was assisting in the late 1980s and early 1990s. A summary of these findings were published in 1995 (Carael, 1995). We see from these data that in certain broad measures of casual sex—namely, the percentage reporting one or more nonregular partners in the past year; percentage of never-married men and women fifteen to nineteen years who reported sexual intercourse in the past year; median age of sexual debut; percentage who were virgins at the time of first marriage or partnership, among never-married men and women age twenty-five to forty-nine; mean interval (in years) between first sex and first regular union; and percentage of men and women reporting commercial sex in the past year—that risk behaviors are noticeably greater in (sub-Saharan) Africa than in Asia (Carael, 1995).

This generalization holds true especially for women. African women are much likelier than Asian women to be sexually active and to have multiple partners (see Figure 2.2).

Figure 2.2
Percentage of 15-to-19-Year-Olds Who Reported Sexual Intercourse in the Last Twelve Months

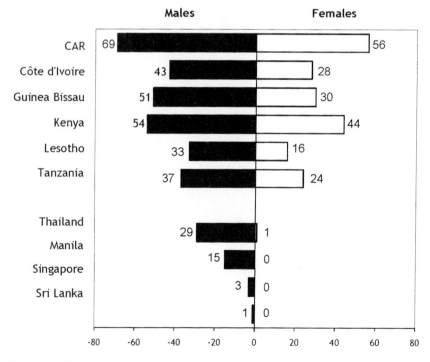

Source: Jim Chin

Given the generally greater likelihood of male–female compared to female–male transmission of HIV, and the possible enhanced biological vulnerability of young women to HIV infection, these clear differences in levels of risk behavior between African and Asian women may go a long way toward explaining the great differences in HIV infection levels between the continents. Epidemiologist Jim Chin, who produced Table 2.4 from WHO/GPA survey data, believes that virtually all variation in epidemics levels can be explained by differences in casual sex, as measured in the various ways mentioned (just as virologists such as Max Essex and Jaap Goudsmit believe that virtually all variation can be explained by viral subtypes, with little or no reference to behavior). However, the viral subtype factor remains murky, while the male circumcision factor has become established as one of the most significant determinants of HIV prevalence levels.

Contrary to widely held beliefs by laymen and experts alike, when we compare levels of premarital sexual activity and multiple partners from the United States or the United Kingdom with those of Africa, there is not much difference. The one difference is that youth, ages

Table 2.4
Estimated Regional HIV and STD Prevalence and a Calculated STD Index

Region	Adults 15-49	# HIV cases in millions	HIV rate %	# STD cases in millions	STD rate %	STD index
Sub-Saharan Africa	273.5	23.40	8.56	32.0	11.9	17.0
Caribbean & Latin America	269.0	1.55	0.58	18.5	7.1	10.1
South & SE Asia	993.5	5.80	0.58	48.0	5.0	7.1
"Western" countries	359.4	1.43	0.40	7.03	1.9	2.7
E Europe & Central Asia	197.7	0.41	0.21	6.0	2.9	4.1
N Africa & Middle-East	171.9	0.21	0.12	3.5	2.1	3.0
East Asia & Pacific	821.7	0.64	0.08	6.0	0.7	*1.0
Totals	3,086.7	33.34	1.08	116.5	3.8	

Source: Jim Chin, "Patterns and Measurement of Heterosexual Risk Behaviors." Paper in progress, 2003. From WHO data.

*The East Asia and Pacific region had the lowest STD rate, and all the other regions are multiples of this lowest rate—that is, the STD rate in sub-Saharan Africa is seventeen times greater than the STD rate in the East Asia and Pacific region. STD and HIV data in the Caribbean and Latin American regions were combined.

fifteen to nineteen, are slightly less likely to be sexually active in Africa. This should give us pause. It has long been assumed by those working in global AIDS that Africans, especially men, have more sexual partners than do Westerners. As early as 1995, papers were appearing attributing the emerging pattern of heterosexual HIV transmission in Africa to promiscuity (Packard & Epstein, 1991). There appears to have been some ethnocentric thinking behind this supposition. Since American AIDS seemed to afflict male homosexuals who had a great many partners, Africans likewise afflicted must also have been having hundreds of partners (Packard & Epstein, 1991). Early studies of African AIDS found associations between infection levels and having multiple partners, and this might have led to the idea that most or all Africans have multiple partners. Sometimes a survey would indeed find that men in special subgroups of Africans, such as long-distance truck drivers or sex workers, in fact reported scores of partners in the past year. Then rumors spread among health professionals that all or most Africans have scores of partners per year, fueled by stereotypes of hypersexed Africans long held by missionaries, writers, explorers, colonial administrators, and the like (see Table 2.5).

I still encounter this stereotypic thinking on the part of health professionals and social scientists, people who ought to know better. There are subgroups of Americans who have scores of partners annually but they are hardly representative of most Americans. Westerners who work in African AIDS ought to be familiar with the growing body of literature showing that most Africans have no greater number of sexual partners than most Americans or Britons, nor are youth in the three areas different in mean ages of sexual debut.

It is also important to remember that levels of casual sex in the majority population make far more difference in generalized epidemics, such as those found in sub-Saharan Africa, than in concentrated epidemic, such as that of the United States. Furthermore, there are other factors in addition to premarital sexual activity and multiple partners, as we currently measure these variables. We must also consider levels and types of STDs, patterns of age mixing, practices that cause lesions in the genital epithelium (anal sex, dry sex), as well as other factors identified in the previous section.

There are in fact a number of epidemiologic factors that combine in what might be called a deadly synergy to determine levels of HIV infection. Some, such as male circumcision, prevalence of STDs (especially HSV-2 it seems), and levels of casual sex seem to be more determining than practices such as dry sex or sex during menstruation. To understand why populations differ so greatly in levels of HIV infection, it is useful to compare Botswana, a country with about 36 percent HIV prevalence nationally, with the Philippines, a country with less

Table 2.5
Percentage of Never-Married Women and Men Who Have Ever Had Sex and Percentage Who Are Currently Sexually Active, by Country, According to Gender and Age Group

	Ages 15-19				Ages 20-24			
	Women		Men		Women		Men	
	Ever had sex	Sexually active	Ever had sex	Sexually active	Ever had sex	Sexually active	Ever had sex	Sexually active
Sub-Saharan Africa								
Ghana	49	23	32	16	88	41	82	43
Mali	34	17	34	14	81	37	71	37
Tanzania	33	18	40	27	77	37	83	49
Zimbabwe	14	4	32	14	54	19	82	36
Asia								
Philippines	1	0	12	3	7	1	41	9
Thailand	3	u	27	u	15	u	68	u
Latin America & Caribbean								
Brazil	22	12	63	31	51	29	93	61
Costa Rica	15	6	42	19	34	11	78	38
Dominican Republic	13	5	48	19	44	16	85	48
Haiti	17	7	46	21	48	11	79	40
Jamaica	37	17	65	25	65	22	89	46
Peru	10	3	45	26	36	11	84	56
Developed countries								
Great Britain	58	u	63	u	84	u	88	u
United States	45	33	55	u	75	57	90	u

Source: Singh, Wulf, Samara, & Cuca, 2000.

Note: Currently sexually active is defined as having had intercourse in the last month, except for U.S. women, for whom it reflects intercourse in the last three months.

Key: u = unavailable

than 1 percent HIV prevalence nationally (both estimates from ante-natal clinic data in 1999, compiled by UNAIDS). The comparison applies only to factors related to heterosexual transmission of HIV.

A country like Botswana has virtually all of the known or suspected risk factors—including unusual ones, such as dry sex—while Philippines has very few, in spite of growing poverty since the economic crisis in Southeast Asia in recent years which has pushed more young women into sex work.

Some Epidemiologic Factors Accounting for High HIV Prevalence in Botswana

- High levels of casual sex, multipartnerism
- Lack of male circumcision
- Low age of sexual debut (16.4 for women) and pattern of young girls having sex with older men
- High levels of ulcerative and other STDs in high-risk populations
- Practice of dry sex
- High consumption of alcohol
- High levels of stigma, fear, and shame associated with AIDS, limiting discussion about AIDS and what to do about it; constraining programs of VCT, school-based preventive education, and indeed all AIDS-related programs; and helping people remain in denial about AIDS and the need to address the problem

Some Epidemiological Factors Accounting for Low HIV Prevalence in the Philippines

- Low levels of casual sex
- Near-universal male circumcision prior to age of sexual debut
- High age of sexual debut (18.8 for men; somewhat higher for women)
- Low proportion of men exposed to commercial sex core groups
- Low levels of ulcerative STDs in high-risk populations
- Low level of CSW customer turnover (average of two to four clients per week)
- Low level bridging between core groups and the majority population
- Few IDUs (but high-risk behaviors found among that group)

For years I have felt that AIDS preventive programs do not reflect fully what we know epidemiologically. For example, no program that I know of addresses risk factors such as heterosexual anal sex or use of vaginal tightening agents, to say nothing of male circumcision. In fact, we tend to use generic prevention programs, as if one approach will suit all populations in all parts of the world.

Which epidemiological factors, or mix of factors, are the most determining? This is one of the most important questions in understanding AIDS. In Chapter 6, we will consider evidence that PBC led to significant decline in HIV prevalence, suggesting that sexual behavior (levels of casual sex, age of sexual debut, sexual mixing patterns) is the most important cluster of determining factors. The Multicentre study supported by UNAIDS was designed to explore explanations for the striking differences in HIV infection levels and rates of transmission. Surveys were conducted in four African cities in four countries: Contonou (Benin), Yaounde (Cameroon), Kisumu (Kenya), and Ndola (Zambia). Results and analysis showed that lack of male circumcision and evidence of genital herpes (HSV-2) seemed to be the main determinants. The only behavioral factor that seemed determining was an early age of sexual debut and a pattern of sexual mixing by age. Condom use was not found to make significant difference (Lagarde et al., 2001).

In their recent paper, Auvert, Carael, Males, and Ferry (2002) concluded, "Early age at first sex is associated with subsequent risk behaviour for HIV. The association of HIV status with younger age at first sex was likely due to an increased number of lifetime partners." Two of the researchers in the Multicentre study later reanalyzed the data from this study and concluded that lifetime number of sexual partners was itself an important determining factor (Auvert & Ferry, 2002). This finding was obscured earlier by the high rates of partners in Yaounde, where HIV infection rates were kept relatively low by a 99 percent male circumcision rate. Unfortunately, a number of abstracts are circulating that conclude, "The difference in HIV prevalence between the four cities could not be explained by differences in sexual behavior" (Buvé, 2002). In fact, an entire special issue of *AIDS* was devoted to papers from this one study.

We now turn to the age of first intercourse, the disparity in ages among those infected in Africa, and related topics.

SEXUAL ACTIVITY AMONG YOUTH

Age of first intercourse—or sexual debut—tends to be younger in Africa than in other parts of the less-developed regions of the world, although this age tends to be rising in recent years. In fact, a pattern is emerging in several countries in Africa in which HIV prevalence is declining among women at antenatal clinics among the youngest age cohort but not among older women. Since there have been few (mostly FBO) efforts to persuade young people to delay age of sexual debut and to avoid premarital sex, decline in HIV prevalence might be due to a rise in age of first sex. It might also be due to partner reduction, changes in sexual mixing patterns, or increases in condom use (Zaba et al., 2002) (see Figure 2.3).

Young people, both male and female, are especially vulnerable to HIV infection. As noted in the following:

Figure 2.3
Support Your Friends

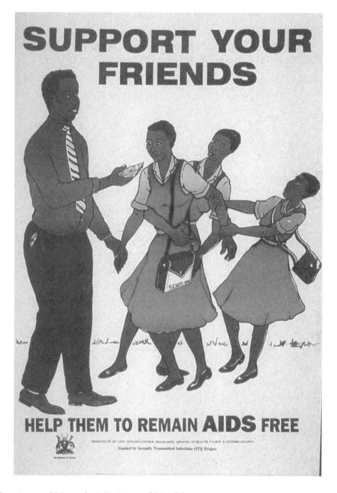

Source: Courtesy of Uganda Ministry of Health

Adolescents often are not able to comprehend fully the extent of their exposure to risk. Societies often compound young people's risk by making it difficult for them to learn about HIV/AIDS and reproductive health. Moreover, many youth are socially inexperienced and dependent on others. Peer pressures easily influence them, often in ways that can increase their risk. (Kiragu, 2001, p. 1)

In fact, youth often have a feeling of invulnerability, even invincibility, when they are actually at highest risk for STDs and unwanted pregnancy. Moreover, the period between first intercourse and first marriage is the time when people tend to be most likely to have multiple partners. Thus, a delay of only one year can have great impact on overall HIV infection rates because it significantly reduces the chances of infection. The briefer the interval between first sex and first marriage, the lower the lifetime number of sexual partners. This crucial bit of evidence, along with the increased vulnerability of young females, is overlooked by those who dismiss abstinence education as a fruitless effort that simply delays HIV infection by a year or two.

It has also been shown that there is a widespread pattern found especially in East and Southern Africa of young women (15–19 years) being infected with HIV in much greater numbers than males of the same age. This is in spite of recent evidence that in Africa, there may be greater HIV transmission efficiency from female to male, rather than male to female, unlike the pattern reported for Europe or the United States (Gray et al., 2001; O'Farrell, 2001). In fact, as the various AIDS epidemics in Africa mature, infection rates among young women are at least twice the rates of those of young men (Kiragu, 2001).

This may be due in part because women are infected at earlier ages (Kiragu, 2001; Laga, Schwertlander, Pisani, Sow, & Carael, 2001). Likely explanations for this are that young females are more vulnerable to HIV infection than older women or men of any age; HIV transmission is more efficient from male to female than female to male; and older men seek younger women as partners, and older men are more likely than younger men to be HIV infected. This is in spite of the fact that even at young ages, men usually report higher numbers of partners than do women (UNAIDS/MAP, 2000).

Several studies since 1994 have suggested that young females may be at increased biological vulnerability to HIV infection. It seems that the younger they are, the more easily they can be infected (Bulterys, Chao, Habimana et al., 1994). This may be because of increased permeability of the vaginal lining in immature females, or microlesions during intercourse, especially if male partners are full adults and intercourse is coerced or forced. "It is highly plausible that the risk of HIV acquisition increases even further during acts of sex in which vaginal or cervical trauma and bleeding are common, such as forced sex or during the loss of virginity" (Laga, Schwertlander, Pisani, Sow, & Carael, 2001, p. 932). Laceration of the hymen at first sexual intercourse may also place young women at special risk of HIV infection (UNAIDS/MAP, 2000). It appears that changes in the female reproductive tract during puberty make the tissue more susceptible to penetration by HIV. Furthermore, "hormonal changes associated with the menstrual cycle often are accompanied by a thinning of the mucus plug, the protective sealant covering the cervix. Such thinning can allow HIV to pass more easily" (Kigaru, 2001, p. 7).

There may be also less mucous production in younger than in older women. Mucus in the female genital tract has four functions as follows:

It acts as a physical barrier, separating semen and other material from the vaginal and cervical walls. It is a lubricant, protecting the surface of the vagina from abrasion during intercourse. It flushes the cervix and vagina in the same way that mucus flushes the respiratory tract, removing foreign material. It has an immune function, that is, mucus contains cells of a separate immune system whose function is to activate the immune responses of the cells in the vaginal and cervical surfaces. If mucous production in young women, and post-menopausal women, is less proficient than in older pre-menopausal women so too will these protective roles be less effective. There will be less of a barrier to viral penetration. It will provide less assistance in minimizing irritation and tearing of the genital membranes and so facilitate viral entry. (Reid & Bailey, 1992, p. 4)

Because young females are more likely than older women to be infected, they are also more likely to be infectious, to transmit HIV to their male partners. It is established that degree of infectiousness, related to degree of viral shedding, is a significant factor determining the likelihood of HIV transmission. In fact, we can see this in the following:

There are two major periods of HIV infectiousness. The first is immediately after HIV infection and the second period is end stage, when high viral loads in blood result in HIV shedding in many body fluids. In between is a latent period of variable duration. (Hitchcock & Fransen, 1999, p. 513)

Given the preference for young women as sexual partners, they are likely to be infected at an early age and to be in a stage of high viral load and viral shedding as men continue to seek them.

Older men are more likely than younger men to be HIV infected; they then infect the younger women that they seek, and these younger women subsequently infect other older men (Laga et al., 2001). In fact, the newly infected young women have higher viral loads and therefore are more likely to infect others than older women who have been HIV infected for longer periods. And if that were not enough, "Men also appear to be less likely to use condoms with young female partners they have selected in this way. The skewed balance of power in relationships between older men and younger girls makes it exceptionally difficult for girls themselves to negotiate safer sex in these relationships" (Laga et al., 2001, p. 932). There is also the male belief found in diverse parts of Africa that sex with a virgin can cure a man of AIDS. This is rarely mentioned in medical journals but such beliefs are often reported in African and other newspapers as underlying rapes and seductions of minors (e.g., Kaiser Daily HIV/AIDS Report, November 2001).

If substantial numbers of such females are not sexually active, this ought to impact overall infection rates, since the high HIV prevalence among females ages fifteen to nineteen years could be critical in provoking and maintaining an explosive HIV epidemic in heterosexually driven epidemics (Buvé et al., 2001). Another way to say this is that if those at highest risk for both infection and for infecting others are not engaging in sex at all—through abstaining or delaying sexual debut—this ought to have a major downward effect on HIV prevalence.

Incidentally, this disparity in infection rates among African youth was recognized early in the epidemic, but it seems that few countries outside of Uganda and Senegal developed special efforts into targeting young females with interventions aimed at delay of sexual debut—into empowering young women to resist the coercion and seduction of older men—in the earlier years of their epidemics. In fact, by at least 1998, Uganda's national plan mentioned the increased biological vulnerability of young females, speaking of "immature vaginas" or "immature sex organs" as a risk factor. This language, which alerts people to a crucial HIV risk factor, is also found in some of Uganda's IEC print material aimed at various target groups including youth.

A study in California found that when male partners are significantly older than girls, there is greater likelihood of early sexual initiation and for initiation to have been unwanted by the girl (Marin et al., 2000). Preadolescent relationships with older partners "are particularly risky because they are associated with unwanted sexual advances and peer norms encouraging sexual activity" (pp. 416–417). The authors of this American study conclude that "interventions are needed that provide young people with a sense of their personal power, the ability to state feelings and needs, and an ability to set limits and personal boundaries" (Marin et al., 2000; Liebmann-Smith, 2001, p. 134). As we will see in Chapter 6, this is precisely what successful youth-oriented programs, such as Life Skills, the Sara Initiative, Straight Talk, and Teen Star aim at doing.

Further evidence of the importance of age of sexual debut come from the UNAIDS Multicentre study. Commenting broadly on the various findings of this study, Carael and Holmes (2001) note the following:

Surprisingly, with the exception of young age at first marriage, young age of women at sexual debut, and large age differences between spouses, most other parameters of risky sexual behaviour (such as contact with sex workers, lifetime numbers of sexual partners, rate of acquisition of new partners and lack of condom use) were not consistently more common in the high HIV prevalence sites than in the relatively low prevalence sites. (pp. S1–S2)

The authors acknowledge that failure to measure differences in what ought to be considered risky sexual behavior findings might relate to the stage of the epidemic. By the time of the present study, those with the riskiest sexual behavior might have already died, leaving those exhibiting less risky behavior.

It is surprising that there has not been more of a program response to findings about the vulnerability of young females. Peter Piot, executive director of UNAIDS, issued the following press release on September 14, 1999, after the preliminary analysis of data from the Multicentre study:

The Joint United Nations Programme on HIV/AIDS (UNAIDS) today released highlights from a research study providing the strongest evidence yet that dramatically high HIV levels in teenage girls are linked to sexual contact with older men. The study found HIV infection rates of 15%–23% among girls 15 to 19 years old, 26%–40% among men aged 25 or more, and just 3%–4% among 15-19 year old boys. . . . The unavoidable conclusion is that girls are getting infected not by boys their own age, but by older men.

The UNAIDS report pointed to additional avenues for prevention. Michel Carael, one of the study authors, observed, "When almost a quarter of teenage girls have HIV and when close to half of them carry the virus that causes genital herpes, the only possible explanation is that they are becoming infected during their first few exposures to sex— maybe even their very first." The press release continues as follows:

"For millions of young African girls in or nearing their early teens, this is an emergency. Prevention just can't wait," said Anne Buve, coordinator of the Multicentre study. "Girls have the right to know the facts—that they are at high risk of becoming infected quickly even if they have just one partner, especially an older man," Dr. Buve stressed. "Parents, schools and communities must make sure that girls have the information, skills and tools to delay first sex and to resist unwanted or unsafe intercourse."

Elsewhere, Carael and Makinwa (2000) recommend programs of "demand reduction" (making sex with teenage girls socially unacceptable) and providing girls with skills and opportunities that reduce dependence on men. As can be seen in Chapter 6, youth-targeted, girl-friendly programs can in fact be developed and implemented and apparently can achieve desired results. There has also been reform of Ugandan laws pertaining to rape and seduction of minors in the direction of tougher penalties.

Researchers recently tested the hypothesis that interventions designed to modify behavior in adolescents may not only reduce the exposure to risk during adolescence itself but may also be protective in later life (White, Cleland, & Carael, 2000). Several studies in the United States, Europe, and the United Kingdom had found that early age of debut was associated with higher number of lifetime partners, either for men or both genders. The authors of the present study analyzed nationally representative data on sexual practices from three countries: Cote D'Ivoire, Thailand, and Tanzania, and one study from Lusaka, Zambia. Through statistical analysis of responses of men ages fifteen to forty-nine, the researchers found that the earlier the age of sexual debut, the greater the probability of having extramarital partners in adult life. The same association was found with reporting a higher number of premarital partners. The researchers also found a clear trend between increased age of sexual debut and reduced number of pre-marital partners (O'Connor, 2001; White, Cleland, & Carael, 2000).

It is unfortunate that women were not part of this study. Still, this research gives further strength to arguments that more resources ought to be directed toward programs targeting youth and aimed at delay of sexual debut and reduction in number of sexual partners.

A study in Namibia provides further evidence that it is necessary to reach youth before they become sexually active. A randomized trial of a fourteen-session, face-to-face intervention emphasizing abstinence and safer sexual practices was conducted among 515 students (median age seventeen years and median grade eleven) attending ten secondary schools located in two districts. Students were randomly assigned to intervention or control groups. HIV risk behaviors as well as intentions and perceptions were assessed at baseline, immediately postintervention, and at six and twelve months after the intervention. There was no significant difference in behaviors between the two groups overall, but the following was observed:

However, analyses conducted among the subset of youths who were sexually inexperienced at baseline (n = 255) revealed that a higher percentage of intervention youths (17%) than control youths (9%, P < 0.05) remained sexually inexperienced one year later. Moreover, in the immediate post-intervention period, among baseline virgins who subsequently initiated sex, intervention youths were more likely than control youths to use a condom (18 versus 10%, P < 0.05) (Bonita et al., 1998, p. 2473)

As we will see in Uganda, a key component of its successful AIDS prevention program was reaching youth before they became sexually active, in primary schools. Delay of debut was and is the primary message—but not the only one—for Ugandan youth.

It may be useful to cite a study from the United States before turning to Uganda. The United States has had one of the highest rates of teenage pregnancy in the developed world. Yet there have been significant and sustained declines in these rates since 1991.[2] A study by the Guttmacher Institute found that about 25 percent of averted pregnancies were due to abstinence and to the decreased proportion of youth with any sexual experience. Trends in the level of contraceptive use were mixed, but there was a significant increase toward greater use of newly available long-acting hormonal methods, particularly injectables. The study concludes as follows:

These findings show that reduction in sexual activity and use of more effective contraceptive methods both played roles in the recent decline in teenage pregnancy rates and birthrates. Both of these behavioral changes were undoubtedly influenced by broader societal changes in policy and programs, and in attitudes and values. We have yet to understand many of these changes and their interconnections. . . . These findings suggest that the best strategy for continuing the declines in teenage pregnancy levels is a multifaceted approach. Programs and policies should aim at encouraging teenagers—particularly those at the youngest ages—to postpone intercourse and at supporting sexually experienced youths who wish to refrain from further sexual activity. At the same time, it must be recognized that most young people become sexually active during their teens, and sexuality education and information should also prepare them to adequately prevent pregnancy and sexually transmitted infection if and when they do have sex. (Darroch & Singh, 1999)

This conclusion seems so reasonable and intuitively correct that it ought to be unnecessary to write a book to argue the case for it. But until donors and other decision makers in AIDS programs look carefully and with an open mind at the evidence for the impact of behavior changes other than contraceptives, drugs, and medical devices, the vast majority of prevention funds will continue to go only to these risk reduction interventions.

A team of UNAIDS researchers also concluded that patterns of sexual mixing by age may contribute significantly to HIV infection rates. They recommend that prevention programs provided to young women and their older partners in high HIV prevalence epidemics aim at the following: (1) reduce early exposure to risky sex, (2) reduce likelihood of transmission per sexual act, and (3) reduce age difference between partners (Laga et al., 2001). This makes sense.

Whatever the interventions, there is now growing consensus that it is crucial to focus on young people and their behavior. UNAIDS Director Peter Piot recently observed the following at a New York press conference:

"In every single country where AIDS had been brought under control it has begun with young people," he said. He noted that Cambodia, Brazil and Uganda have made progress in cutting AIDS infection rates by zeroing in on

people who are just becoming sexually active. "So success is possible," he
said. "This is a problem with a solution. And we know it works." (Anonymous, 2002)

SOME TRENDS IN YOUTHFUL SEXUAL
ACTIVITY IN AFRICA

The DHS has been asking questions about age of sexual debut and
first marriage since the 1980s, in its standard demographic/family planning module, since these two ages are considered proximate determinants of fertility. When there are DHS data from the same country for
more than one year, such as age of sexual debut, and proportions sexually active before marriage, as well as proportions reporting multiple
partners, the behavioral trend is most often in the direction of less risk,
even if change is marginal. Trends in percentage of men and women
ages eighteen to twenty-four and twenty to twenty-nine who have ever
had sex are shown in Figures 2.4 and 2.5 (Mahy & Gupta, 2002, p. 17).

Figure 2.4
**Percentage of Women Ages 18–24 Who Reported Having Had First Sex
before Age 18, by Relative Date of Survey**

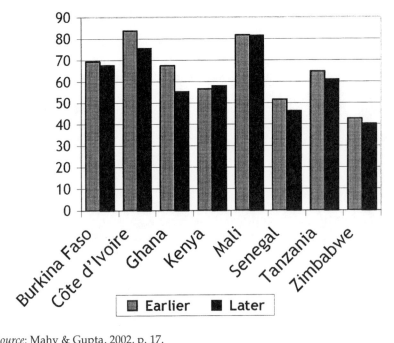

Source: Mahy & Gupta, 2002, p. 17.

Figure 2.5
Percentage of Men Ages 20–29 Who Reported Having Had First Sex
before Age 20, by Relative Date of Survey

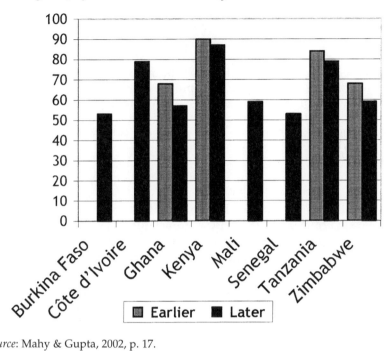

Source: Mahy & Gupta, 2002, p. 17.

The question must arise: If partner reduction, abstinence, and delay have significant impact on HIV seroprevalence, and if there have been positive changes of this sort reported in national surveys, especially in countries with relatively high HIV infection rates, why hasn't there been more impact on national seroprevalence? It must be kept in mind that changes in measures, such as average age of first sex, have been marginal. Also, there are biological and other factors that also determine seroprevalence. And there probably has been some impact, especially in young cohorts. By 2000, UNAIDS reported that HIV prevalence for Africa as a whole seemed to have stabilized—to have not continued the pattern of rising every year. (On the eve of the XIV International AIDS Conference in Barcelona, UNAIDS was denying what they had said two years previously and were asking for vast increases in cash donations, telling the world that infection rates were far from being stabilized in Africa or anywhere else.)

Even in South Africa, considered an AIDS basket case by many due to the explosive infection rates from the early 1990s and the lack of government response, as well as having the highest number of HIV infections in the world, we see the beginnings of change and impact on prevalence among youth and in the age of debut. According to UNAIDS:

Teenage prevalence declined from 21 percent to 18 percent, prevalence in women in their twenties remained unchanged at 27 percent, whereas trends in those aged 30 and over rose from 17 percent to 20 percent. The decline in teenage prevalence occurred in most provinces, with the exception of West Cape (a low prevalence province) and North West and Free State. Age at first birth rose between 1998 and 1999, suggesting that the decline in HIV prevalence was very likely due to an increase in age of first sex among teenagers. (UNAIDS/MAP, 2000, pp. 14–15)

This prevalence rate (among women under twenty) fell to 15.4 percent in 2001 (UNAIDS/WHO, 2002).

What all this suggests is that youth ought to be targeted in AIDS prevention efforts, and that PBC—especially delay of sexual debut—ought to be emphasized with youth. Given their special vulnerabilities, it is especially important to keep young females from becoming sexually active at early ages, and out of the pool of infectables. This also protects older men from HIV infection. More supporting evidence for these recommendations can be found in particular in Chapters 6 and 7 on Uganda and Zambia, and there is description and discussion of how to implement interventions aimed at PBC in youth, based on experience and success, rather than mere consensus.

NOTES

1. I am indebted to Dr. Saifuddin Ahmed for this concise formulation.

2. In fact, the proportion of unmarried U.S. teenagers ages fifteen to nineteen who had ever had intercourse began to decline in 1988 (Abma & Sonenstein, 2001).

PART II

WESTERN APPROACHES TO AIDS PREVENTION IN DEVELOPING COUNTRIES

3

"Behavior Change" and the Problem of Ethnocentrism

An experience I had at a recent international health conference drama-tizes the problem I am seeking to define in this chapter. I was attend-ing a session on AIDS prevention. Most in the audience seemed to be from Africa or Latin America–Caribbean. Four speakers were sched-uled but only one showed up due, we were told, to problems related to travel. The North American speaker gave his presentation about what he felt was needed to prevent AIDS. He spoke only about MSM transmission and he used the word "homophobia" about a dozen times. I got the feeling most in the audience understood little of what was being presented. Since no other presenter came, there was time for questions and answers—too much time, about ninety minutes.

Yet the audience had no questions or comments. And there was still ninety minutes to fill. People might have left, but no one rose to leave. It was an awkward situation. The session moderator knew me and perhaps because I was sitting near the front of the room, she asked me if I would like to open up a discussion about AIDS prevention. So I commented that patterns and dynamics of transmission were quite different in American cities and African villages, and since most people in the room appeared to be from developing countries, perhaps they would like to hear a bit about primary behavior change findings in Uganda. Members of the audience quickly came to life and made com-ments like, Why do we not hear more about delay of sexual debut and partner reduction? Why don't we involve religious groups and school-teachers more? How can we prevent seduction of schoolgirls by older men? How can we get husbands to stop running around and then in-fecting their wives? Just as the audience had no comment about the presentation they had just heard, the presenter had no comments about what the audience began to speak about animatedly.

This illustrates not only the very different types of epidemics we have in the world and therefore the different responses needed to address them, but also a clash of cultures and values between the West and Africa and other resource-poor areas of the world (some contrast the North and the South). Audience members from places like Kenya and Haiti (as I recall) thought it was exactly the right response to promote fidelity and abstinence, while this is usually thought by Westerners to constitute unwarranted infringement in people's lives.

Consistent with experience at this conference, I have found that PBC usually seems to make sense to audiences from Africa and the Caribbean, whereas discussion of this is likely to provoke controversy with Western audiences. Westerners are particularly resistant if they have spent little or no time actually living in a developing country.

The very term "behavior change," widely used synonymously with condom adoption in AIDS prevention circles, suggests that outsiders know what is best for resource-poor countries. There is also the implicit assumption that Africans are misbehaving and need to change their behavior, even though in fact sexual behavior in many African societies is conservative by American standards.

"Behavior change communications (BCC)" replaced the earlier term IEC (information, education, communication) in order to put more emphasis on the bottom line, changing behavior. But the term assumes that behavior is harmful before donor-driven programs show the poor masses what their behavior ought to be. It does not suggest that the behavior of some groups might be already low risk, and so it merely needs to be reinforced and encouraged. Certainly among some religious, conservative groups of Africa, sexual behavior prior to any interventions is less risky than that of the outside experts who have come to change behavior. From this consideration, the earlier term IEC, still used in Uganda's own programs, seems preferable because it does not smack of donor paternalism.

IS BEHAVIOR CHANGE ONLY RISK REDUCTION?

It can be argued that condom adoption is a form of behavior change because it involves a new behavior (and technology). For a man who has had multiple sexual partners for years and a history of STDs, beginning to use condoms is indeed a change of behavior. But it can also be argued that condom adoption does not really qualify as a fundamental or primary form of behavior change because it allows continuation of previous, high-risk sexual behavioral patterns by conveying a feeling of protection from the consequences of those risky behaviors. Looked at this way, condoms are really a risk reduction solution for people who don't change their high-risk behavior.

It is useful to make a distinction between risk reduction and risk avoidance in considering HIV prevention strategies. Promotion of condoms is an example of the first; promotion of sexual abstinence or mutual fidelity to a single uninfected partner is an example of the second. Risk or harm reduction approaches assume that behavior is difficult or impossible to change, therefore, efforts ought to be made to mitigate the consequences of risky behavior that are likely to occur despite efforts to change it. Risk avoidance assumes that behavior can change. Richens has suggested primary behavior change to denote risk avoidance strategies that involve fundamentally different ways of behaving, such as abstinence, delay of debut, and monogamy or faithfulness to one partner (or to all spouses in a polygamous union). I have found that people seem more likely to adopt the term PBC than risk avoidance, possibly because the latter sounds too much like risk reduction and people forget which is which. Moreover, risk avoidance practiced imperfectly—as in partner reduction but not mutual monogamy—is a type of risk reduction, yet it is not the same as condom use since it involves a different, arguably more fundamental, behavioral change.

The model used in AIDS prevention is primarily an infectious disease model rather than a risk behavior model, whether we speak of risk reduction or prevention. There is a parallel with smoking and health. Until quite recently, public health and tobacco industry efforts were aimed at (1) trying to filter out amounts of tar and nicotine and (2) producing less harmful tobacco, rather than stopping smoking; in other words, behavior change. It seems clear that most health benefits were achieved only when significant numbers of people quit smoking altogether. The parallel is imperfect. Obviously people need to procreate, but they do not have to have multiple partners.

Programs of harm reduction began to develop in the drug treatment field, where some felt that the Alcoholics Anonymous or Narcotics Anonymous model required too much radical behavior change too soon, namely, complete abstinence all at once as the first step. The harm reduction idea was to meet the addict where he was, injecting drugs in shooting galleries or in his home. The idea was not to scare the addict away by asking him to do more than he is willing to do. Provision of clean injecting equipment (for injecting drug users) and condoms (for those at risk for sexual transmission of HIV) is a type of harm reduction. These actions may be regarded as technological fixes, or quick fixes, to complex problems involving human behavior. Technological fixes never really address the cause of a problem. Still, the harm reduction philosophy suggests that it is better to reduce harm or mitigate risk than to scare the addict away by attempting to change his behavior.

The solutions adopted by AIDS risk reduction involve medical technologies, that is, drugs or devices manufactured by pharmaceutical companies. In other words, a medical solution is offered for a problem defined medically rather than behaviorally, and this has an appealing internal logic. Those who have recognized some of the shortcomings of condoms and pills have put their hope in female condoms and vaginal microbicides such as Nonoxynol-9 gel. I have been someone who has put hope in the latter, especially because it would be a female-controlled method. Alas, studies have not yet confirmed the *in vivo* efficacy of vaginal microbicides.

Risk reduction has always been the dominant approach in prevention of sexually transmitted AIDS in the United States. This was due in part because the disease first developed among gay men and IDUs. The first group was not responsive to public health educators passing what appeared to be moral judgment on their behavior, nor did they want to change their behavior. And the behavior of IDUs was thought for the most part to be unchangeable. The risk reduction approach to AIDS prevention quickly spread to other major international programs and donors, in part because the United States quickly became the largest donor to fund such programs. Another factor was that gay men with AIDS prevention experience in U.S. cities were prominent among the first experts in international AIDS prevention. Condom use was widely believed to be the best solution to sexually transmitted AIDS in the United States; it was even believed to have been responsible for reducing HIV infection rates among gay men in some key cities where infection levels among gay men reached extremely high levels.

The argument against seeming to pass judgment on harmful behavior is that it drives away the people we need to reach. The example often given is again the drug addict. However, successful antismoking efforts in the United States, among other programs, show that one can address underlying harmful behavior in ways that do not shame or produce undue stigma on smokers. I would suggest that with IDU addicts, we can and should provide clean needles. But even in this case we do a disservice to the addict and to society if that is all we do. We should also provide options for detoxification and rehabilitation, for stopping the behavior harmful to the IDU and to society. And this can certainly be done in ways that do not create any more shame and social stigma than already exist. In fact, treatment of addiction in America today is not particularly shame or stigma producing. Among celebrities, it may even be a badge of honor. In America, addiction treatment for the most part follows the disease model; it should not be regarded as shameful that one gets a disease.

Therefore there seems to be no valid reason to shun (or not fund) programs that prevent rather than merely reduce risk on the grounds that risk avoidance necessarily produces stigma, or drives away the people we want to reach with our prevention messages. True, there may be a great deal of stigma associated with AIDS in much of Africa and elsewhere, but interventions that promote PBC in fact are acceptable and conform to prevailing social and religious norms, whereas condom promotion and STD treatment are likely to generate shame and stigma.

It seems to me that those who control global AIDS prevention funds have made the fundamental error of trying to apply risk reduction solutions to majority populations. Meanwhile, it has missed the significance of locally developed (e.g., Ugandan, Jamaican) interventions that have had significant impact in majority populations. We still read and hear comments on a daily basis, such as "HIV prevalence in Nigeria is increasing rapidly. Increased condom use is the most viable solution to slow down or reverse this trend" (Van Rossem, Meekers, & Zkinyemi, 2001, p. 252).

Until very recently, there has been little change in mainstream, official thinking about where AIDS prevention resources should go. Peter Piot, who was recently interviewed at the Sixth International Conference on AIDS in Asia and the Pacific meeting in Melbourne, Australia (October 5–10, 2001), described AIDS prevention as

a combination of the "how" and the "what." The "what" goes from condom promotion to public information and harm-reduction programs, but the "how" is also important. That is a matter of political leadership, which is something that is lacking in many countries. (From the report of the interview posted by the listserve SEA-AIDS)

I agree with the need for political leadership but not with putting all our resources into risk reduction and awareness programs, as is implied here by the most senior global AIDS official. AIDS prevention should employ harm reduction approaches but should also try to change high-risk behavior or prevent it before it becomes established.

One of the problems that have constrained the development of effective AIDS prevention strategies is that AIDS appeared in the middle of the sexual revolution in the West, a time when the availability of contraceptives and other factors had led to greater sexual freedom than in the past. Traditional norms and values that influenced sexual behavior were being replaced by new values that full sexual expression was healthy for both straight and gay people. In a review criticizing a book (by a gay man) that challenges the risk reduction/condom approach, award-winning AIDS journalist Mark Schoofs declares, "The first principle of behavior change is not to impose outside norms but to build on indigenous ones" (Schoofs, 1997). Yes, but does this necessarily mean we should not try to modify or change indigenous norms if they are harmful or deadly? What if rape is common, including rape of preadolescent girls in the belief that this will cure HIV infection? Should we respect indigenous norms and leave them alone in this case?[1] Moreover, isn't the West imposing its norms on Africa by insisting that Africans rely on Western technological fixes and not even directly address risky sexual behavior?

It is clear that there is a bias in international AIDS programs favoring condoms and other technological forms of risk reduction. In the ABCs of AIDS prevention, to which lip service is paid, we quickly see that the vast majority of prevention resources have gone to condom promotion, and more recently, to the treatment of the treatable STIs, another risk reduction approach. Few in public health circles really believed—or even believe nowadays—that programs promoting abstinence, fidelity, or monogamy, or even reduction in number of sexual partners, pay off in significant behavioral change. This has only begun to change in the past year, and so it is still too early to know if the Western consensus paradigm will yield any ground to more balanced, culturally appropriate and—as will be seen in the next section—effective approaches to prevention.

Risk reduction approaches are both needed and appropriate for high-risk groups, both in the North and the South. Condom provision and STD treatment are as needed for CSWs, soldiers, and truck drivers in Africa just as they are anywhere else. Indeed, CSWs and their clients are more willing to use condoms than other groups. A recent study in Nigeria concluded, "Men's condom use is highest in commercial sex, inconsistent in casual relationships, and lowest in marriage" (Messersmith et al., 2000, p. 46). In fact, we already know this is true for most of the world. The right kind of condom promotion and provision can lead to high user rates (over 90%) among CSWs and their clients, and this certainly ought to impact HIV prevalence rates. Truck drivers along the trans-Africa highway in southern Uganda have also been found to adopt condoms quite readily (Gysels & Whitworth, 2001). Another report, apparently of the same study, concluded, "Most drivers claimed to use condoms during casual sex, and this was confirmed by the CSWs. General use of condoms is encouraging, particularly given the context of a culture generally opposed to condoms" (Gysels, Pool, & Bwanika, 2001, p. 373).

But this is not all we should be doing. In fact risk reduction interventions seem not to have had great impact among majority populations in Africa, as Chapter 4 demonstrates. Another approach seems to be especially needed for the parts of the world where HIV is not concentrated among core transmitter groups. I am certainly not against condom use. But I question the approach of "condoms for everyone, everywhere at all times and for all occasions." People are not the same. They differ in ways we routinely measure: region (country, culture, language), age, sex, religion, education, political orientation, rural or urban residence, degree of HIV risk behavior, and the like. Condoms may be the best solution for CSWs who plan to remain in that line of work. It may not be the best solution—nor their promotion the best intervention—for primary school students who have never experienced sexual intercourse. They may not be the best intervention for twelve to fifteen-year-old students because (1) another intervention (e.g., delay of first sex) may be more likely to be adopted, as we have seen in countries like Uganda and Zambia; (2) another intervention may be more cost-effective; and (3) another intervention may be more protective against HIV infection.

A DOUBLE STANDARD OF BEHAVIOR CHANGE

In an interesting critique of AIDS programs in Africa, Gausset (2001) notes that there have been two phases to Western studies of African sexuality, the first being during the colonial period when observations were made by missionaries, travelers, anthropologists, and colonial administrators. Gausset observes, "In general, African sexuality was studied only in as far as it was different from our own. It has been from the beginning, described as wild, animal-like, exotic, irrational and immoral" (p. 510). Early descriptions amounted to what could be called ethnopornography. There was a reaction to this by anthropologists such that studies focusing on African sexuality became rare after the 1950s. However, with the rise of AIDS, there again seemed to be a need, in fact a life-or-death urgency, for accurate information on sexuality. According to Gausset, citing Fasin (1999),

The state of "anthropological emergency", and the desire to save lives lowered the level of ethical, theoretical and methodological self-control of the researchers. . . . Like the first studies of African sexuality, it was once again the "exotic, traditional, irrational and immoral practices" that were the focus of the research. (p. 511)

In their search for explanations for Africa's explosive HIV infection rates, anthropologists—but also others with no training in ethnographic fieldwork—began to search for explanations in African culture. There was emphasis once again on the exotic, even the lurid: dry sex practices or use of vaginal drying agents or implants; injection of monkey blood into human pubic parts; multiple sexual partners; inheritance of widows whose husbands had died of AIDS; premarital sex; wife sharing; circumcision and scarification rituals practiced on a large scale with the same knife; the sugar daddy phenomenon; beliefs that sex with a virgin, even a baby, could cleanse one of AIDS (Kaiser Daily

HIV/AIDS Report, January 2001);[2] extremely high STD rates; and reports that some men were actually proud to have an untreated STD. The list could go on. The tendency to blame African culture can even find its way into African national AIDS program documents, including in Uganda. "Early researchers were looking for things to blame, and identified African cultural practices as culprits" (Gausset, 2001, p. 511). The implied or stated solution to soaring HIV transmission rates was to stamp out these dangerous, dysfunctional cultural practices; that is, ban dry sex and polygamy, discontinue coming-of-age rituals and widow inheritance, and arrest sugar daddies.

Even if such public health interventions might reduce HIV transmission, we must remember that this may appear to Africans to be another example of cultural hegemony: White Americans advising Black Africans to renounce their heritage. Why? Because (largely) American research suggests this would be good. It should be realized that many or most Africans believe that AIDS comes from the West, that it originated in America. Africans are also becoming aware through films, videos, magazines, and the like that homosexual anal intercourse, self-injection with narcotics, and suburban wife swapping clubs are among the exotic practices of the West. Perhaps they have also noticed that public health programs do not normally target these cultural practices for annihilation; instead, we hear of far less draconian solutions, such as safer sex. In the West we tend not to talk about the need for people to stop being homosexuals or drug addicts, at least unless we are religious conservatives. We instead provide such people with condoms and clean needles.

I agree with Gausset to some extent that there is something of a double standard in AIDS prevention between what we preach for Africa and other less developed areas and what we preach for ourselves. This diminishes the authority and credibility of the major donor organizations with non-Western people when they hear that the solution to AIDS is to abandon African culture, use condoms always, submit to mass treatment for STDs with a new drug, or submit to mass circumcision. I happen to believe that one of the most draconian sounding solutions proposed for AIDS prevention—mass male circumcision—might in fact bring down national HIV infection rates significantly. But Westerners must remember how this idea sounds to Africans.

On the other hand, I don't agree with Gausset completely, since, as I point out in several places in this book, those who work in public health are loathe to appear to make value judgments about sexual behavior. Therefore they are more comfortable promoting condoms and treating STDs than advocating having few partners, whether the audience is African or American.

IS THERE REALLY A BIAS TOWARD CONDOM-DRUG APPROACHES?

The strongest evidence of bias toward medicalized risk reduction approaches is found in resource allocation for AIDS prevention: Virtually all funds go to condoms in one way or another, with what is left over going to STD treatment. Unfortunately, neither USAID, the World Bank, or other donors divide up their budgets in ways that can be tied easily to separate A, B, or C interventions. There are certainly large budget items (under commodities) for condoms and drugs. And there are $100 million projects dedicated to condom social marketing, and none supported by major donors dedicated to abstinence, delay of sexual debut, or fidelity or partner reduction. Still, there may also be small components within other projects that relate to A or B interventions. But often they are simply there in name to deflect criticism that AIDS prevention equals condom promotion, a charge periodically made by African political and religious leaders.

A USAID official, apparently in response to a request, recently made a search for language such as "abstinence," "delay of sexual debut," "monogamy," and "partner reduction" in the official language that describes various USAID–supported projects. Language associated with A interventions showed up a couple of dozen times, usually in association with school or youth AIDS prevention programs. Abstinence/delay interventions seem always to be subcomponents of broader projects that promote condoms, improve STD treatment, or simply educate people about AIDS. There seem to be no separate budgets for A and B components. I know from experience that sometimes A and B language is only there to mollify possible critics, and that few if any resources actually go into such interventions. Yet other times, and more recently, part of project resources may actually go to promotion of abstinence along with condoms, as happened in the HEART project in Zambia.

There was little evidence from the internal USAID language search that resources go to interventions related to fidelity, monogamy, or simply partner reduction. Such language rarely shows up even in formal project descriptions.

I searched the abstracts of papers presented at the most recent Global AIDS Conference in Barcelona. "Condoms" came up 777 times, compared to sixteen for "faithfulness" or "fidelity" and seventy-four for "abstinence." However, many or most of the abstinence abstracts were about abstaining from drugs, and many others just used the word in passing without evidence of any sort of an abstinence intervention.

I received the following note, quoted with permission, from the founding and (at this writing) current chairman of the Kenya National AIDS Control Council, Muhammad Abdullah (October 31, 2002):

I am sure you are aware that at times help comes with strings attached. We received US $10 million aid but it had to be [used] only [for] condoms. We had two options: to accept all the US $10 million worth of condoms or refuse. If it was our choice, we would have spread this help to other forms of prevention as well and particularly advocacy for behaviour change in schools. The ministry of education is looking for help to print its syllabus, and book aids to help the teachers and the children to learn about HIV infection and how to prevent it. No one wants to help to print books and teaching aids. . . . So you can see the mismatch in emphasis between the needs perceived by locals and those of our collaborators. We have adopted an attitude that anything that helps is welcome, even if it is not priority, since we may not get what we call priority [help] if we insist on having it our way.

This speaks for itself. Although we cannot quantify it adequately, few funds actually go to behavioral or primary prevention interventions or to any interventions other than condoms or drugs. The few hundred thousand dollars of USAID funds that went to religious groups in Uganda in the mid-1980s, some WHO funds that supported these efforts earlier, and the HEART youth campaign in Zambia described in a later section, are exceptions.

Another powerful piece of evidence is that there were no program impact indicators (at least in USAID, the largest bilateral donor to international AIDS programs) relating to fidelity (partner reduction) or abstinence (or delay of debut) until 1996 and 2000, respectively. This is discussed later in this section.

As recently as May 2002, there was a review of the cost and effectiveness of HIV/AIDS interventions in Africa. Data were analyzed from twenty-four studies in Africa. Every intervention consisted of drugs or condoms. There was no mention of interventions that address PBC, no doubt because there are so few of these that they are not noticed (Creese et al., 2002).

In June 2002 an article in the *New York Times* announced that a major report was about to be released by the United Nations. The report would tell us, the article warns, that in spite of the devastation of the AIDS pandemic and all the effort that has gone into AIDS prevention, there has been little behavior change: Condom use remains very low in less developed countries. This may be true if we are considering Africa and our definition of behavior change is restricted to condom use.

The *Times* article, which was based on interviews with UNAIDS experts, clarifies what is meant by behavior change in the following:

Even where people are beginning to take notice, their precautions may be inadequate. Many men and women said they were limiting sexual activity to one partner as a way to avoid infection, but only a minority—fewer than 8 percent of women and 15 to 25 percent of men—said they had begun using condoms with those partners. In societies where men may have several wives or extensive premarital or extramarital sexual contact, most men are not using condoms, carrying the risk to all involved. (Crossette, 2002, p. 6)

Here we have it spelled out once again: Monogamy is not the answer—using condoms is. In fact, this article assumes that people in monogamous relationships ought to be using condoms regularly, which of course people do not do anywhere unless perhaps we are talking about the minority of, say, African discordant couples who have been tested and counseled (although even a tiny minority of these may use condoms, according to studies in Rakai). This *Times* article ignores what we know about condom use, namely, that it usually occurs with high-risk, irregular partners and not among married couples or regular partners, and as usual it dismisses monogamy as inconsequential.

Evidence for the condom–drug bias can unfortunately be detected easily in national AIDS programs in Africa and everywhere. For example, the national AIDS program of Mozambique lists the ways to prevent AIDS by avoiding HIV infection. This advice can be read (in Portuguese) at http://www.cncs.org.mz/sida/index.html. Mozambicans are told to use a condom every time in every type of sexual relation. This is followed by advice to not forget male and female condoms; always use new needles and razors; don't share needles; and don't share personal objects where there might be contact with blood, such as razors, toothbrushes, and the like. No mention of sexual behavior or any need to change it.[3]

This list is typical of AIDS prevention programs in Africa. The advice looks like it was copied from a pamphlet used in New York, except that there is no mention of homosexuality. It is of little use to most Mozambicans. They are not likely to use a condom in commercial sex, let alone in every type of sexual relation. When the main advice given is not feasible, there may not be much hope that the other admonitions will be followed. Advice about sharing needles will seem as alien as condoms, or more so, to the great majority of Mozambicans. This list of ways to prevent AIDS is a perfect example of how preventions designed by Americans for high-risk, urban groups have little relevance to the rural masses of Africa.

Surveying published and unpublished literature, it is hard to find any report that credits partner reduction, delay of debut, or abstinence as significant behavior changes, or as anything that influences HIV prevalence rates. One has to search through a tangled thicket of obfuscation, denial, or benign neglect to discover this for oneself, as we have already seen in several examples.

An article in the *Daily Nation* (Kenya), posted on the U.N. Integrated Regional Information Network Web site (September 24, 2001), reported findings of a survey commissioned by the Media Institute and carried out by Strategic Research and Public Relations, with financial support from USAID. The report began, "A significant number of Kenyans had not changed their sexual behaviour in spite of massive public awareness about HIV/AIDS." What proportion in the survey had not changed their sexual behavior? 12.3 percent, meaning nearly 88 percent, reported they had changed, a bit higher than our 1998 survey in the Dominican Republic (see below). Changed in what way? Unsurprisingly, "38.6 percent of them had abstained from sex and 27.6 percent had reduced the number of sexual partners they had." This article went on to give no credit for this type or magnitude of change, but instead suggested that condom use in Kenya was not enough. This is the usual bias we encounter, namely, to overlook behavioral changes unlinked with condoms and to imply (or state) that only condom use qualifies as real behavioral change.

This condom or risk reduction bias is pervasive. Even though I think I understand many of the apparent reasons for this bias, it remains hard for me to understand how researchers can collect and analyze data from places like Uganda and not notice or comment on the importance of abstinence/delay (reported by 25–35% in the past year) or fidelity or zero grazing (reported by 93% in the past year, if we add the abstainers) (DHS/Uganda, 2000). These findings go without comment while much is made of the 49 percent of men and women who reported condom use with their last nonregular partner. Yet only 6.9 percent of the sexually active reported more than one partner. Virtually all behavioral surveys related to AIDS exhibit the same lack of interest in any behavior change unrelated to condoms or drugs.

PROGRAM IMPACT INDICATORS

Another measure of bias in how AIDS prevention is conceptualized and implemented can be found in the program indicators that donors use. The major donors and players in international AIDS (USAID, UNAIDS, WHO, CDC) use essentially the same indicators. Impact indicators measure progress toward achieving specific objectives. Those who implement AIDS prevention programs are held accountable to the extent that programs achieve progress as measured by these indicators. If there are no indicators, for example relating to abstinence, then a program is not held accountable for achieving any measure of abstinence. Put another way, if there are no X impact indicators associated with an AIDS or other health program, it is doubtful that project time or resources are devoted to X. Put yet another way, if there are several indicators relating to Y and Z, then we know immediately that project time or resources are devoted to Y and Z.

Individual projects funded by the major donors do not choose their own impact indicators. The donors agree in advance on these and then ensure that virtually all projects and programs they support seek to achieve the same types of objectives, that is, use the same impact indicators.

USAID's recent handbook (year 2000) of indicators for HIV/AIDS programs emphasize condoms first, then knowledge of HIV/AIDS, and then sexual behavior (most of which are in fact more condom-related indicators). Of the seven sexual behavior indicators, four are in fact condom related, two are MSM related, and one is CSW related. For Pattern II countries, only risky sex in the last year and sex with a CSW are of major relevance. The first indicator is the proportion of men or women who have had sex with a nonmarital, noncohabiting partner in the last twelve months. If multipartnerism is indeed driving the pandemic, then this is a much-needed indicator that—I think—was only borrowed from WHO in about 1996 (and then in draft form, as I recall). The Demographic and Health Surveys apparently starting asking questions, or at least one question, about casual sexual partners in 1994.

Since casual sex, or having multiple partners, drives the AIDS pandemic, it is difficult to understand why there were no program indicators related to it until 1996, or why the major U.S.–funded, AIDS-related survey waited until 1994 to ask a question about it.

The WHO/GPA has been conducting population-based surveys on sexual behavior since 1988. It seems that USAID, through its major contractors, overlooked the need to ask about casual sex or multiple partners for many years. WHO/UNAIDS apparently tried to persuade the DHS over some years before DHS added questions about sexual behavior (M. Carael, personal communication, October 24, 2001). This information is consistent with the lack of USAID performance indicators relating to partner reduction and abstinence or delay of debut prior to about 1996. UNAIDS, which grew out of the WHO/GPA, adopted indicators of this sort earlier than USAID.

For another type of evidence we can consider the DHS. These surveys are used by USAID–supported HIV/AIDS programs to monitor and evaluate AIDS programs, therefore the questions asked reflect not only the interest of USAID and the many organizations that receive USAID funds but also the allocation of project or program resources. We can begin by considering where emphasis lies in the current questionnaire. The word "condom" is used in questions twenty-nine times, if a few female condom questions are included. (By contrast, the Uganda Ministry of Health managed to only use the word condom to respondents five times in its most recent population-based KABP survey.) Yet there is only one question in the DHS about age of first intercourse (How old were you when you first had sexual intercourse [if ever]?), and one about having multiple partners. Neither "abstain" nor "absti-nence" appears in any question. I cannot help wondering if twenty-nine mentions about condoms sends a signal to the respondent that the interviewer is interested in condoms, especially relative to other answer options. This might prompt more condom answers than another survey instrument would.

For a decade or so, the DHS also asked a related pair of questions about (1) if the respondent had changed behavior due to AIDS, and if so, (2) in what way. The second question allowed respondents to offer information not specifically asked for or prompted. What resulted was a great deal of hitherto untapped expression of PBC. Yet in 2000, the administrators of the DHS decided with colleagues from UNAIDS that these questions were not useful and so dropped them from the questionnaire.

An indicator capturing the age of sexual debut was adopted in USAID's handbook of indicators for HIV/AIDS (2000). As it happens, both age of marriage and age of sexual debut are considered "proximate determinants of fertility," therefore DHS surveys have been getting these data in its fertility (family planning) module for a number of years. Yet it seems it was only in 2000 that USAID adopted this as an AIDS-related indicator, as indicator A1 under the rubric, Sexual Behavior among Young People. As of this writing, there seems little awareness among those working in AIDS with USAID funds that age of debut has become a program indicator. Yet because it is, it seems likely that targeting this behavior in prevention programs will become more common.

This indicator ought to capture the phenomenon of young people delaying sexual debut. Yet this is not as easy as it sounds. If one simply asks respondents how old they were when they first had sex, data only come from those who have had sex. It misses what may be a large proportion of youth delaying sex at the time of interviewing. We end up with a lower figure than if we somehow captured those not yet sexually active—which can be a substantial proportion in countries such as Uganda and Senegal.

The Measure project, which conducts the DHS surveys, recently improved the wording of how median age of sexual debut is measured. The following is Measure's description:

This measure is constructed from data on current virginity status among young people, not from retrospective questions about age at first sex. In household or special surveys focusing on young people, respondents are asked whether or not they have ever had penetrative sex. A curve is plotted according to the percent who say they have had sex by each single year of age. The age at which the curve exceeds 50 percent is taken to be the median age at first sex. On average, people reporting they are a certain age will be six months older than that age. (For example those who say they are 15 will range from those who turned 15 on the day of the survey to those who will turn 16 the following day. Assuming an even age distribution, they will be on average 15.5.) Half a year should therefore be added to the exact ages used in the calculation of the median age at first sex.[4]

However, as of this writing, the DHS is still calculating median debut age from retrospective questions about age at first sex. A May 8, 2002 e-mail to me from the Measure project explained that they hoped the new measurement would be adopted in the future. This would be an improvement.

USAID also has indicators intended to measure HIV and STD incidence and prevalence, policy, and political commitment to AIDS, all appropriate indicators.

There are also four indicators related to treatment of STDs, reflecting its interest in technical, medical solutions that involve export of drugs and commodities. This number suggests that STD treatment is exceeded only by condoms and basic AIDS education in importance, judging by the associated number of indicators in the current manual. Predictably, the STD indicators are of limited use in places such as Africa, home of the world's highest HIV infection rates, since they measure people who present at health care facilities. There is ample evidence that many or most Africans either self-medicate or present their STDs at the huts of traditional healers, and thereafter receive herbal medicines rather than STD drugs.

The third indicator in this category relates to drug supply at STI clinics, another medical intervention based on clinic attendance and the distribution of commodities that flow from North to South.

It should be remembered that local USAID–funded programs have the latitude to develop their own programs even if they go beyond the current list of HIV/AIDS indicators for monitoring and evaluation. This happened in Uganda as early as 1992 when programs targeted partner reduction and delay of sexual debut. Yet such programs are much more likely to be included if indicators related to them are already in the agencywide handbook of indicators. With the new directive from the overall administrator of USAID in May 2002 (see below), the stage ought to be set for the development of prevention programs that aim at PBC.

NEWEST BEHAVIOR CHANGE PROGRAM INDICATORS

Current UNAIDS indicators, which can be found on the Measure (DHS) Web site, http://www.measuredhs.com/hivdata/ind_tbl.cfm, are as follows:

8   Sexual behavior

8.1   Higher risk sex in the last year

8.2   Condom use at last higher risk sex

8.2.1 Condom use at last sex with spouse or cohabiting partner

8.2.2 Condom use at last sex with anyone

8.3   Commercial sex in last year

8.4   Condom use at last commercial sex, reported by client

8.5   Condom use at last commercial sex, reported by sex worker

8.6   Higher risk male–male sex in last year

8.7   Condom use at last anal sex between men

9   Young people's sexual behavior

9.1   Median age at first sex among young men and women

9.2   Young people having premarital sex in last year

9.3   Young people using a condom during premarital sex

9.4   Young people having multiple partners in last year

9.5   Young people using a condom at last higher risk sex

9.5.1 Young people using a condom at last higher risk sex of all young people surveyed

9.6   Condom use at first sex

9.7   Age-mixing in sexual relationships

Under the category of "Sexual behavior" (code 8), there are nine indicators, of which six measure condom use and two measure commercial sex or male-to-male sex. Under the next category, "Young people's sexual behavior," there are eight indicators of which four measure condom use. There seems to be some recognition that more other-than-condom measures are needed for young people. This represents some progress over a few years ago.

Then there is the so-called HANIG indicator for casual sex, recently adopted by the DHS: "The percent of respondents who have had sex with a non-marital, non-cohabiting partner in the last 12 months of all respondents reporting sexual activity in the last 12 months." This indicator fails to capture either those who are delaying/abstaining (a crucial measure of risk behavior, especially among youth, in whom USAID, UNAIDS, UNGASS, and others are now especially interested) or those who have only one partner. It assumes that if a couple does not cohabit, they are at higher risk, even if the couple is mutually faithful and monogamous.

Programs have been officially promoting A, B, and C for years, even if the money and program indicators relate to C . Programs have not been urging Abstain, Be faithful, Cohabit! I am not sure where or how the interest in the possible riskiness of noncohabitation arose, but to measure it and not multiple partners is to diminish even further the importance of multiple partners and any programs that have actually promoted sticking to one partner or "zero-grazing."

If we are indeed interested in multiple partners, questions about numbers of partners are more useful. We need simply ask married and unmarried men and women how many partners they have had, pure and simple, avoiding problems over how we define partners. When we do this we see that 98–99 percent of Ugandan and Dominican women (see below) report only one partner in the past year. These data seem to shed light on why HIV prevalence is declining or at least stable in these two countries. And they serve as a measure of impact of preventive programs actually promoted: fidelity, or stick to one partner.

While this book was in progress, the Bush-appointed administrator of USAID sent a cable to all field missions in March 2002, identifying new prevention and behavior change indicators: median age of sexual debut, number of nonregular partners, and condom use for nonregular partners. It is not certain whether new DHS questions capturing number of nonregular partners will be added or amended so that data on this, rather than on cohabitation, will result.

There are a few inchoate signs that thinking may be changing. In a recent *Population Reports* focused on youth, the summary urges that prevention programs go beyond merely offering information "to fostering risk-avoidance skills as well, such as delay of sexual debut, abstinence, and negotiation with sex partners" (Kiragu, 2001, p. 2).

However, most AIDS prevention programs to date, perhaps especially in Africa, seem to proceed on the assumption that there is only one realistic preventive strategy to AIDS, namely, condoms. Typical of this thinking is an article of over 10,000 words about AIDS prevention in Ghana and published recently in a major journal. I am singling it out because, first, it was based on qualitative, in-depth research, which ought to tell us something a little deeper than surveys based on instruments with precoded answers. Second, it was published in 2002, which illustrates that none of the findings assembled for the present book have penetrated the condom paradigm for many or most who work in international AIDS.

The article repeats all the reasons we have heard for years about why condoms are not used more than they are: "The high value placed on fertility, the negative association of condoms with prostitution, and the women's limited ability to influence decision-making in this area" (Mill & Anarfib, 2002, p. 325). How many hundreds or perhaps thousands of papers and conference abstracts have said the same thing?

We can't help but be pushed toward the conclusion that here is another population of irrational Africans who just don't know what is
good for them. At one point, Ghanaian participants in the study are
asked what they themselves think is needed to prevent AIDS. As with
respondents to surveys such as DHS and WHO/GPA and UNAIDS,
Ghanaian women in the present in-depth study mentioned responses
such as "abstinence in sexual relationships before marriage to having
fewer partners and 'not roaming from man to man'" (Mill & Anarfib,
2002, p. 325) . For those who have learned the lessons of Uganda and
other countries successful in reducing AIDS, this sounds both reasonable and familiar. Yet there is no comment in the present article about
informants' suggestions that partner reduction might have value. And
as for abstinence, the authors note, "Although the men concurred with
the notion of abstinence before marriage, they admitted that, for some
men, it was not possible" (Mill & Anarfi, 2002, p. 325). For these authors,
"some men" is apparently equivalent to all men (and women) because
these other-than-condom notions are never mentioned again. Discussion returns to what these, and indeed most, AIDS researchers no doubt
believed in before going through the bother of research: condoms.[5]

In a parallel example from South Africa, a new U.S.–funded project
in the eastern Cape is described in an AIDS newsletter. The author
describes what Africans themselves are doing to respond to AIDS,
which is promoting abstinence until marriage for youth. But then the
U.S.–funded project which employs the author arrives and supports
something else, namely condoms and VCT. We might think the outside project would to some extent want to take the opportunity to build
upon what people themselves are already doing (i.e., on the endogenous response to AIDS), but apparently not. The author implies that
these Africans need to be brought up to speed. She observes, "Young
women in Chief Dlamini's communities feel they are helping their community and nation by abstaining from sex." But this is what they are
getting from the project: "Through social marketing campaigns, young
people feel it is 'cool' to wear branded condoms while the thousands
visiting public clinics now have access to free condoms without consultation. Finally, for the growing numbers who want to know their
HIV status, VCT sites are increasingly available" (Urdaneta, 2003).

The title of this article is "Best Practices: What Do We Know about
Prevention Programs that Work?" It is not hard to guess which type of
programs the author thinks are the only best practices. Of course she
only reflects the dominant paradigm. A recent 221-page "Summary of
Best Practices by UNAIDS" (Pisani, 1999) identified almost every activity associated with AIDS prevention except interventions aimed at
partner reduction or abstinence. This is an egregious example of consensus-based, as distinct from evidence-based, thinking.

For a particularly egregious illustration of Western consensus-based AIDS thinking, the UNGASS Indicators Task Force recently finalized its recommendations to the U.N. general assembly for global HIV prevention and care program indicators. These indicators, like those already used by UNAIDS and USAID, will help define the measurable outcomes that future programs, for example, those funded under the GFATM and other major international donors. A group of experts met during 2002 to decide upon the recommended behavioral indictors for HIV/AIDS prevention. They were announced during the global AIDS conference in Barcelona. There is only one official indicator: the proportion of youth using condoms.

In spite of some progress on the part of USAID and UNAIDS in recent years in defining indicators that are more evidence based, UNGASS has apparently reaffirmed the reduction behavior change to condom use, period. This action by UNGASS may provide the mandate and yardstick for, for example, country programs funded by the GFATM, to continue business-as-usual condom programs, and to call this AIDS prevention for youth. It is particularly troubling that this single indicator seems about to become enshrined, considering the focus of UNGASS on youth. We have several clear examples from Africa and elsewhere that (1) HIV prevalence rates tend to decline first among youth; (2) abstinence and delay of debut are often the behavior changes largely responsible for this decline (as occurred in Uganda, Senegal, Zambia, and even, it seems, as is beginning to happen in South Africa); and (3) when abstinence/delay of debut and fidelity/partner reduction are promoted through schools, faith-based peer education programs, and the like, such behavior changes are more likely to occur.

Some people are already worrying that the millions allocated through the GFATM will not produce results, but probably not for the same reasons I have been discussing. An executive of an AIDS NGO posted on Break-the-Silence list serve, "Under the GFATM-Government arrangement it is difficult to ensure that funds are allocated to programs that are working, not to programs with great objectives that are failing" (Burgess, 2002a). He goes on to say the following:

Few are as disappointed as I am at the terrible performance of development and emergency interventions over the past twenty or thirty years. This is not about bad lazy people . . . the problem is great people working very hard in institutions and organizations that have become slaves to ineffective systems and processes and procedures. It is time we broke out of this vicious situation, and created a virtuous loop of positive feedback based on accountability and performance criteria. (Burgess, 2002a)

I agree, even if my diagnosis may differ as to why many of us have become slaves to ineffective systems.

I have probably written more about impact indicators than any sane person wants to read. Many other examples of bias against PBC are sprinkled liberally throughout this book. In fact, it is time to confront the question, Why is there such a strong bias? As I asked at the beginning of this book, if there is evidence that PBC has been a major contributor to reduction of HIV infections, or *the* major one, why have so few experts recognized this? This is a difficult question with no simple or single answer. But it is an important one. I have spent quite a lot of time thinking about it in recent years.

WHY IS THERE A BIAS TOWARD CONDOM-DRUG APPROACHES?

To better understand the evident bias in favor of risk reduction and against PBC, it may be useful to outline the main probable reasons at this stage. The global response to HIV/AIDS was developed disproportionately by Americans, and secondarily by Europeans. It is therefore useful to understand the perceptions and values that underlay the initial response to AIDS in the United States. And to understand this, it is useful to consider American perceptions and values in the 1960s and 1970s, just prior to the emergence of AIDS. Of this period, social historian Peter Allen notes the following:

Old scourges like syphilis and gonorrhea were now seen as minor nuisances that could be cured with a couple of shots. . . . Prophylactics, contraceptives, and abortion were increasingly socially accepted and easy to obtain. Coupled with these factors was a series of social movements that drastically changed people's concepts of the meaning and place of sex in their lives: the sexual revolution, feminism, and the beginnings of the modern gay and lesbian movement. Suddenly, much of the population felt much freer to be sexually active than it had in decades, and the accidental consequences of sex—pregnancy and infection— seemed more remote than they had ever been. Sex outside of wedlock was safe; it was readily available; it was viewed as liberating; and—perhaps most important of all, in the consumer culture of the United States—sex was fun.

Into this petri dish of social change dropped the virus that would come to be known as HIV. This microscopic particle would reveal the flaws in many of the assumptions that had governed recent views of sex, disease, and many other parts of life. The freedom and openness with which men and women viewed casual sex, the safety with which many viewed heterosexual marriage, the strength of national borders, and the belief that science could control the threats of the natural world—all of these comfortable assumptions were challenged and weakened by the power of a diminutive parasite that was not really even alive. (Allen, 2000, p. 120)

USAID relied to a large extent on AIDS experts from the American gay community to guide the earliest international programs. There was a perception that these experts had the answer because by the mid-1980s, there seemed to be evidence that American gays were changing their behavior. The behavior change was said to be widespread condom use, and to a lesser extent, nonpenetrative or safer sexual practices. It was also the case that gays had fought for years to develop their own lifestyle of sexual freedom, and they did not want anyone, even other gays who worked in public health, to tell them they should have fewer partners, to be monogamous (Rotello, 1997). One of the gay-lesbian movement's "earliest and most basic objectives, especially for gay men, was sexual freedom: the right to have sexual lives that were untrammeled by the conventions and limitations of society's norms. . . . For many, it meant the freedom to enjoy sexual relations with many partners, either on a continuing basis or just in passing" (Allen, 2000, p. 125). This value became embedded in AIDS prevention programs designed for developing countries, even though prevention programs were already underway in countries like Uganda and Senegal that emphasized restriction of sexual behavior, having fewer sexual partners.

Soon the mantra around the major international AIDS prevention donors was, The condom is the only weapon we have in the war against AIDS. The first director of the WHO Global Programme on AIDS described sexual behavior change as an achievable goal, and described the approach as risk reduction and involving condoms, even several years into the global program (Merson, 1993). If there was any language about the dangers of having multiple partners, it tended to come from local educators who had not yet heard, or believed, the "only weapon we have" message. Or it might have been language meant to assuage local religious leaders or school authorities, but it rarely reflected donor priorities in funding or impact indicators.

In addition to condoms, American AIDS prevention advisors also thought of ways to promote masturbation and oral sex to Africans and others, to liberate them from outmoded and perhaps repressive sexual norms, especially homophobia. What Americans and Europeans forgot when designing these responses to AIDS in Africa and other less-developed parts of the world is that these cultures were still largely bound by tradition and religion; they had not undergone the sexual revolution, and certainly not the gay-lesbian revolution, of the West.

Even though it was increasingly recognized through a growing body of research that having multiple sexual partners drove all sexually transmitted epidemics, there was little talk of designing programs to discourage multipartnerism ("promiscuity" was quickly dropped from the public health vocabulary). It must be remembered that President Reagan's wife had suggested to "just say no" as the solution to AIDS in America. This phrase became a rallying cry for gays, lesbians, liberals, and most of us in public health, something to be opposed at all costs since it was seen by many of us as a code phrase for compulsory heterosexuality and premarital chastity, total rejection of condoms, a compete ban on all abortion, discouragement of all contraception, rejection of women's rights (and perhaps restriction of women's roles to domestic chores), and diversion of AIDS funds to those judged innocent of sin, not to mention hatred, intolerance, and repression, and, perhaps, teaching creationism in schools. Few Americans or Europeans designing AIDS prevention interventions at that time had enough experience in Africa to realize that a phrase like "just say no" or "zero-graze" had no such associations for Africans. It made a great deal of sense for the presidents of Uganda and Senegal to develop prevention programs in the mid-1980s, before most donor-driven programs began, that discouraged multiple partners.

Put simply, a great deal of the early design of prevention programs for generalized epidemics were done by experts in a different kind of epidemic, namely, those driven by core transmitter groups. That is, those with experience in reaching high risk groups (MSM, IDU, CSW) in developed countries of the West strongly influenced the design of the first programs aimed at majority populations in resource-poor countries of the less-developed world. These early programs defined the model and the paradigm of prevention. It must be acknowledged that there were no other experts around at the time, so it is not my intention to assign blame with benefit of hindsight. But understanding this goes a long way toward helping us understand how risk reduction interventions became the standard approach for all epidemics, early in the pandemic. It is largely a matter of incompatibility between cultures and epidemiologic patterns.

I was conducting research related to contraception and sexual behavior in the mid-1980s in the Dominican Republic when the first team of Americans arrived in that country to design the first U.S.–funded AIDS prevention project. The team spent its time visiting brothels, gay bars, nightclubs, and other places associated with AIDS of the American pattern. I wondered at the time if this team was interested in the broader population or only in certain high-risk groups. Perhaps we didn't know at the time what HIV transmission pattern would come to characterize the Dominican Republic. But it would have been safe to guess that the Dominican pattern might develop at least somewhat like those developing in Africa or at least in Haiti, since the Dominican Republic is situated on the same island as Haiti, and HIV was already in the general Haitian population.

Why has the issue of Pattern I solutions for Pattern II problems not been recognized sooner? Part of the answer lies in arrogance on the part of donor organizations, but there are many other contributing reasons, such as reliance on an infectious disease model, awe of technological solutions, stereotyping of African sexual behavior, and the like. It did not help that we dropped reference to these different global patterns a few years ago. We can find evidence of pattern confusion among leading AIDS experts today. For example, anthropologist Richard Parker wrote, "In all societies, regardless of their degree of development or prosperity, the HIV/AIDS epidemic continues to rage, but it now affects almost exclusively the most marginalized sectors of society" (Parker, 2002, p. 343). This is true in the United States and possibly in Brazil, but not in Africa.

In fact, one might expect that anthropologists would have recognized that the type of AIDS prevention being exported from Washington and Geneva was inappropriate to the cultural and epidemiologic realities of Africa and the Caribbean. But anthropologists did not notice or speak out on this issue, and my own attempts to bring this to the attention of American academic anthropologists working in AIDS were usually met with silence or criticism. But the cultural and epidemiologic mismatch was harder to ignore in Africa itself. A South African anthropologist recently published an article in the *Mail and Guardian* newspaper called, "South Africa: Prevention Means More Than Condoms" (Leclerc-Madlala, 2002), which criticizes the U.S.–funded LoveLife campaign along the lines of this present chapter. She points out that the slick, multimedia campaign that has found its way into nearly every South African home has little relevance for Black South Africans. The idea behind the campaign is to make condom use seem hip: "The youth are portrayed as middle class, sophisticated, and seem likely to spend their weekends enjoying multi-racial camaraderie in suburban rave clubs. Wittingly or unwittingly, the thrust of our national HIV/Aids prevention effort speaks primarily to a narrow band of privileged youth" (Leclerc-Madlala, 2002, p. 19). She goes on to point out that her country should be looking not to Beverly Hills for answers to AIDS, but to Uganda, where people changed their behavior—and not for the most part by using condoms. She concludes, "As unlikely as it may sound, Uganda's experiences suggest that the promotion of abstinence before marriage and mutual faithfulness in relationships may be the keys to halting the spread of Aids in Africa" (Leclerc-Madlala, 2002, p. 19).

Reflecting on the overall response to AIDS in Africa, Tangwa of the University of Yaounde recently observed, "The response to the HIV/AIDS pandemic in Africa has so far ignored important traditional African values and attitudes toward disease and commerce. These values and attitudes are significantly different from the libertarian, market-driven, profit-oriented values and practices of important sectors of the Western world. To deal with this epidemic, the world should consider respect for, and possibly even adoption of those African values" (2002, p. 217).

Turning to other reasons to explain bias, many professionals who work in AIDS prevention have backgrounds in population and family planning. For that matter, the DHS organization developed out of this same background and preexisting expertise. This predisposes international AIDS professionals to think of AIDS solutions that involve contraceptives. USAID, as well as the World Bank and various U.N. organizations such as UNFPA, had extensive experience in condom and other contraceptive promotion and distribution, prior to the appearance of AIDS. Confirming this orientation, USAID often comments that it has a comparative advantage in the condom supply and promotion part of AIDS prevention. Other major donors could also make the same comment. Family planning backgrounds predispose AIDS experts to be suspicious about working with religious leaders or organizations because there is a long history of antagonism between family planners and certain religious groups, notably the Roman Catholic Church, and more recently, the religious right in America. Some of my family planning colleagues fear that any questioning of contraceptives, including use of condoms for AIDS prevention, is part of a larger agenda, or indeed plot, to cut off funding for all contraception and to oppose the advancement of women's rights.

And yet if one believes on providing a full range of options and choices in family planning, then surely the same full range ought to be offered in AIDS prevention. And those who work in family planning know that the condom is one of the least effective methods of preventing unwanted pregnancy. How could the paradox have escaped them that the same method is considered the most effective method of preventing HIV infection? In fact, as shown in Chapter 4, HIV is more likely to get through latex than sperm, even if the chances of becoming HIV infected in a single act of penile-vaginal intercourse are fairly low compared to becoming pregnant.

Mindful of the full disclosure one expects these days about any possible author bias, I ought to add that I also have a background in family planning, including condom and other contraceptive social marketing programs. I even earned a bit of fame for my work in oral contraceptive social marketing in the Dominican Republic and in showing that condom use had risen as a result of an effective AIDS prevention program in the same country. I say this to show that, if anything, I share the same assumptions and viewpoint as most international AIDS professionals. It was only when I first went to Uganda briefly in 1993 that I began to think that PBC might be important.[6]

AIDS, including its prevention, has become a billion-dollar annual industry. The U.S. budget alone for global (excluding domestic) AIDS activities is projected at $884 million for fiscal year 2003 (this was before President Bush's February 2003 pledge of $10 billion new money for global AIDS). It would be politically naïve to expect that those who profit from this industry would not be inclined to protect their interests. Those who work in condom promotion and STD treatment, as well as the industries that supply the devices and drugs, do not want to lose market share, so to speak, and so they may go out of their way to ignore, disguise, or discredit findings that show something else is working to bring down HIV infection rates.

Furthermore, it is tempting to rely on quick technological fixes to complex problems involving complex human behavior. Condoms and STD drugs can be procured, promoted, distributed, and—more important—all this can be counted easily. Thus the donor has good ready-made monitoring and evaluation units of measurement in condoms and drugs, and these units are familiar from decades of family planning programs.

Those who work in public health tend to look at problems in a medical way, in accordance with their training. There are also various types of behavioral scientists working in AIDS prevention, but it is safe to say that the problem of AIDS has been highly medicalized rather than seen as a behavioral challenge involving sociocultural variables. Once a problem is medicalized, the solutions become drugs and medical technology and the means become health facilities and medical personnel.

With AIDS, it seems easier to work with a medical or a medical-technological solution than one involving intimate forms of behavior and their determinants. People with various types of health training are more comfortable with medical and technical solutions than with dealing with behavioral, social, cultural, or economic issues. Specifically, health personnel feel uncomfortable making value judgments or moralizing about someone else's behavior. This is partly due to lack of training in this area, partly due to the premises of risk or harm reduction philosophy (if you moralize, you drive the patient away), and partly due to it simply being more comfortable for the health worker to avoid these difficult issues.

Health professionals for the most part believe that dealing with sexual behavior is awkward at best, although they are more likely to comment that it is more realistic and even ethical to refrain from moralizing, or even seeming judgmental, about sexual behavior. This attitude developed in the United States early in the AIDS epidemic, before American experts went to Africa or elsewhere in the developing world to confront AIDS. And understandably, it seemed to make little sense for health professionals to seem to pass negative judgment on the sexual behavior of gay men or the drug or sexual behavior of IDUs. That would only alienate the very people that needed help, perhaps making them inaccessible.

Turning to yet another reason, for those who have long been extolling the advantages of condoms (i.e., most who work in AIDS prevention), it may be very difficult to acknowledge that PBC is an essential, but overlooked, factor in reducing AIDS epidemics. Professional reputations and egos are at stake. People don't want to admit that they may have completely missed something vitally important for years. As a book that reviews great debates in the history of medicine shows, new ideas threaten egos as well as current funding priorities to such an extent, the wonder is that any new ideas are adopted in medical science at all (Hellman, 2001). In one of many examples, Ignaz Semmelweis (1818–1865) lost his job and ended his days in an insane asylum for having the effrontery to suggest to doctors that they wash their hands before delivering babies. The parallel with questioning the AIDS prevention paradigm may be justified: The lives of many babies and mothers were certainly lost before hand washing, and many lives may have been lost to AIDS in the past two decades, by failing to promote a full range of effective means of prevention. No one wants to feel responsible for the latter.

Next is the issue of sexual stereotyping. Many AIDS professionals simply do not believe—even if they would never say it publicly—that Africans could or would ever change their sexual behavior significantly. This may be due to racial and ethnic stereotyping of sexual behavior, which in its worst form depicts African men as unable to control sexual urges. Westerners often have an exaggerated notion of how many sexual partners Africans have—meaning most Africans, or Africans in the majority population.

As already noted, the AIDS prevention paradigm for Africa and indeed the world was largely developed in the United States for high-risk groups, such as gay men, IDUs, and sex workers. It certainly seemed that these groups were unlikely and indeed unwilling to fundamentally change their sexual behavior, and so risk or harm reduction made sense. In the minds of most Western AIDS experts, Africans were no more likely to reduce numbers of sexual partners than high-risk Americans. Thus when evidence of significant behavior change emerges, such as in Uganda, it is disbelieved or ignored.

An experience I had in Uganda will illustrate this last point. A Ugandan health educator and I were in the office of a Western AIDS expert. She was explaining why it was not necessary to have an abstinence component in a prevention project she was implementing, even though a portion of donor organization funds had been allocated for this very purpose. "Ugandans," she said, "are the most promiscuous people in the world and they would never change their sexual behavior. So it would be a waste of money to promote abstinence."

I was shocked that she would say such a thing in the presence of a host country national, even if it were true. But it wasn't. So I asked her about the research that even then, in 1998, pointed to significant change in sexual behavior, especially in partner reduction and delay of sexual debut. It turned out that she was unaware of the published research from the country she was living and working in.

A cynic might suggest that we face a pro-condom, antibehavior change bias because no one makes money if someone in a developing country simply remains faithful to a spouse and therefore does not need male or female condoms or STD treatment. Certainly the marketing of condoms (rather than the cost of condoms per se) has become a multimillion-dollar industry, as to a lesser extent has the treatment of STDs. A dozen or so for-profit organizations, and several large and successful nonprofit organizations, have been thriving on contracts and grants from USAID and other donors over the past nearly twenty years. However, the social marketing, BCC, IEC, and related skills of these organizations could be put to use selling programs such as Life Skills that promote PBC. This is discussed further in Chapter 11.

But before leaving this point, it does seem that A and B programs may not be regarded as real interventions in the minds of many AIDS professionals. Because abstinence and fidelity do not require sale of commodities, our commodities-oriented mentality may unconsciously discount such programs. A colleague active in international AIDS programs wrote an e-mail that recounts a recent discussion she had with a U.N. official about funding for A and B interventions. It stated the following:

He stated that everyone accepted that A and B are HIV prevention alternatives. I mentioned that if they wanted the church to believe that they were considered legitimate partners with a legitimate intervention then international donors should be providing the church with equal funding for A and B programs. At that point he looked me in the eye with complete sincerity and said, "but you have to pay for condoms." I informed him that good A and B promotion would require programs that would also cost. He genuinely seemed surprised. (D. Brewster-Lee, personal communication, July 4, 2002)

The e-mail writer, of course, is right that A and B promotion involves costs, but it is also true that we know less about the range of such costs, largely because there has been so little experience in funding such programs. I deal with the issue of designing and funding A and B interventions in Chapter 11.

Finally, Gorna has analyzed the AIDS prevention paradigm from a women's or feminist perspective. She notes, "In addressing HIV prevention to women there is a tension between the need to focus on long-term societal change and the need to develop short-term protective measures" (1996, p. 294). The latter, of course, refers to condom promotion. By focusing on this, the status quo is maintained and there is less need to address women's inequality and oppression. Unfortunately, short-term measures have a way of becoming entrenched, or becoming the only proven intervention. Even Gorna seems to question in the following the possibility of a solution or intervention that goes beyond technology:

The contexts within which sex happens are sufficiently diverse and complicated that it would be logical to expect a range of technologies to reduce the risk of HIV transmission. Not so. To date there is but one method which is proven: the latex male condom; and one which can be recommended: the polyurethane female condom. This reduction of HIV prevention to condoms is bizarre when compared to the range of contraceptive technologies available for women. (1996, p. 296)

Note this author's use of "technologies," as if solutions must lie in these. The title of the chapter where this quote appears is "Just Say No?" which suggests that the author considered behavior change nondependent on technology and rejected it, perhaps as unrealistic for today's women. And what about fidelity or partner reduction? Again we see evidence that many people define non-condom behavioral options as consisting of abstinence (only). People either have sex and use technology, or they do not, and of course abstinence is unrealistic. This either–or thinking has interfered with giving fair consideration to the options that people are likely to report due to concern with AIDS, namely, fidelity or partner reduction and delay of debut. Too often discussion about possibilities that go beyond condoms is preempted by a sarcastic, Just say no?

MASTURBATION AND NONPENETRATIVE SEX

There is another prevention option beyond ABC that seems to have developed in the United States but seems not to have been promoted very much in Africa, namely, nonpenetrative sex. In this option, people at risk are taught to substitute such practices as oral sex, mutual masturbation, and other nonpenetrative practices that lead to sexual satisfaction. This has felicitously been called "outercourse" as distinct from intercourse (Gorna, 1996). Feminist Robin Gorna doesn't believe nonpenetrative sex has been promoted much even in the West. She says in the following:

The fact that "safer sex" was invented by gay men means that there are inevitable restrictions with its methodology for women. By the time it was translated to vaginal sex, the concept "safer sex = condoms" was well-established, and it would (and will) take a lot to shift the orthodoxy. (1996, p. 302)

Some Americans with experience in U.S. gay communities and who were among the first outsiders to bring AIDS prevention ideas to Africa early in the epidemic were surprised to learn that such practices were relatively rare in Africa, or at least seemed to be. With this discovery, some AIDS educators thought they could and would revolutionize African sexual behavior once these options of safer sex were taught, thereby greatly reducing HIV transmission. Some even saw their work as liberating Africans from their outmoded sexual taboos, bringing the sexual revolution to Africa, as it were.

In spite of some efforts to promote (or legitimize) masturbation and nonpenetrative sex, there does not seem to be much evidence of results, at least in Africa. Barton, citing two Ugandan studies (Busulwa, 1995; Okuma et al., 1994), commented, "Although various forms of solitary or mutual masturbation and fondling have been described, they do not appear to be significant alternatives to penetrative coitus at the present time" (1997, p. 36). Busulwa's qualitative study of sexual beliefs and practices in the Jinja district, Uganda, in fact found evidence of individual and mutual masturbation, as well as male and female homosexual practices. For example, there is a phenomenon called "darlingism" that refers to girls in boarding schools who get female lovers (Busulwa, 1995, pp. 54–59). This researcher also describes a "rare" nonpenetrative sexual practice in western Uganda called *kakyabali* (Busulwa, 1995, p. 57).

Qualitative research in Zimbabwe concluded, "Types of sexual behaviour other than penetrative vaginal sex are uncommon and considered deviant. Safe sex messages from the West therefore are inappropriate in the Zimbabwean context" (Vos, 1988, p. 5).

It has been hypothesized, "Young men who have an open acceptance of masturbation as a healthy form of sexual expression, will, on balance, be less likely to be involved in high-risk sexual behaviors" (Clark, 2001). This may be true and if so, efforts should be made to legitimize masturbation. In South Africa, a popular jazz musician who has performed with the group, Stimela, has been targeting youth with this message as a means of AIDS prevention. According to the following news posted on af-aids@healthdev.net, May 9, 2002):

Ray Phiri and what he calls his "One Armed Struggle Regiment" were in Harare recently to give us the message, "Play with yourself," referring to masturbation as a way of safeguarding against contracting HIV. The name One-Armed Struggle Regiment is derived from the act of masturbation as usually practised by men (using one hand).

Phiri sees masturbation as an effective and cheap way of maintaining one's sexuality and achieving sexual satisfaction while avoiding infection. He emphasised that masturbation is not a sin and dismissed the myths around the subject, where young people have been told things such as that they will grow hairs on their palms or go blind should they engage in the activity. Men should use it instead of seeking out casual partners or when their wives don't feel like having sex. (http://archives.Healthdev.net/af-aids/msg00356.html)

Likewise, South Africa's foremost youth AIDS awareness campaign, LoveLife, has run an AIDS prevention advertising campaign that encourages young people to try "sucking, licking, and kissing a person's genitals" as an alternative to penetrative sex, according to Deutsche Presse-Agentur (June 14, 2002; posted on af-aids@healthdev.net, June 28, 2002). This predictably provoked controversy, even the comment from the South African deputy president that such practices were wrong and unnatural.

Still, such efforts are rare throughout Africa. The promotion of oral sex, mutual masturbation, and related practices may in fact be seen as a projection of Western, urban sexual norms and values, whether gay or heterosexual, onto rural Africans. These are the values of the Western generations that grew up with contraceptives (and cars). And if values are rooted in American gay experience, these developed during or after a successful struggle for alternative lifestyles. Some in the gay community believe in an "anything goes" sexual expression that takes as a given that sexuality should be expressed and enjoyed to the utmost, and there need be little or no worry about consequences. In the AIDS era, this value persists in safer sex, which is often taken to mean any pleasurable sexual act that is less likely to transmit HIV than penetrative sex.

In fact, anyone who disagrees with "anything goes" sexuality might be accused of having a phobia. In a book about AIDS and sexuality, in a section on anilingus, "fisting," and sadomasochistic practices that provoke bleeding—all for and by women—the author suggests that anyone who disapproves of such sexual expression is a victim of "germophobia" or "erotophobia" (Gorna, 1996, p. 232). The book's foreword is by the highly respected late Jonathan Mann, former director of the WHO/GPA. My concern is twofold. First, these modern, Western, urban values tend not to be found in Africa, and any campaign designed to modify behavior ought to be made compatible with prevailing rather than foreign values and attitudes. Second, in societies where rape, seduction of minors, and coerced sex is common, the promotion of free sexual expression by outside experts might exacerbate these problems. In any case, the norms, values, and sexual behavioral patterns in rural Africa are not as many Western experts imagine them to be, and behavior change messages involving condoms or mutual masturbation need to remember who their target audience is and return to the basic principles of cross-cultural communication.

There is some cultural precedent in Africa for at least one type of safer sex behavior. For example, among at least some Nguni groups, young men used to be taught to practice nonpenetrative thigh sex. In focus group discussions I conducted among South African traditional healers in 1992, I found that "healers commented that in former times, elders took boys to the bush to educate them about proper sexual behavior. This included instruction in 'thigh sex' (*ukusoma, ukufema, ukujuma*), or other intercourse where there is no penetration, intended for youth and the unmarried" (Green, Zokwe, & Dupree, 1995, p. 507). Other researchers in southern Africa have likewise reported that nonpenetrative or nonvaginal (intercrural) intercourse used to be taught (Armstrong, 1987) or permitted (Ames, 1974) in the past, but that such practices are rare or nonexistent nowadays. Nonpenetrative has sometimes been mentioned as a traditional form of pregnancy avoidance in West Africa (e.g., Caldwell, 1968) and East Africa, namely, Kenya (Leaky, 1931; Southall, 1960). In all societies where these practices were found, there were strong sanctions against premarital pregnancy. The adolescent age group sometimes collaborated with elders in monitoring premarital behavior because the behavior of an individual reflected upon the group, for example, Bantu-speaking groups in South Africa (Steyn & Rip, 1968).

In 1974, a group of Zulu nursing students described the following nonpenetrative practices of the (unspecified) past, which were part of instruction accompanying coming-of-age rites:

Traditionally, the instructress was an older girl, age 19–20, who instructed, answered questions, and supervised the ritual seclusion of the pubertal girl. At age 17–18, the girls were permitted to choose a steady boyfriend with teaching about "ukusoma", a legitimate form of heavy petting (intercrural coitus). Boys during this time were also receiving instruction about the importance of preserving the girl's virginity. Girls were periodically examined for virginity, and transgressions by the boy would result in severe chastisement by the elders. Ukusoma was supposed to be limited to once per month, with marriage in the near future to avoid excess emotional and sexual strain. . . . In the urban situation, boys can more readily persuade the girls to accede to full vaginal intercourse and not waste time with this "soma business". (Cheetham, Sibisi, & Cheetham, 1974, p. 41)

We see evidence here of the breakdown of traditional practices and cultural mechanisms for preserving premarital virginity and avoiding pregnancy. Indeed, more recent surveys in South Africa were finding that teens knew little about sex, pregnancy, menstruation, and other topics covered in rites of passage instruction. One study found that "only 31% of the young women understood the relationship of menstruation, sexual intercourse, fertility, and conception" (Craig & Richter-Strydom, 1983, p. 239). This study found the following:

Family, schools, and the public media were all inadequate in their presentation of these topics. Currently, parental sex education for girls seems limited to the caution to "stay away from boys or they will bring shame to you." Open social control has been replaced by ignorance and secrecy. (p. 239)

In a systematic survey my colleagues and I conducted among seventy traditional healers from diverse parts of South Africa some years later, we observed the following:

We asked healers if any people in their area practiced thigh sex or other non-penetrative intercourse. Only 13 (19%) said yes, usually with the qualification that the practice had become increasingly rare, 42 said no, and 15 did not know. In some urban areas such as Capetown, healers commented that the practice is "unknown" among younger people. A number of healers in the predominantly rural Tsonga "homeland" commented that people were no longer interested in thigh sex (*mantanga*), one noting, "even the youngest want penetrative sexual intercourse."

Thigh sex was reported to be common only in the Swazi self-governing area of KaNgwane, where healers sometimes encourage the practice when a wife is menstruating. (Green, Zokwe, & Dupree, 1995, p. 507)

I noted at the time the potential that might be exploited for promoting safer sex, at least with this group, referring here to nonpenetrative intercourse. However, I have not seen evidence that there has been much promotion of this type of safer sex, nor any significant behavior change in this direction. Nor have I seen evidence that a more Western, urban, liberated style of sexuality has been very much promoted in most of Africa, nor has this been adopted by Africans as a way to avoid HIV infection. As seen in evidence cited already, the most commonly reported response to threat of AIDS in open-ended questions has been to have fewer partners. This is not to say that other safer sex options and possibilities might not work as well.

As for teaching masturbation as a form of safe sex, I suspect that Africans and others do not have to be taught about this by Americans.

ABSTINENCE: A POLITICAL LIGHTNING ROD

Primary behavior change, and even the ABC approach, has been framed by Western AIDS experts as politically loaded abstinence and thus rejected. In other words, the political meaning of abstinence in the United States has blinded Western AIDS experts to the appropriateness of the PBC response in Africa.

What is the background to this? A very polarized liberal-conservative argument has developed in the United States in recent years, one in which the issues are pitched as the "condoms only" people against the "abstinence only." This is most unfortunate and it weakens the cause of putting some reasonable portion of prevention resources into programs that promote delay of debut or partner reduction. Those who suggest such a strategy are suspected of having a hidden, right-wing agenda that secretly seeks to put funds into abstinence only. The argument about "abstinence only" is a straw man. It may be compared with the following illogical syllogism:

Exercise and proper diet are necessary for good health;

Exercise alone is not enough.

Therefore there should be no exercise programs.

Not only do professionals working in AIDS and broader reproductive health feel suspicious of anyone who questions the condom solution, most Americans seem to feel the same way. The following letter to the editor in *USA Today* is typical:[7]

Condoms will save millions of lives by preventing HIV/AIDS and other sexually transmitted diseases. Abstinence is honorable, but not a reality when looking at a massive world health problem that is killing millions of people every year. Graham should come out of the Middle Ages and into the 21st century and help defeat this terrible disease. (March 7, 2002)

Many an AIDS expert has likewise told me that abstinence sounds wonderful, but of course, this is not a realistic option—especially in Africa. The unspoken assumption or implication here is that Africans are more sexual than the rest of the world and that they could never control their sexual behavior. If I point out that this is racial stereotyping and, in fact, at odds with existing data, my colleagues might say something like, Well, you know, in the tropics, in these little villages, there is little else to do but have sex. It's all they have for recreation. If I mention the evidence about delay of debut or partner reduction, many immediately think this is a trick to weaken their critical judgment. Or it is a Trojan horse that will be used to slip abstinence-only programs through their defenses and into AIDS prevention.

The behavioral change that was probably most responsible for Uganda's 66 percent decline in HIV prevalence, partner reduction, is not mentioned. Anything that is not condom or pill related becomes abstinence.

To get around this use of, and reaction to, the "A" word, I sometimes point out that even if one doesn't believe in abstinence or fidelity behavioral change, it might make sense to embrace these to some degree if only for public relations. The fact is that many or most African leaders remain to be convinced that condoms are a good thing to promote to the general public, as distinct from high-risk groups. This is true for all levels of leaders, down to the villages. It should be "Anthropology 101" to approach behavior change interventions in ways that are culturally acceptable, even apart from effectiveness considerations. A leading sociologist recently put it the same way. He argued that men in particular need to stop having multiple sexual partners, and unless they do, "they will continue to be infected and pass on HIV to their wives and girlfriends, and through them, to their children. This is not some kind of a moralistic or socially conservative, pro-abstinence and monogamy message. This is Sociology 101" (Etzioni, 2003, p. 9). He further notes that "the main burden of making the required tough changes, must be carried by local leaders and the people involved," not foreign experts.

The views of President Museveni of Uganda and his wife are discussed in Chapter 6. Zambian former president, Frederick Chiluba, recently questioned the use of condoms in AIDS prevention and commented, "I don't believe in condoms myself because it is a sign of weak morals on the part of the user. . . . If you cannot abstain from casual sex then try to regulate yourself" (*Bay Area Reporter*, January 11, 2001). King Mswati III of Swaziland went further and tried to impose a five year sex ban as a solution to AIDS in his country (*African Eye News Service*, September 17, 2001), which actually means he is trying to promote delay of first sex among youth. And ex-President Moi "urged Kenyans to abstain from sex for at least two years to try to curb the spread of AIDS." In fact, this plea might have been to appease conservative religious powers in Kenya, according to the following news report:

The government's plan to import (300 million) condoms ran into swift opposition from both Christian and Muslim religious leaders who believe the government should be more actively promoting abstinence. The Secretary-General of the Council of Imams and Preachers of Kenya, Sheikh Mohamed Dor, said the country was "committing suicide" importing so many condoms, a move he said would encourage young people to have premature sex. (Reuters, July 12, 2001)

This is the position of many—but certainly not all—religious leaders in Africa.

These desperate-seeming pleas and edicts and condemnations from African leaders seem ludicrous, dictatorial, judgmental, and perhaps frightening to Westerners. What's the matter with these backward moralizers? Are they out of touch with reality? Perhaps they are not entirely out of touch. Their reaction suggests that they would prefer to promote the behaviors that Africans say in surveys they are turning to: delay of debut, fewer partners, monogamy, and abstinence. And these behavioral changes seem to be having impact on HIV infection rates, while it is harder to demonstrate this for condoms, at the level of population, in Africa (see Chapter 4).

The term "abstinence" has particular baggage with it in the United States. It is almost impossible to separate the idea from the liberal-conservative battle over what should be promoted in American schools. Abstinence is more baggage free in Africa and perhaps elsewhere in resource-poor countries, yet American AIDS experts working in these areas bring their values and opinions with them. It is probably fair to say that most Western public health professionals become wary when encountering words such as abstinence and faithfulness. They sound judgmental and moralistic. Many fear that such an approach leads to stigmatization of those who do not or cannot follow the dictum, for example, powerless women. Would they become outcasts if they cannot abstain? And abstinence in particular sounds like something impossible to achieve, especially in the case of teenagers with raging hormones.

As will be seen later, Uganda has probably had the greatest behavioral change in the direction of abstinence and faithfulness of any country, and at the same time it significantly reduced AIDS-associated stigma and raised the status of women.

Abstinence seems to be somewhat more acceptable when it is phrased as delay of sexual onset or debut. In Uganda, the English word "abstinence" tends to imply stopping something that has already begun, according to several Ugandan informants. Therefore, Ugandans used the term "delay" more often than abstinence. It would almost seem worth dropping the "A" word, as I suggested in an interview published in the *New York Times* on February 2, 2003. Incidentally, in spite of this interview, and an op-ed article I wrote in the *New York Times* on Uganda's ABC approach, an editorial appeared in the *Times* on March 28, 2003 ("AIDS Funding and Politics") reducing the issues once again to abstinence versus condoms. The editorial makes it clear that the first choice means being against pro-choice and family planning, and that it is bizarre to question the condom solution to AIDS.

Yet even if we dropped the "A" word because of American politics and perspectives, we would still need measurement tools to capture actual behavior trends in Africa. And not only for delay of debut. We need something that describes what some call "secondary abstinence," namely, not having sex for a period of time (often measured by surveys these days in twelve-month periods) after people have been sexually active. This is a phenomenon that deserves recognition and monitoring. For that matter partner reduction is more acceptable than faithfulness, fidelity, or even monogamy, because it sounds more objective and less moralistic.

Going beyond semantics and politics—which is often difficult to do in actual conversations—what is the evidence that abstinence is an achievable goal? Recent reviews of studies in the United States do not provide strong evidence to show abstinence interventions lead to sustained behavior changes. There are studies that show a link between abstinence interventions and delay of sexual onset and reduced sexual activity in youth, but it is not clear how long these effects prevail, and not all such studies are of sound design, or have adequate follow-up periods (Jemmot & Fry, 2002). Research does demonstrate that some form of comprehensive sex education, or "abstinence-plus" programs, can achieve positive behavioral changes among young people and reduce STDs, and that these programs do not encourage young people to initiate sexual activity earlier or have more sexual partners (Collins, Alagiri, & Summers, 2002).

One problem in implementing programs that nominally promote both abstinence and condoms to youth in resource-poor countries is that many such programs, especially those with funding from major international donors, are not truly "abstinence-plus." Most or all of the emphasis tends to be on the condom option, which is not surprising since this is where most international prevention funds and program indicators are allocated.

As we will see in Chapter 6, various groups in Uganda, including the Ministry of Education, seem to have found the right "abstinence-plus" approach, at least in an African context. We can judge by the results: high and increasing proportions of young people ages fifteen to nineteen delaying first intercourse, and high levels of condom use as well as monogamy or fidelity among those who are sexually active. The section on Zambia below provides evidence of youth programs that have successfully promoted both abstinence and condoms, even though there may be a degree of incompatibility inherent in a message that promotes both.

In sum, the political meaning of abstinence in the United States has blinded the global community to the appropriateness of this response, or the related response of partner reduction, in Africa, even when Africans themselves have developed such responses and they have worked stunningly well.

NOTES

1. Elsewhere I have summarized the debate over how far cultural relativism should go in public health (Green, 1999a).

2. A study conducted by the University of South Africa at the Daimler Chrysler factory found that 18 percent of those surveyed believed that having sex with a virgin would cure AIDS (reported on af-aids@healthdev.net, April 9, 20002).

3. In July 2002, I served as a member of a World Bank mission to Mozambique. The Mozambican national AIDS council (and especially the Ministry of Health) proved willing to modify the national AIDS strategy in the direction of a more balanced ABC approach.

4. Available at: http://www.measuredhs.com/hivdata/ind_tbl.cfm.

5. A recent qualitative study of bus drivers in Ibadan, Nigeria, did not filter out information in this way. The author concluded, "Most of the young drivers were unwilling to consider the use of condoms or partner reduction. However, adult drivers preferred partner reduction to use of condoms" (Akintola, 2002, from abs.).

6. My condom research was mentioned or discussed favorably in the *Journal of the American Medical Association*, as well as in some forty American and foreign newspapers. I was interviewed about it on National Public Radio ("All Things Considered"), and my research was published by the American Association for the Advancement of Science (in its special book "AIDS 1988"). In contrast, my first paper on the impact of PBC was rejected by four major journals, an experience shared by some of the others who have even implicitly raised any question about condoms being the only, or main, solution to AIDS. Peer reviewers have commented that raising any question about condoms endangers public health.

7. Call me a lowbrow if you must; I read this at the doctor's office.

4

Questioning Condoms

ARE CONDOMS THE ANSWER TO AFRICAN AIDS?

There are thousands of journal articles and conference papers that tell us explicitly or implicitly that condom use is the most effective means for preventing the sexual transmission of HIV, assuming they are of good quality and are correctly and consistently used—three major assumptions in resource-poor countries. Yet there is also general agreement that AIDS prevention has not been very effective, especially in Africa where most HIV infection is sexually transmitted and where the greatest proportion of global HIV infections occur. The answer for most who work in AIDS is to redouble efforts to distribute condoms. Or to test and counsel people, and then give them condoms. See Figure 4.1.

Yet it's time to look more closely at the evidence for condom effectiveness, especially in Africa. Here we encounter issues that do not arise to the same extent in developed countries, such as problems of distribution and affordability of condoms, as well as transportation, storage, and hygienic disposal. Condoms also have a relatively high failure rate in Africa, due to incorrect use but also to the poor quality of condoms often found in poor, tropical countries. In fact, quality may deteriorate from incorrect or simply lengthy storage in hot warehouses or shelves of clinics or shops. Or condoms can be of good quality but the wrong size for the local population. In any case, condoms can tear, slip off, and become lodged in the vagina (Darrow, 2001). And cheap as condoms may be through social marketing programs, they cost at least a few cents each, which if used often, amounts to an expense of some consideration for the poor. Sometimes cost as well as lack of availability are cited to explain nonuse of condoms.

Figure 4.1
It's Raining Condoms

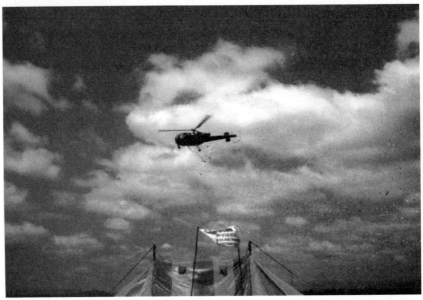

A helicopter in a Southern African country drops hundreds of packets of condoms on a crowd of dignitaries below at the launch of a U.S.–funded AIDS project. (In fairness to the United States, this was not an American idea. The local defense force was so grateful to have U.S. funding for a military AIDS project that to show their gratitude, they arranged to have condoms rain from the sky, believing that the Americans present would be delighted.)

Furthermore, condom use depends upon the cooperation of men; African women are in no position, or at least a weak position, to insist that their partners use a condom, especially if the woman is far younger than the man, a pattern widespread in southern and East Africa and elsewhere. And then there are problems of regular, consistent use of condoms during each sexual act with a partner who might be infected. This has been a problem even among well-educated American and European gay men at high risk for HIV who have been saturated with AIDS prevention information, and availability or affordability are not serious issues (Davidovicha et al., 2001; Rotello, 1997).

If condoms are to be available for consistent use, they need to be constantly resupplied. This is a formidable problem in rural Africa. As Uganda's President Museveni put it, "In countries like ours, where a mother often has to walk twenty miles to get an aspirin for her sick child or five miles to get any water at all, the question of getting a constant supply of condoms may never be resolved" (Museveni, 2000, p. 252).

PRODUCT SAFETY OF CONDOMS

I hesitate to write a section on this topic because experience shows that those who raise any sort of question about the safety and reliability of condoms become highly suspect and are often the target of accusations of having a religious or moral agenda rather than a concern for public health. But if we are serious about promoting the public health, we must put aside biases and preconceptions and look at available evidence with open minds.

Let us begin with the issue of the permeability of latex to HIV. A recent *Population Reports* declares bluntly, citing six sources, "Laboratory tests show that no STI, including HIV, can penetrate an intact latex condom" (Gardner, Blackburn, & Upadhyay, 1999, p. 13). Using somewhat more guarded language, the recent NIH study of condom effectiveness, based on a review of 138 peer-reviewed articles, reported that male latex condoms provide a "highly effective barrier to transmission of particles of similar size to those of the smallest STD viruses" (Cates, 2001, p. 231).

However, the head of the laboratory of the U.S. FDA, where many of the early AIDS-related lab tests were conducted, recently wrote me the following:

I was intrigued to hear recently of a new (?) emergence of interest in the federal health research community about the notion that condoms might be partially permeable to (HIV and other) viruses. I thought this question had already been clarified in research published by our laboratories 10 years ago, in which that kind of phenomenon was demonstrated and quantified (at least approximately). Our initial publication reported laboratory simulations using HIV-sized fluorescent beads to test permeability and found that latex condoms reduced exposure by a factor of about 10,000 compared to the unprotected case. Subsequent published studies by other researchers in our labs used actual viruses (though not HIV) and found somewhat greater reductions in exposure. It should hardly be surprising that some such permeability, albeit small, exists since condom pores can be significantly larger than the HIV virus. (Herman, 2002)

He wrote me because I had toured this FDA lab in 1988, when I was working in contraceptive social marketing and this research was underway. Another interpretation of why the issue was never resolved, or the FDA research ignored, is that it is difficult to promote condoms as a safe method of AIDS prevention if there is any question about HIV leakage. And so, the AIDS establishment simply ignored any such evidence. Or in the case of the *Population Reports* previously cited, simply denied that there is any evidence of leakage. The CDC follows suit on its Web site with the following:

Myth #2: HIV can pass through condoms

A commonly held misperception is that latex condoms contain "holes" that allow passage of HIV. Although this may be true for natural membrane condoms, laboratory studies show that intact latex condoms provide a continuous barrier to microorganisms, including HIV, as well as sperm.

The Global Health Council, in a recent posting about condoms on its Web site, uses more cautious language in its overall assessment of condoms in the following:

In laboratory studies simulating normal conditions, latex condoms have been shown to be highly impermeable to HIV, the virus that causes acquired immunodeficiency syndrome. While condom leakage rates are of concern, breakage and slippage are further factors that can contribute to method failure in routine use. Failure of condoms can also result from inconsistent or incorrect use of the device (user failure). (C. Murphy, 2002)

Whatever we know from studies in American laboratories, real life conditions are not usually well simulated in laboratory studies involving condoms. And in developing countries, the quality of condoms may not be up to that of the new, high-quality condoms tested in America. In fact, there are so-called "leaker" condoms in which small holes are detectable by the water leak test but marketed anyway because of the "finite acceptable quality level" of the testing procedure (Carey, Lytle, & Cyr, 1999). As these authors argue, there is more viral transmission due to condom breakage than leakage.

How often do condoms break during normal use in Africa? A study of condom breakage in Ethiopia among literate men measured the number of condoms broken while opening the package, putting the condom on, or during intercourse or withdrawal. Of 143 participants, 26.6 percent broke condoms (Mekonen & Mekonen, 1999).

That may be called product failure. What about user failure? The *Population Reports* just quoted cites a U.S. study which shows "incorrect use accounted for about one-fourth of unwanted pregnancies" (Gardner, Blackburn, & Upadhyay, 1999, p. 14). The article continues: "Breaks or tears can result from incorrect use such as unrolling the condom before putting it on, trying to put on the condom the rolled rim held toward the body rather than away from it, snagging the condom with fingernails or rings, and reusing condoms" (p. 14).

Another U.S. study of the failure rates of condoms and other temporary contraceptive methods for pregnancy found the following: "The average failure rate for the entire 24-month period is 19 percent. Thus, one in five women who begin using a reversible method become pregnant within two years if they do not change or discontinue methods for other reasons" (Ranjit et al., 2001, p. 19).

But there is a problem extrapolating to HIV. First, HIV can get through pores and tears in latex easier than sperm can. But more important, there is only a narrow time window when a woman is fertile. Yet one can become HIV infected throughout the menstrual cycle. Therefore whatever the failure rate of condoms in contraception, it should be higher in HIV prevention.

Most studies about user failure have been conducted in the United States, where user failure ought to be less than Africa and other resource-poor countries. The U.S. studies found that breakage is less likely among older and married couples, and most likely among sex workers and men with their unmarried girlfriends (Gardner, Blackburn, & Upadhyay, 1999). In other words, during acts of intercourse in which disease transmission is most likely. One recent study of condom use among sex workers in China found that "a substantial proportion" of sex workers experienced condom failure, namely, 20 percent slippage and 13 percent breakage (Qu et al., 2002, p. 267). The practice of dry sex (use of astringents, herbs or other implants to make the vagina drier and tighter), reported in parts of central and southern Africa and the Caribbean, is thought to contribute to condom breakage (Gardner, Blackburn, & Upadhyay, 1999; Runganga, Pitts, & McMaster, 1992; Van de Wijgert, 1997).

Penis size may be associated with breakage, although circumference may be more important than length (Smith et al., 1998). Condoms come in various sizes and there are measurable differences by populations. Sometimes condoms intended for one population are sold in areas where another population predominates. This can lead to slippage, if condoms are too loose, or breakage, if they are too small and tight.

Regarding slippage, "Studies report that condoms slip off the penis completely in about 1% to 5% of acts of vaginal intercourse and slip down the penis without falling off in 3% to 13%. Rates of slippage during anal intercourse range from less than 2% to 21% (Gardner, Blackburn, & Upadhyay, 1999).

There are also problems if the wrong type of lubricant is used with a condom. For latex condoms, lubricants must be water based and not oil based. Mineral or vegetable oils, found in common products such as petroleum jelly, skin lotion, and cooking oil lead to breakage. Many people use these products to lubricate condoms, even in the United States (Gardner, Blackburn, & Upadhyay, 1999). Avoiding use of such lubricants may be a difficult message to convey in Africa, and people would likely use whatever is handy, if they used a lubricant at all. If a lubricant is not used, a condom is more likely to break (Gorna, 1996).

And if sex is nonconsensual, it is less likely that the vagina will lubricate naturally. As noted previously, there is a great deal of nonconsensual sex, especially first-time sex and especially when older men have intercourse with young women and girls. In any case, in such encounters, condoms seem to be less often used than in other encounters characterized by less age differential between partners.

In recent years a second condom has been on the market. The male polyurethane condom is stronger, though less elastic, than latex, and resists both oil-based lubricants and the harmful effects of ozone. Some men find it does not reduce sensitivity as much as latex condoms. Polyurethane is usually odorless and transparent, attributes that some condom consumers prefer. Moreover, some people are allergic to latex. However, a recent randomized, controlled study found that both breakage and slippage of polyurethane condoms are at least six times higher than latex condoms (Frezieres et al., 1998).

In the comments to follow, we return to conventional latex condoms.

SUPPLY AND DEMAND

A vast number of qualitative and quantitative studies throughout Africa have documented the reasons why condom use remains low despite a variety of educational and marketing strategies. One is that condoms are associated with commercial sex and promiscuity, giving condoms "a sordid image" (Cohen & Trussel, 1996, p. 150). As a result, spouses and those in stable relationships often shun condoms because to insist upon or ask for one would be interpreted as a sign of mistrust between regular partners. In addition, many Africans simply do not believe that condoms can protect against AIDS, in spite of all the IEC they have been exposed to (Cohen & Trussell, 1996).

Other reasons for weak demand for condoms include the following:

- They reduce pleasure
- They reduce the spontaneity of sex
- They are often seen by parents, school officials, religious leaders, and the like as encouraging promiscuity, as tacit approval of sexual license
- Women in particular fear that condoms will become stuck in their wombs or otherwise injure their health
- They prevent pregnancy, and it is common in Africa to want many children

Regarding the last, there are always occasions when they are not used for the simple reason that people want and need to have children. Pronatalism may be so strong in parts of Africa that even among unmarried, teenage girls, the desire to have babies may outweigh the desire to protect themselves against HIV infection (Magnani et al., 2002). A recent review notes the following:

HIV prevention strategies are incompatible with conceiving children, and the high prevalence of HIV means that transmission commonly occurs as a direct result of attempts toward reproduction. In this context, the availability of therapy to reduce vertical transmission of HIV is also a critical health consideration but one destined to increase the number of "AIDS orphans" already so visible throughout sub-Saharan Africa. (Cohen & Eron, 2001)

One summary pointing to obstacles to condom promotion in southern Africa put it as follows a few years ago:

The failure of vending machines in Botswana . . . rumours that the USA is providing sub-standard condoms to Zimbabwe, beliefs that condoms are part of the South African government's efforts to reduce the rate of black population growth, or that condom use is all part of some other kind of conspiracy against Africans, or simply men's unwillingness to recognize the risk and the issue of trust between partners in a steady relationship . . . all these factors make condom programmes difficult to introduce. (Barnett & Blaikie, 1992, pp. 162–163)

Such problems of condom demand or acceptability can be found not only in Africa but throughout the developing world and beyond. A recent *Lancet* article reminds us that "Massive increases in condom use worldwide have not translated into demonstrably improved HIV control in the great majority of countries where they have occurred" (Richens, Imrie, & Copas, 2000, p. 400). However, this is a rare admission.

A recent analysis of condom supply in Africa seems to shed considerable light on both demand and supply. The authors obtained condom data from UNFPA and USAID, and supplemented this information with interviews with key informants knowledgeable about condom provision in Africa. They found the following:

Provision of condoms by donors remained surprisingly constant (400–500 million per year) over the past five years. The numbers fell from just over 600 million in 1995 to about 340 million in 1998 before rising again to just over 500 million in 1999. In addition, by 1999 roughly 210 million condoms were purchased by countries' own funds. This amounts to a total of about 724 million condoms or only 4.6 condoms per man aged 15–59 years in sub-Saharan Africa. (Shelton & Johnson, 2001, p. 139)

This means that as AIDS exploded in southern Africa, reaching the highest levels anywhere, ever, condom provision remained stable, or actually declined. This is in spite of the donor organization preference for condom promotion and provision over other preventive interventions (e.g., STD treatment, promotion of partner reduction, or absti-nence/delay). When we consider that all this promotion amounts to only 4.6 condoms per man, per year, it is not surprising that condoms seem to have made little dent on the explosion of HIV in sub-Saharan Africa. It is also hard to avoid the suspicion that demand for condoms remains low in spite of all the resources that go into promotion (IEC, Behavior Change Communications, social marketing). Those of us who have worked in condom social marketing know that if more demand were actually there, donors would increase, not reduce, the amount of condoms going to Africa. Certainly, overall funds available for address-ing the AIDS crisis have increased substantially in recent years.

A study by the AIDSMark project (of Population Services Interna-tional [PSI] and subcontractors) analyzed survey data from six Afri-can countries and concluded that the main reasons for not using condoms have to do with demand: with trusting their partner and therefore seeing no need for condoms, or with dislike of condoms. They conclude, "Most participants did not identify lack of availability and cost as barriers to condom use" (Longfield et al., 2001, p. 9). Al-though the word "participants" is used here, those surveyed amount to 16,767 respondents.

Reflecting on 4.6 condoms per year per African man, do we now put twenty-two times as many funds as are spent at present into condoms (to bring the number up to about 100, which is considered couple-year protection in contraception circles), or do we try something else in addi-tion to condoms? Would a level of ten condoms per year per African man be better than the current average of 4.6? In fact, that is the average num-ber of condoms available per man in Zimbabwe, a country with one of the highest HIV prevalence rates in the world: 25 percent (see below).

CONDOM AWARENESS

Even condom awareness, which ought to be the precursor to con-dom use, seems unrelated to success in AIDS prevention in Africa. Judging by DHS survey findings among adolescents in sub-Saharan Africa (Gupta & Mahy, 2001), there is no relationship between levels of contraceptive awareness in general, or condom awareness in the context of AIDS (as measured by a correct answer to the question, Do condoms prevent AIDS?) and either HIV seroprevalence levels or success in seroprevalence stabilization. If anything, there is an inverse relation-ship. The countries with the highest levels of adolescent (ages 15–19; in some cases, 20–24) awareness are Zimbabwe, Kenya and Côte d'Ivoire, which all have high HIV infection rates relative to other countries in their respective regions. Côte d'Ivoire, for example, has the highest rate in the West Africa region, 10.76 percent in 1999, according to

UNAIDS. In fact, the condom measure is really one of belief in condom efficacy for AIDS prevention. Those countries where belief among young women in condom efficacy is lowest (Senegal, Mali, Burkina Fasso, Ghana) stand out as countries of low HIV seroprevalence.

Likewise, a survey in Lusaka, Zambia, found in its statistical analysis that "knowledge of contraceptives, in general, and condoms, in particular, was associated with higher probabilities of ever having had sex and number of partners in the last 3 months" (Magnani et al., 2002, p. 81).

CONDOM AVAILABILITY

If we look at levels of condom provision or availability in Africa, we find the kind of relationship we don't want to find. In Table 4.1, we take the total number of condoms donated by the major donors between 1989–2000. We then calculate the average annual number of condoms that reached a country and divide this by the number of males ages 15–59. This gives us the average annual number of condoms available per male, as shown in the fourth column. Unfortunately, it seems that the higher this number, the more HIV infection we find in that country, which is shown in the fifth column (Spearman's rank order correlation = 0.87, p = 0.003). True, it could be argued that condom availability does not necessarily mean condom use. But over a twelve-year period, there ought to be some relationship between the two, unless we know that condoms are being used as children's toys or for some other unintended purpose.

Actually, according to the calculation by Shelton and Johnston (2001), provision in the six countries with highest levels of condom availability (Botswana, South Africa, Zimbabwe, Kenya, Togo, and Congo) averaged about seventeen condoms per man ages 15–59, the highest in Africa. The first three of these countries have HIV infection among the highest in the world, and Kenya's rates are high by East African standards (and would be even higher without male circumcision, practiced by a significant proportion of the national population).

It might also be argued that the higher the country's HIV infection levels, the more condoms it needs to import, and so high levels of condoms per man reflect primarily that. But over a twelve-year period, one would expect to see some downward pull on HIV prevalence if condoms are capable of reducing prevalence at the population level. Ought we to wait another twelve years before we even ask this question?

Taxpayers might reasonably ask at what level of availability do condoms begin to pay off. One somewhat evasive answer we hear is that there would have been even more infections in high-prevalence areas had there been no condom use at all. This may be true, but the question of when we see measurable payoff on the population level persists.

Table 4.1
Average Number of Condoms per Male 15–49 in African Countries for
Which Data Are Available

Country	Average annual condoms 1989-2000	Males 15-59 1995 (in thousands)	Average annual condoms per male 15-59	HIV Prevalence (%)
Benin	4,065,408	1,263	3	2.45
Botswana	2,436,232	356	7	36
Cameroon	10,378,900	3,280	3	8
Ghana	9,901,068	4,424	2	3.6
Kenya	42,391,034	6,666	6	14
Senegal	5,513,517	2,091	3	1
South Africa	76,284,892	11,645	7	20
Tanzania	27,217,215	7,603	4	16
Uganda	16,702,846	4,740	4	6
Zambia	12,131,695	2,280	5	20
Zimbabwe	29,149,405	2,826	10	25

Source: D. K. Tiagai International.

Moroever, there is an assumption that condom availability is desirable and makes a difference in AIDS prevention. This assumption is embodied in the USAID program impact indicator defined as "total number of condoms available for distribution nationwide during the preceding 12 months, divided by the total population aged 15–49." This indicator was formerly the WHO/GPA Prevention Indicator 2.[1] Condom availability sounds like a reasonable objective, and perhaps at some point there will be data that show or suggest a causal relationship between levels of availability and lower HIV prevalence.

CONDOM USE

What about reported condom use and its relationship with levels of HIV prevalence? As Willard Cates (2001) reminds us, "it is not possible to evaluate condom effectiveness using the ideal study design—a prospective, randomized controlled trial. In populations at high risk for STDs, for ethical reasons individuals cannot be randomized to a group that is not to use condoms" (p. 231). However, we do have natural experiments, since some people use condoms and others do not. We need only look at multicountry data that show no relationship, or the wrong type of relationship, between either condom availability and use, and HIV infection, to question the assumption that condom availability, and use (which is supposed to follow from availability), are the best intervention for AIDS prevention.

For example, in addition to high condom availability, Zimbabwe may have the highest condom user rates in Africa. We are told, "Zimbabwe is one of the few African countries that have made substantial efforts to involve men in contraceptive use" (Adetunji, 2000, p. 196). And it was recently called "the African country that has best understood the importance of condom use" (Ezzell, 2000, p. 96). Yet Zimbabwe has one of the highest HIV infection rates in the world, 25 percent in 1999.

Table 4.2 is based on recent DHS data showing reported condom use at last higher risk sex, condom use at last sex with a spouse or cohabiting partner, and condom use at last sex with anyone. As with condom availability, there is no association between condom use and lower HIV prevalence rates. If anything, we see a trend in the opposite direction. Since inconsistent condom use has not been found to provide significant protection against HIV infection at the population level (Hearst & Chen, 2003a), it seems more useful to look at a measure that might approximate (but is not the same as) consistent use, namely, condom use at last sex with anyone. The countries that report 20 percent or more are (in order of highest) South Africa, Zimbabwe, Kenya, Burkina Faso, and Zambia, all with high rates of infection compared to other countries in their respective regions of Africa (e.g., Burkina Fasso at 6.5% in 1999 was high compared to most other countires in West Africa).

As with condom availability, condom use is an official program impact indicator used by USAID and UNAIDS. "Condom use at last sex with anyone" is UNAIDS indicator 8.2.2. The other two measures in Table 4.2 are also program impact indicators, in fact the ones that generate most interest and discussion when it comes to behavior change. They guide the allocation of hundreds of millions of dollars. They assume, of course, that the higher the use, the lower the HIV prevalence, at least at some point. This has not happened yet.

For further findings on condom use in Africa, data were gathered in a randomized community trial in Rakai, Uganda. Condom usage information was obtained prospectively from 17,264 sexually active individuals ages fifteen to fifty-nine years over a period of thirty months. HIV incidence and STD prevalence was determined for consistent and

Table 4.2
Reported Condom Use, African Men

Condom use at...	last higher risk sex	last sex with a spouse or cohabiting partner	last sex with anyone
Benin 1996	21	4	9
Burkina Faso 1999	57	8	21
Cameroon 1998	29	5	16
Côte d'Ivoire 1998	49	6	-
Ethiopia 2000	30	0	5
Ghana 1998	-	-	15
Guinea 1999	33	3	14
Kenya 1998	44	8	21
Malawi 2000	39	6	14
Mali 1996	36	3	10
Mozambique 1997	-	4	6 -
Nigeria 1999	-	-	14
Rwanda 2000	51	1	6
South African National HIV Prevalence, Behavioural Risks and Mass Media: Household Survey 2002	-	-	30
Tanzania 1996	32	4	11
Togo 1998	38	6	19
Uganda 1995	36	3	9
Uganda 2000-2001	59	4	15
Zambia 1996	40	8	20
Zambia Sexual Behaviour Survey 2000	39	-	-
Zimbabwe 1999	70	7	28

Source: DHS/Measure Web site (http://www.measuredhs.com).

irregular condom users, compared to nonusers. Only 4.4 percent reported consistent condom use and 16.5 percent reported inconsistent use during the prior year. Condom use was higher when reported by males, and younger, unmarried, and better educated individuals, and by those reporting multiple sex partners or extramarital relationships. The authors found the following:

Consistent condom use significantly reduced HIV incidence [RR, 0.37; 95% confidence interval (CI), 0.15–0.88], syphilis (OR, 0.71; 95% CI, 0.53–0.94) and gonorrhea/chlamydia (OR, 0.50; 95% CI; 0.25–0.97) after adjustment for sociodemographic and behavioral characteristics. Irregular condom use was not protective against HIV or STD and was associated with increased gonorrhea/chlamydia risk (OR, 1.44; 95% CI, 1.06–1.99). (Ahmed et al., 2001, p. 2171)

The authors observe that "inconsistent condom use may actually be an 'enabling' process allowing individuals to persist in high risk behaviors with the false sense of security" (Ahmed et al., 2001, p. 2177). Whatever factors may be operating, there have been numerous findings showing a relationship between condom use—probably inconsistent use—and higher rates of STD and HIV infection.

A 1970 study was conducted among university students in Kampala (N = 789), using a handed-out questionnaire and a convenience sample (those who attended lectures on sexual hygiene). Of 685 men who returned the questionnaires, 370 (54%) reported a history of one or more STDs, compared to 5 out of 99 women. In comparing male groups with STD and no STD reported, "occasional condom use" was reported by 18.3 percent of the "VD group" compared to 10.1 percent of the "non-VD group" (Arya & Bennett, 1974, p. 56).

A survey in rural Zimbabwe (N = 9,843, of whom 44.9% were under age twenty-five) likewise found the following:

Women whose most recent partner had other partners and women who had consistently used condoms with their most recent partner had elevated risks of infection.

Further restriction of the analysis to respondents who had had sex in the previous two weeks did not change the effects of personal and behavioral factors; however, HIV risk was elevated among those who had used condoms consistently with their most recent partner (2.0 for both men and women) and rose slightly with each year by which the respondents were younger than their most recent partner (1.04). (Rosenberg, 2002, p. 230)

I am quoting exact wording to avoid accusation of distorting findings. The main risk factors identified by analysis of these data were "cumulative number of sexual partners," early age of first intercourse, and a pattern of young females having sex with older men (Rosenberg,

2002, p. 230). The first solution proposed by the author, while politically correct, does not follow from the study's findings: Get men to stop having unprotected sex (i.e., use condoms) (p. 231).

Other studies have likewise found higher rates of STD or HIV infections among inconstant condom users than among condom nonusers (Darrow et al., 1989; Hearst & Chen, 2003a; Mann et al., 1988; Mbizvo et al., 1994; Saracco et al., 1993; Taha et al., 1996). And, of course, condom use is inconsistent far more often than it is consistent, virtually everywhere. Contemplation of the implications of these two findings should give us pause, to say the least.

There is often an assumption that lack of condom use in a population is a risk factor for HIV infection. Even in the United States, a study has found an association between homosexual condom use and an increased risk of seroconversion (Samuel et al., 1993, cited in Brody, 1997). Likewise a study of gay men in the Dominican Republic found "among men who had not tested positive for HIV before that study, consistent condom use during receptive anal intercourse carried 3.3 times the odds ratio of incident seropositivity (marginally missing the .05 significance level) of never using condoms" (Tabet et al., 1996, cited in Brody, 1997, p. 155). This may be because condom nonusers were less likely to engage in risky sex.

Indeed, none of this is to say that use of condoms causes AIDS, only that condoms might give men a somewhat greater sense of security than warranted by actual condom effectiveness. This might lead to more risky sexual behavior than men might practice if condoms were not available. The situation might be comparable to people using sunscreen, but then exposing themselves to sunlight longer than they would have if sunscreen did not exist and thereby increasing their risk of skin cancer. As Richens, Imrie, and Copas (2000) conclude, "A vigorous condom-promotion policy could increase rather than decrease unprotected sexual exposure, if it has the unintended effect of encouraging greater sexual activity" (p. 400). This phenomenon has been called "risk compensation." The theory of risk compensation states that the extent to which condoms or seat belts or sunscreen reduce one's feeling of vulnerability, this will be matched by the extent to which one lowers one's guard and engages in risky behavior (Richens, Imrie, & Weiss, 2003).

Of course there are several possible explanations for the relationship between condom use and higher HIV or STD infection. The range of explanations and the possible causal associations include the following:

1. People who know or suspect they are HIV+ are more likely to use condoms (effect–cause).
2. People who would have more partners anyway are both more likely to use condoms and more likely to be infected (effect–effect).

3. Condom promotion might encourage higher risk sex (cause–effect).

4. Failure to separate out commercial sex (in its various forms) from the data.

5. Failure to fully adjust for other possible confounders. (Hearst, 2003; Hulley et al., 2001, pp. 125–130)

To disentangle causal factors, it is useful to have longitudinal data for a cohort of individuals so that at least the sequence of events can be observed over time. Hearst and his colleagues hope to be conducting research of this sort soon. Condom use also needs to be accurately categorized as consistent or inconsistent. Self-reporting on this may not be very accurate. It is safe to say that most condom use is inconsistent everywhere. This is true even in the United States, where condoms are available and widely known (Catania et al., 1992).

One recent study was conducted in the African country with the highest condom use (Zimbabwe) among the population perhaps most likely to access and use them (men in their early twenties at two technical colleges in the capital city, Harare). The survey found that 24.6 percent reported using condoms every time. Use of marijuana and "the situational influences of bars" negatively affected "quality of condom use" (Zvinavashe & Rusakaniko, 2000, p. 158). So it would seem that even if we believe self-reporting in this case, best-case, consistent use seems to be more often the exception than the rule. And if we introduce alcohol or drugs, or coerced sex, consistent and proper use is diminished further.

How much more protective are condoms when used consistently? A Cochrane review meta-analysis was recently conducted of effectiveness when condoms were used consistently. The reviewers identified 4,709 studies, of which fourteen met the strict criteria for inclusion in the meta-analysis. The authors concluded the following:

This review indicates that consistent use of condoms results in 80% reduction in HIV incidence. Consistent use is defined as using a condom for all acts of penetrative vaginal intercourse. Because the studies used in this review did not report on the "correctness" of use, namely whether condoms were used correctly and perfectly for each and every act of intercourse, effectiveness and not efficacy is estimated. Also, this estimate refers in general to the male condom and not specifically to the latex condom, since studies also tended not to specify the type of condom that was used. Thus, condom effectiveness is similar to, although lower than, that for contraception. (Weller & Davis, 2002)

This last sentence prompts the observation that condoms are widely accepted to be one the least effective methods of contraception, yet they are considered by many experts to be the most effective method of AIDS prevention. This is an interesting paradox.

The following report sympathetic to condom promotion concurs with the Weller and Davis (2002) meta-analysis: "Overall effectiveness for reducing sexual transmission of HIV through consistent use of condoms is approximately 80%. Estimates of condom effectiveness range widely from 94.2% (best case scenario) to 35.4% (worst case scenario)" (Gardner, Blackburn, & Upadhyay, 1999).

It is likely that where condoms are most needed—in higher-risk encounters in Africa—failure rates are closer to the worst case than the ideal scenario. Indeed in real-world, Third World situations, where use may not be correct, or condoms may be of poor or deteriorated quality, made of nonlatex, or the wrong size, protection may actually be less than 80 percent, even when use is consistent, which is rare. This prospect is not very reassuring. It means that with repeated exposures to an infected partner, such as a man visiting a sex worker in Nairobi or Johannesburg once a month, the man will likely be infected within five months, even with consistent condom use. And most use is inconsistent.

A recent UNAIDS review of condom effectiveness found roughly 90 percent effectiveness in the best studies of serodiscordant couples using condoms consistently (Hearst & Chen, 2003a). However, this figure is derived only from cases in which couples know their HIV status and are probably highly motivated to change behavior. Thus, for most of Africa and elsewhere, actual condom effectiveness would be more like the 80 percent Cochrane figure, or lower.

Condom effectiveness is not just an issue in Africa. A prospective study of condom use in Baltimore found no differences in STI infection rates among those who reported using condoms 100 percent of the time versus 0 percent of the time (Zenilman et al., 1995). This study provoked a great deal of controversy and published comments. The results were so startling that most letters to the editor decided there must have been something wrong with the methods of the team at Johns Hopkins University that conducted the research. It seemed to occur to no one that less than 100 percent condom effectiveness and continued risk behaviors could have accounted for the results. (In the methods section, we read, "Previous attempts to validate condom use have focused on . . . collecting used condoms from sewers.")

A Ugandan leader of a youth group concerned with AIDS wrote me the following:

Abstinence is a better approach than throwing condoms around and expecting people to use them all the time. The fact remains that sex without a condom does not feel the same as with a condom. Once, twice, thrice with a condom and then one time without it. What (happens) next? Better sexual feeling and no return to the condom. On the other hand, self-esteem will create in people the value of abstinence that in turn will lead to more careful decision making, particularly in the area of sexual intercourse.

Let researches be continuously carried out among rural folks in Africa to find out how often they (really) use condoms. Maybe from that information efforts can be put together for a new approach to promote both abstinence and condoms. Maybe it should be an approach promoting abstinence without necessarily appearing to be fighting condoms, on one hand, and on the other hand, another approach promoting condoms . . . but presented clearly *with all the facts* (Ssemwogerere, personal communication, April 11, 2002. Italics mine)

My comment is that fidelity, monogamy, or partner reduction may be the behavioral response that has the greatest impact on HIV infection rates at the population level, more than abstinence. The evidence for this is strongest in Uganda (see Chapter 6).

A NOTE ON CONDOM USE MEASUREMENT

One of the many reasons condoms have become the primary AIDS prevention intervention is that they are relatively easy to count and to monitor. Therefore whatever their limitations, at least we should have good, clear data on trends in condom use. But this is not really so. Major surveys such as DHS, WHO/GPA, and UNAIDS have moved, over the years, from asking about condom use ever, to condom use with last nonregular partner, to condom use with last nonregular, noncohabiting partner. Other surveys have asked about condom use in the last six months, three months, or one month. Or about condom use with the last partner of whatever type. The time frame of condom questions about use with last partner has also varied from the past six months (e.g., the 1993 Kenya DHS) to the past twelve months (e.g., the 2000 Uganda DHS).

In fairness, the DHS and other surveys make these changes in the hope of improving the measurement of condom trends, usually or often after consultation with various international health experts. But the result is that it is difficult to measure change in even the intervention into which most AIDS prevention resources have gone.

I agree with the following Internet posting about USAID–funded AIDS research in Africa:

In accounting and financial reporting, one of the basic rules is to use the same measurement methods in both the current year and the prior comparative years. This makes it possible to get valid trends. Data that are flawed but consistent from year to year can be used to give quite reliable trend line information and certainly can give indicators that progress is being made. One of the criticisms of the current data is that the data collection and analysis methods change from year to year and trends relate not only to real trends but to changes in methodology. (Burgess, 2002b)

THE CUMULATIVE RISK FACTOR

One of the shortcomings of studies of condom effectiveness is that cumulative risk over time is not usually factored into estimates. However, a group of researchers recently reviewed studies of condom failure and then conducted mathematical modeling to better understand interactions between factors contributing to these outcomes. The authors conclude, "One's risk of infection increases with increasing numbers of *unprotected* sexual acts with an infected partner. Similarly, our calculations indicate that one's risk of infection increases with increasing numbers of *condom-protected* sexual exposures. Based on our models, the *relative risk* of infection in condom users also increases with increasing numbers of exposures" (Mann, Stine, & Vessey, 2002, p. 348).

The authors continue with the following:

Our findings also call into question the validity of studies that attempt to measure the effectiveness of condoms in preventing STD transmission but fail to measure the number of sexual acts (exposures) of participants. Future studies of condom effectiveness must measure the number of sexual acts in which study subjects participate. (Mann, Stine, & Vessey, 2002, p. 347)

This ought to conform to common sense: Whatever the risk of exposure per episode of sex with an infected partner, that risk will increase steadily with continued episodes of intercourse with an infected partner, or partners. The authors caution, "General statements about condoms being '80%, 90%, or 99% effective' for preventing STDs must be avoided. For such statements to be accurate, the number of exposures to a particular STD must be specified" (Mann, Stine, & Vessey, 2002, p. 348). The authors urge that we keep in mind the concept of cumulative risk: "As the number of uses of any imperfect prevention intervention increases, the cumulative potential for intervention failure also increases" (Mann, Stine, & Vessey, 2002, p. 348). Fitch and colleagues (2002) point out that an intervention that is 99.8 percent effective for a single episode of intercourse can yield an 18 percent cumulative failure rate with 100 exposures.

The modeling study by Mann, Stine, and Vessey (2002) was regarded as important enough to be accompanied by an editorial (subtitled, "the Positive Spin") by Ward Cates, president of FHI. Cates (2001) had recently published a defense of condoms after release of the 2001 NIH report. In the present editorial, Cates concedes, "The authors correctly conclude, on the basis of an assumed level of condom breakage/slippage, that even consistent use of condoms will lead to measurable levels of STD transmission over time, especially for organisms with high transmission coefficients" (p. 350). However, he also criticizes some of the assumptions used in the model, namely, the authors' assumption of continuous sexual exposure to an infectious partner. Cates assumes that this refers only to sero-discordant couples, and he notes that some of the STDs under consideration are often detected and cured. This means that the situation might be self-correcting and the risk of infection reduced or eliminated: "For a curable STD, antibiotic treatment would render the infected partner noninfectious. Thereafter, condoms should be unnecessary if both partners remain uninfected. For a noncurable viral STD, knowledge of discordancy could provide added motivation for more consistent condom use" (p. 350).

However, the editorialist does not consider the possibility of multiple partners. If the infected person is engaging in casual or regular sex with multiple partners, there is less likelihood that there would be treatment of curable STDs (in more than one partner) or that knowledge of partner's sero-status might lead to all partners using condoms. In other words, the cumulative risk of being infected eventually is increased when more than one partner is involved. I agree with Cates and everyone else who argues that condoms are far better than no condoms, but I take the cumulative risk findings of Mann and colleagues to be further evidence of the need to reduce number of sexual partners, to change behavior in a more fundamental way than condom adoption can accomplish.

If higher levels of risky behavior associate causally with higher levels of HIV infection, this would seem to strengthen the argument that interventions are needed to lower the levels of higher-risk sexual activity. Adding condoms to high-risk behavior does not seem to have much impact on the consequences of the behavior. Condoms evidently do not protect against HIV infection as well as they are supposed to.

CONDOM USE IN HIGH-RISK SITUATIONS

It has been found that genital herpes is a major cofactor in HIV transmission (Carael & Holmes, 2001). Therefore prevention of herpes ought to be a priority in AIDS prevention, particularly in populations where herpes is prevalent. Unfortunately, while condoms may reduce the risk of acquisition of HSV-2 in women, they do not seem to in men. This may be because, even when used correctly, "condoms fully cover the skin of the penis, from which the virus is shed, but do not protect men against exposure to all female genital sites from which the virus may be shed. . . . Contact with vulvar or perianal areas, the most common sites of viral shedding in women, may be a factor in the lower effectiveness of condoms in transmission from women to men" (Wald et al., 2001, p. 347; Rosenberg, 2001).

Of course, chances of HIV transmission are enhanced in the presence of a range of STDs, particularly those of an ulcerative type. Therefore it is especially important that condoms be used when someone knows he or she has an STD. Yet often this does not happen. Men and women in Nairobi (where condoms and condom information are relatively available) were found to wait approximately a week after the appearance of STD symptoms before they sought treatment, and during this time only 22 percent of men and 18 percent of women said they used condoms during intercourse (Fonck et al., 2001).

It is true that in some of the AIDS success stories considered in this book, such as Uganda, Jamaica, and Thailand, condom use reported by sex workers is over 90 percent, at least in capital or major cities. That is an accomplishment and it ought to block much of the transmissions that would otherwise occur. And reported male condom use with nonregular partners may now be at the 50 percent or higher level in several African countries, including Uganda. But what about other high-risk situations?

As noted previously, condom use in Africa can be very low even when someone knows he or she is HIV infected. In a Rakai study already cited (Ahmed et al., 2001), only 6.3 percent of discordant couples reported occasional condom use, and only 1.2 percent reported consistent use, in spite of condom promotion by a U.S.–funded project (Gray et al., 2001). These findings appear not to be an extreme example so much as they are illustrative of the reluctance of Africans and others to use condoms when in married or stable relationships.

Even in Thailand, famous for its 100 percent condom policy for AIDS prevention, and for its highly developed family planning program, condom use for contraception among married couples has never exceeded 2 percent (Knodel & Pramualratana, 1996).

In spite of what is known about their effectiveness, condoms are promoted as if they were 100 percent safe in resource-poor parts of the world. Reviewing condom messages from the United States in the mid-1980s, there were almost always warnings about condom effectiveness, such as: Condoms cannot guarantee you won't be infected, but they will certainly improve your chances. But in Africa and other resource-poor areas, we simplified to: Use Protector! Rely on Shield condoms! Rely on Trust or Sure condoms! I do not remember ever hearing or seeing in Africa, the Caribbean, or Asia any messages equivalent to the ones we have used in America. Perhaps this is because condom social marketing programs seemed the most cost-effective way to promote condoms, and perhaps prevent AIDS. And in mass marketing there is little use for equivocation. We did not want to confuse the message. I have heard marketers say they have a hard enough task getting Africans to use condoms, so any mention of problems with condoms would result in even lower user rates.

But what about Africans and others who believed condoms were 100 percent effective, used them as directed, and then became infected? This is an ethical issue, a serious human rights issue. The case could be made that health officials from rich countries have withheld information that would allow people in poor countries to make an informed choice, a choice that has life or death consequences.

Such thoughts may already be in the minds of some Africans. I was visiting a high school in Uganda in December 2002 when a student asked, "If condoms are not 100% protection, why are they promoted in Uganda?" And the following was posted on af-aids on September 24, 2002, by Rose Mlay:

Last week we had a discussion with youths (grade 9–12) in one of the secondary schools in Tanzania. They were quite bitter with us (health care providers) that why don't (we) comment when the media advertise that condom is a complete preventive measure for AIDS. "Why do they lie to us and you just keep quiet" these youths said. They went on saying that even (a) 1% risk of condom use should constantly be communicated because to the individual, it is 100% (risk). The question is how safe is this new approach? Is it a problem in other places or it is only in Tanzania? (parentheses mine)

Note that condoms were still referred to as a new approach in 2002.

None of the foregoing is to suggest that condoms do not have their place and should not be promoted. The risk reduction interventions for sexual transmission of HIV, namely, condoms and treatment of STDs, should be emphasized with high-risk groups, such as CSWs and their clients, soldiers, truck drivers, men in factory hostels geographically separated from their wives, and the like. But the current approach of the supplying and promoting the maximum number of condoms to the maximum number of people has simply not been found to work very well with majority populations in Africa or anywhere. And it is not a substitute for primary behavior change, for fundamentally altering risky behavior patterns. Therefore AIDS prevention programs should not bet all their money, or even most of it, on the condom solution.

Globally, condoms may be most effective in averting HIV infections in Pattern IV countries, such as those in Southeast Asia, especially during the earlier stages of local epidemics. In a country like Thailand, HIV and STDs were very concentrated among CSWs and their clients. Cambodia may have the highest HIV infection rates in Asia (2.8% of sexually active women in ANC clinics), although there seems to have been a recent decrease in HIV seroprevalence there. The sale of condoms in Cambodia is said to have increased from nearly 100,000 in 1994 to 11.5 million in 1998 (Sharma, 2001).

As in Thailand, there has been a great deal of condom promotion in Cambodia. But also like Thailand, there has been primary behavior change, for example, significantly fewer men going to CSWs. In the early news about Cambodia's apparent success, one only heard about high condom use. Later Cambodia's National HIV/AIDS Center reported survey results showing the following:

The percentage of soldiers who said they had visited a prostitute in the previous month dropped from 47% in 1999 to 20% in 2001. The proportion of police officers who reported visiting a prostitute within the previous month dropped from 37% in 1999 to 18.5% in 2001, while the proportion of motorbike taxi drivers who visited a prostitute dropped from 34.5% to 8.5% within the same time period. (Kaiser Daily HIV/AIDS Report, 2001)

These are significant behavior changes that would be especially high impact in an epidemic driven by infections among CSWs and their clients. The online report did not state that these results were published. Indeed, most of the publicity about Cambodian AIDS has to do with condoms. The following listserve posting from SEA-AIDS reports:

Foreign aid workers have built this country's first Condom Cafe to mark World AIDS Day on Saturday. Built in downtown Phnom Penh, it is a lead taken from similar cafes in Australia, Thailand, Vietnam, and elsewhere across the Asia-Pacific region. "We need to identify children who will become orphans and integrate them with uncles or aunts, with foster parents, and stop them from going onto the streets, we have to find a solution," (Sebastion) Marot said.

He said the Condom Cafe would be informal and lively, designed to attract kids who are already on the streets "and yes, the walls will be covered with condoms." (November 30, 2001)

It is relatively easy to persuade men to use condoms with CSWs. If there is widespread, consistent use of condoms among such men, many infections ought to be averted. In a later stage, when HIV bridges to the majority population (men infected by CSWs typically infect their wives), condoms are much less likely to be used, especially on a regular basis. Therefore condoms are less likely to make much difference in HIV infection rates in later stages of Pattern IV countries. This is because of reluctance almost everywhere to using condoms with spouses or regular partners. This is also true with men who have sex with men (Hospers & Kok, 1995). In fact, a recent study of gay men in

Amsterdam showed that men are more likely nowadays to become HIV infected from their steady partners, as distinct from casual partners, because they are less likely to use condoms with steady partners (Davidovicha et al., 2001).

Condoms will not always be used even in commercial sex situations. I was involved in an ethnographic study of CSWs in Tanzania in the mid-1990s. We were trying to establish an information base for developing an effective STD prevention and control program for brothel-based female sex workers in the town of Morogoro. At the time of interviews, a great deal of AIDS preventive education and condom promotion was going on. We gathered a great deal of information about condom attitudes and use. The following conversations were recorded, transcribed and translated from the Haya language; the English translation preserves the idiom of English as it is spoken in Tanzania, and "SW" stands for "sex worker" (Green, Nkya, & Outwater, 2000–2001):

Interviewer: Have you heard of condom?

SW1: Yes. That is not something new to me. Even here I have them.

Interviewer: Can I see them?

SW1: Yes, here they are (one box shown).

Interviewer: Do you know how to use them?

SW1: Yes. It is a sock to cover men when we are doing our business.

Interviewer: Why do you think men put that condom on?

SW1: Because the doctor says we should use that to prevent us from pregnancy, STDs, and AIDS.

Interviewer: If it is for prevention for AIDS, why are people dying every day?

SW1: Well, we are not using condoms as we are supposed to.

Interviewer: When a customer comes, do you ask them to use condoms?

SW1: Most of our customers don't like condoms because they say they don't enjoy the business with condom on.

Other sex workers claimed they used condoms, as in this following exchange:

Interviewer: You told me that in the old days you didn't use condoms. When did you start using condoms?

SW2: I started using condoms when people started talking of AIDS.

Interviewer: Do all of your customers like condoms?

SW2: Not all the customers like condoms. There's a certain man called (X) who used to pay as much as 1,000 shillings as long as you would go without a condom. Now why do you think he gives so much money? Is it not that he is already contaminated and because he wanted to spread the disease to other people? Because people who are safe, they really like the condom. Some even want to use four condoms (at once) so as to be on the safe side.

Even if sex workers insist that their customers use condoms, it may be unrealistic to expect that women who live from hand to mouth will refuse the customer and forego money, as illustrated in the following narrative segment:

SW3: Another problem is that condoms do burst. When they burst the customers throw nasty words to us.

Interviewer: Now what happens when your customer refuses to use the condom and he's already inside your house?

SW3: Well, you have to observe whether he has abnormality or not and if he doesn't have any abnormality then you'll do it without the condom. So, in other circumstances you have to agree without the condom, because if you insist on the condom, they run away, they go to my friends who don't use condoms, and I don't get any money.[2]

It appears that even among those who used the condoms, use was not consistent. In fact, we found that these Tanzanian CSWs often used condoms for single-time or first-time customers. However, such customers were decreasing in 1994, replaced by more regular sex partners. Within these relationships, condom use was rare (Outwater et al., 2000). In any case, as just suggested, condom use may have come too late. Almost all the 200 sex workers in the study group tested positive for HIV and most had died by 2001.

Even though condoms are more likely to be adopted by CSWs than others, it is still an uphill battle in Africa. For example, a study of CSWs and their clients in Durban, South Africa, found strategies to cope with the possibility of HIV infection other than condom use, such as the following: "(1) denial of risk, (2) fatalism, (3) economic rationalization, (4) partner categorization through selective condom use, (5) purposeful ignorance of HIV status, and (6) abnegation of responsibility for practicing safe sex" (Varga, 2001, p. 351).

The problems and evidence we have been considering have been related to condoms used for vaginal sex. There may be even more problems when condoms are used for anal sex. These problems are better known in MSM sex in the West. For example, one early study sought to estimate condom failure rates during anal intercourse in homosexual men in Amsterdam, The Netherlands. Based on interviews about recalled condom experience, condoms tore or slipped off in 8 percent (117/1,468) of cases (van Griensven et al., 1988).

But we are still constrained by lack of specific trials that would establish the effectiveness of condoms in anal sex. These have not been undertaken, purportedly because condom manufacturers believe such trials would be "bad for the family image," and because running a trial would place people at risk (Gorna, 1996, p. 296). We ought to know more about condom use in anal sex because heterosexual anal intercourse is quite common in several developing countries, and MSM anal sex is also quote common among men (such as in Latin America) who do not ordinarily define themselves as gay or bisexual (Halperin, 1999b).

IMPLICATIONS OF CONDOM FINDINGS FROM AFRICA

To summarize the condom-related findings thus far from Africa, from what we know about condom failure as well as about the protection provided by both inconsistent and consistent use, it seems statistically quite likely that a condom user engaging in casual sex or sex with partners likely to be infected will eventually become HIV infected if he or she continues to engage in risky sex. This may be why Gordon warned earlier in the pandemic that "This makes condoms ineffective for lifelong protection from HIV-infected sexual partners; therefore, in general, condoms provide inadequate risk reduction for the individual" (Gordon, 1989, p. 5). Fourteen years after this was written, we can add that condoms do not seem to provide adequate protection at the population level either, at least not in Africa.

Some researchers, such as those already quoted in the Rakai study, advise that "programs must emphasize consistent condom use for HIV and STD prevention" (Ahmed et al., 2001, p. 2171). However, even if that could be achieved (which in itself is unlikely) that may only delay HIV infection by weeks, months, or a few years at most. Consideration of these findings about condoms makes reduction in the number of partners and later sexual debut more effective and more realistic ways to reduce the incidence and prevalence of HIV in majority populations as distinct from high-risk groups. This is especially true in parts of the world where condoms are not readily available and may be of poor quality.

Maybe the various studies cited here are not to be taken as typical. But there are now enough studies or unpublished data suggesting an unexpected and unwanted association between (1) knowledge of condoms, belief in condom efficacy, condom availability, and actual condom use; (2) risky sexual behavior; and (3) HIV actual infection that we should at least discuss the possible significance of these findings. Yet in none of the studies cited have we found any discussion at all. It would seem that researchers are disinclined to call attention to these findings, let alone contemplate their meaning in writing.

There are not many scientists critical of condoms who find their way into peer-reviewed medical literature. Richens and his colleagues are an exception. They note the following:

There are three ways in which a large increase in condom use could fail to affect disease transmission. First, condom promotion appeals more strongly to risk-averse individuals who contribute little to epidemic transmission. Second, increased condom use will increase the number of transmissions that result from condom failure. Third, there is a risk-compensation mechanism: increased condom use could reflect decisions of individuals to switch from inherently safer strategies of partner selection or fewer partners to the riskier strategy of developing or maintaining higher rates of partner change plus reliance on condoms. (Richens, Imrie, & Copas, 2000, p. 400)

These authors go on to cite studies that show how AIDS prevention messages emphasizing condom use can actually lead to the practice of more high-risk behavior and higher rates of STDs. Yet the condom mindset that prevails among the major donor organizations still seems to filter out both recognition of condom shortcomings and consideration of other-than-condom possibilities. And so the donor organizations continue to scold Africans for having unprotected sex, with the implication that Africans are irrational or backward, forgetting how infrequent condom use is in America and the West.

CONDOM USE IN PATTERN I COUNTRIES

What about condom use in Pattern I countries, in the United States and the West? It is widely believed that by the mid-1980s, gay men in places like San Francisco and New York had adopted condoms on a significant scale. Yet Gabriel Rotello (part of the gay community himself) doesn't believe that condom use was ever very high or very consistent among gays, even during the height of fear that swept gay communities in the mid-1980s. The highest HIV seroprevalence level reached in any cohort of gays was 73 percent in San Francisco in 1985. Other peak levels were between 40 and 60 percent in New York and a few other large cities. From his analysis, Rotello (1997) concludes that condom use by those in the first wave of infected men kept the high water marks from being even higher, but accounted for less HIV decline than saturation. He does not believe that partner reduction contributed much to saturation because there was not much of this due to the following: (1) Gay men felt that they had suffered and struggled for many years to achieve the sexual freedom that they enjoyed by the 1980s in America—they were not going to give this up easily, and (2) AIDS prevention education placed emphasis on condom use and safer sex rather than partner reduction. Rotello notes, "The condom code seeks to contain transmission by lowering the level of infectivity per sexual contact, but it ignores the enormous role played by the contact rate itself" (p. 194).

But why specifically aren't condoms used more often and more consistently by gay men? Rotello (1997) rejects the explanations of lack of education about condoms, lack of availability, remaining "in the closet," and the like. He documents mistakes or unintended lapses on the part of men who normally use condoms; deliberate decisions to have unprotected sex with certain people such as a regular partner, and even deliberate decisions to periodically forego condoms to take a break from protected sex, with the decision aided by mood altering drugs or alcohol, the use of which seems to be relatively high among fast-lane (Rotello's term) gay men. And some men get drunk or high precisely in order to have unsafe sex without fear, inhibitions, and diminished sensation.

Rotello found that even AIDS educators who preached the value of condoms themselves went on holidays from using them. More recently, the *New York Times* (Goode, 2001) described a gay AIDS educator who advocated condoms by day, yet by night, at least periodically, the educator was having unprotected sex with unknown men. The AIDS educator is HIV positive and did not disclose his sero-status to his partners. True, this may be an extreme case, but it lends credence to Rotello's findings that gay men may not use condoms as often and as regularly as was and is supposed.

A recent study among New Yorkers, both gay and heterosexual, found that more than 40 percent of those with multiple partners did not use condoms the last time they had sex, according to what city officials said was the most comprehensive survey ever conducted of the city's sexual habits (Pérez-Peña, 2003). However, it is not lack of condom use but multiple partners and the independent risk factor of anal sex that are behind the high HIV infection rates in the gay community.

Incidentally, Rotello's (1997) book provoked great controversy within the gay community. Judging by the reviews I have read, the controversy was not over Rotello's analysis of condom use but rather over his suggestion that gay men—at least highly sexually active, fast-lane urban gays—developed values and behavioral patterns that led to self-harm, as well as built-in mechanisms that resisted critical self-examination and more fundamental change in sexual behavior, such as having far fewer sexual partners. Rotello refers to this as the multipartnerist ethic of the gay sexual revolution.

If Rotello is right that condom use among America's first and still foremost HIV-infected core group did not use condoms as often and as consistently as is believed, this is both significant and disturbing. The first international AIDS prevention programs (e.g., the WHO/GPA, the USAID–funded AIDSTECH and AIDSCOM projects) were strongly influenced by American gay men who were believed to have discovered the best approaches (at least at the time) to prevention from the success of condom and safe sex (or safer sex) programs in places like San Francisco and New York. Such leadership and beliefs—seldom challenged at the time or even since—set the stage for the predominance of condom promotion as the cornerstone of AIDS prevention in Africa and elsewhere in the developing world.

The evidence suggests that whatever condom use really was among American gay men in the 1980s and early 1990s, it probably became less frequent after the availability of HAART, or ARV drugs. The Multicenter AIDS Cohort Study in 1999 found that gay men were engaging in unprotected receptive anal sex, due to safer sex fatigue. "A message of complacency has arisen in the gay community and the majority population," a researcher commented to Reuters Health. "We've been telling gay men for the last two decades that they need to use a condom each time they have sex, so any kind of suggestion that this is not so important anymore, provides justification for people who want to relax and experience the sexual liberation of the 1970s" (Ostrow et al., 2002).

We who work in public health seem so fearful of appearing judgmental, let alone moralistic, that we often end up never giving the advice that is most needed in sexually transmitted HIV: have fewer sexual partners. Mark Schoof (1997), in criticizing Rotello for making just that suggestion to American gay men, asks with a note of sarcasm, "Should prevention workers print posters saying, 'Reduce your number of partners'? Well, Mr. Schoof, only if you wish to achieve a 66 percent decline in HIV infection, like Uganda." Just as if we want to reduce the rate of lung cancer, we must at least mention cigarette smoking, and probably advise quitting or at least cutting down on numbers of cigarettes. We cannot simply rely on new, improved filters. The astonishing thing is that the idea of partner reduction still astonishes people who ought to know better. Of course a partner reduction intervention must be more than a few posters; it should be at least as comprehensive as the condom programs we currently find everywhere.

As Rotello (1997) acknowledges, advice on partner reduction can lull men into thinking that merely reducing partners or entering a monogamous relationship will keep them safe. But, of course, condom use can also lull men into a false sense of security. We should admit, however, that the first possibility is hypothetical, whereas there are data to show that the second possibility is a real problem, as the research of Ahmed and colleagues (2001) and Rosenberg (2002) suggests. Richens, Imrie, and Copas (2000) note that "increased condom use could reflect decisions of individuals to switch from inherently safer strategies of partner selection or fewer partners to the riskier strategy of developing or maintaining higher rates of partner change plus reliance on condoms" (p. 400). In fact, the false sense of security argument is often used to counter suggestions for any new or different intervention, such as programs to facilitate or promote male circumcision.

WHAT SHOULD THE ROLE OF CONDOMS BE?

The best evidence of condom effectiveness in resource-poor areas is among certain high-risk groups, such as CSWs or soldiers. Attributing national HIV prevalence declines to condom use seems most justified in Southeast Asia, notably in Thailand and Cambodia. As noted, it is relatively easy to persuade CSWs, their clients, and those who operate sex work establishments to use condoms. It is far more difficult to achieve widespread condom use in the majority population, although it is still easier among strangers or casual partners than among married or steady couples.

In view of this and all the findings reviewed in this chapter, what should the role of condoms be in Pattern II parts of the world? Condoms should be targeted more carefully and deliberately to populations where they will be used and among whom they will have the greatest impact. We need to rethink the strategy of condoms for everyone, every time, especially in generalized epidemics. They should be strongly promoted among CSWs and clients, among soldiers and police, among truck drivers, traveling businessmen, bar maids, and any other groups found or suspected to be at high risk. Condoms should also be promoted in one-off situations, that is, in casual sexual encounters. This is not the place to go into details of marketing and promotion strategies, but obviously condoms ought to be available in places where casual sex is likely to occur, including at night since such encounters are often unplanned and unanticipated.

It seems programs quickly reach a point of diminishing returns when putting resources into mass condom promotion to the majority population. Rates of condom use remain quite low in the general populations of Africa, although this is masked by use of statistics that refer only to condom use with casual partners. As will be seen with Uganda (in Chapter 6), national condom use (measured as condom use during last intercourse with any type of partner) is still only about 8 percent or less, or nearly 11 percent of the sexually active population (Macro Uganda/DHS, 2001), and we still know nearly nothing about consistent, correct use. Yet it is quite high (50% male and female rates combined) in situations of casual sex, and very high (over 90%) among urban CSWs and their clients.

Instead of putting all or most of our resources into trying to raise the ever-use rate among majority populations in countries like Uganda, it would be far more cost-effective to target condom programs to high-risk groups and situations, and to direct primary behavior change interventions to the majority. This targeting of interventions would be more efficient economically and programmatically. It would reduce the possibility that mass condom promotion might actually encourage riskier sexual behavior, as a few researchers are beginning to consider might be the case. And it would avoid the backlash typically encountered when condoms are—or seem to be—the only intervention, especially for youth. For example, during a recent AIDS conference in Zimbabwe, delegates from quasi-religious organizations strongly denounced what they called, "the wholesale indiscriminate promotion of condoms" to young people, charging that, "this had actually led most youths to experiment with it." Bishop J. H. Banda from Zambia criticized what he termed "the condomisation of the mind" in Zimbabwe (allAfrica. com, October 3, 2002). Fifty percent of new HIV infections in Zimbabwe are among those under age eighteen.

FEMALE CONDOMS

In heterosexually driven epidemics, it is males who typically determine whether or not condoms are used. And there are varying degrees of male dominance in all societies. Moreover it is men after all who must wear a condom. There is a great deal of male (and some female) resistance to using condoms. For these reasons, there has been great interest in some other methods of protection against HIV and STDs, and for that matter, pregnancy, that women can control. I have long been an advocate of female-controlled methods (e.g., Green & Monger, 1989).

A female condom was introduced in 1992 by the Chicago-based Female Health Company. By 2001, the female condom was available in over sixty developing countries. Some forty-five countries were distributing over 4.5 million female condoms, pushing the total number sold over the last eight years to over 35 million (Crossette, 2001).

UNAIDS, USAID, and other donors are now promoting female condoms along with male condoms. The underlying reason is sound: Women suffer disproportionately from HIV and other STDs, especially younger women and women who are coerced into sex. There is greater viral concentration in sperm than in vaginal secretions, meaning women are at least four times more vulnerable to infection than are men. There certainly is a clear need for a means of protection controlled by women. However, it is not clear how acceptable female condoms are and how often they are actually used.

Before major investment in distribution or marketing, studies were conducted to assess its acceptability, primarily to women. I happened to be marginally involved in one of the early studies to determine acceptability, in an east African country that must remain nameless. By the time of my involvement, groups of women had been paid to attend seminars during which they were taught about the advantages of the female condom, over a period of many weeks. Later, these same groups were renamed "focus groups" and the participating women were surveyed to measure what they thought about the female condom. Not surprising, approval rates were very high. Politeness and the wish for more such income earning opportunities virtually ensured it. And this was quite apart from the issue of quantifying and projecting findings from focus group populations who, of course, do not constitute a random sample. Perhaps this was considered fast track research, since it was done in the name of AIDS prevention.

Other research related to the female condom does not seem particularly useful, for example, the survey in Zambia that concluded, "Users of female condoms are more likely to be female" (Meekers, 1999, p. 3). Of more use is the same author's finding, "These findings suggest that the female condom is not being used for protection in high-risk situations, but rather for protection in relatively low risk acts" (p. 3).

On the basis of all the issues we have reviewed about the male condom, we should not be surprised that there are also problems of cultural acceptability, supply and distribution, price, and the like with female condoms. Regarding the last, a UNAIDS spokesperson admitted that "the price of the female condom is still very high and this is a major obstacle to wider acceptance and use particularly in developing countries. . . . In some countries, it is up to 10 times the price of a male condom" (Crossette, 2001, p. A6).

In fact, the female condom can cost thirty-three times more than a male condom in Zimbabwe. This has led to problems associated with reuse. A recent news report shows the following:

The high cost of the female condom is forcing Zimbabwean women, particularly commercial sex workers, to reuse the device to save money, despite the risks associated with reuse, AIDS activists have warned.

Recent workshops between the Women's AIDS Support Network (WASN) and commercial sex workers have revealed that many of the women were reusing the condom after cleaning it with substances such as beer, urine, water and detergents. (Posted on gender-aids@healthdev.ne, October 8, 2002)

For some, the solution to the dangers of reuse and cleaning the female condom ineffectively or dangerously is to have another information campaign. But lack of purchase power cannot be overcome by more information. Therefore the WHO and UNAIDS convened consultations in June 2000 and July 2002 to deal with the reality of reusing female condoms. While it did not recommend reuse, it developed a protocol that recommends the female condom not be reused more than five times, and that it be sterilized in a weak bleach solution (1:20 parts water), rinsed then in water, and patted dry (Serenata, 2002).

A study in urban Zambia, where female condoms were promoted and sold at a highly subsidized price by a social marketing project, concluded the following:

These findings show that there are substantial barriers to adoption of the female condom in Lusaka, where the female condom has been mass-marketed. More intensive counseling/education about the female condom, especially about insertion, is likely to be extremely important in sustaining women's intentions to use the method and in motivating them to use it. (Agha, 2002, p. 3)

There are also questions about effectiveness. Studies suggest about 5 percent of women relying on the female condom will have an unintended pregnancy in the first year. If the device is not used correctly or consistently, the unintended pregnancy rate seems to be about 21 percent (Trussell & Kowal, 1998). Since viruses can penetrate latex easier than sperm, we can expect higher failure rates for HIV and certain other STDs.

Some studies that have attempted to measure effectiveness of the female condom in preventing STDs in developing countries have shown positive results (e.g., Fontanet et al., 1998; Soper et al., 1993). Others, such as a community intervention trial in rural Kenya, suggest that the availability of the female condom, along with the male condom, does not affect STD rates compared to the availability of the male condom only (Feldblum et al., 2001).

All this is to say that medical technology has not provided easy solutions to preventing AIDS. This is not to say we should give up on technical solutions, only that we should be more open to behavioral solutions, especially if they have proven effective.

NOTES

1. See http://www.measuredhs.com/hivdata/ind_tbl.cfm for list and description of current USAID indicators.

2. Many of these conversations with sex workers were published in *Global AIDSLINK*, vol. 63 and 64 (2000–2001), edited by E. C. Green, L. Nkya, and A. Outwater, "Narratives of Sex Workers in a Tanzanian Town."

5

The ARV Issue

As we question the Western approach to AIDS prevention, it will be useful to briefly consider the current hot topic in global AIDS, namely, ARV drugs. ARVs are relevant to AIDS prevention because when we focus resources and attention on treatment, we divert them from prevention. Furthermore, as we look at the problems inherent in ARV programs in Africa, we should be cautioned by noting the same kinds of cultural bias that have led to disappointing results in medicalized condom–drug prevention strategies.

A glance at the program of the 2002 XIV International AIDS Conference in Barcelona proves that interest has largely shifted from prevention to treatment. The great majority of papers were on technical, medical treatment solutions to AIDS, especially bringing ARVs to poor countries. There was also great interest in vaccines, another technical, medical solution. As a summary of the conference put it, "A major theme of this year's conference was that because treatment works, we must export medication, expertise, and technology to treat patients in resource-poor areas of the world. The United States and Western Europe have led the way" (Valenti, 2002, p. 1). The subtext here is that prevention has not worked. To the extent that prevention was discussed at the conference, it was still focused on condoms, although there was renewed interest in microbicides. If global AIDS efforts were too technological-medical before Barcelona, they promise to be even more so in the future.

An article posted on the internet (Charles & Bolye, 2002) about the ways to prevent AIDS in Africa reflects the new thinking. It covered

ARVs, Nevirapine to prevent mother-to-child transmission, vaccines, and the newest microbicides. There was no mention of behavior change, nor for that matter, of condoms.

Consistent with this view, there were preconference pronouncements by high UNAIDS officials to the effect that prevention has not worked, citing low condom-use statistics as evidence. Even before the conference, it seemed that the global donor community had largely given up on prevention. Having decided that prevention has failed, the thinking seemed to go, we must consolidate our losses and now turn our attention to treatment (or vaccines). True, there were still countless papers about male and female condoms, and some on VCT. In fact, in his closing speech, Nelson Mandela called VCT, "The single most important prevention tool that we have, because it is the one that is most likely to change behavior."[1] Most VCT programs put their behavior change emphasis on condoms.

But the shift of interest away from prevention was quite clear. The problem, in my view, is that the donor community has failed to recognize what has worked in prevention. Instead of looking at a full range of behavior change, they have looked only at the part that has been well-funded condom use. And even the most ardent condom supporters could not claim by mid-2002 that many condoms were being used correctly and consistently, especially in Africa, where we find most of the HIV infections. The contribution of primary behavior change (partner reduction, delay of sexual debut among youth) was not given consideration at Barcelona, although it was occasionally discussed in the hallways, usually to be denounced as a right-wing plot the true aim of which was to ban all contraception and keep women enslaved in kitchens forever.

In the current UNAIDS global report, always released on the eve of a biennial global conference, we heard the following about success in prevention:

Despite all the grim statistics, there are some success stories. Through aggressive interventions, Uganda has managed to reduce its HIV prevalence rate from 8.3% in 1999 to 5% by the end of 2001. Zambia, Poland, and Cambodia have also successfully implemented campaigns that have reduced their infection rates. (Reuters Health, July 2, 2002)

Why not mention that national HIV prevalence has fallen in Uganda from 21 percent in 1991? Would that make prevention seem too achievable, too workable? Would it cause more attention to be paid to what actually worked in Uganda? By minimizing Uganda's achievement, and not mentioning Senegal, the world could now turn its attention to the more expensive and profitable drug solution.

The real winners in the shift away from prevention are the drug companies and consulting firms conducting business as usual. If donors were to begin to promote delay of sexual debut or partner reduction, and this caught on, they would stand to make no profits. This is unlikely to happen any time soon. Meanwhile, as priorities shift from condoms and treating STIs on a relatively limited basis to mass ARV treatment, starting with prevention of mother to child transmission (PMTCT) programs and then expanding to programs for all infected people, the drug companies (which largely sponsor the biennial global AIDS conference) stand to reap great profits. Of course, provision of ARVs for all who need them makes great humanitarian sense. And, of course, any of us who may be infected would want these drugs for ourselves.

It is also true that the drug companies stand to reap great profits. However cheap the price of ARVs become, the drug companies will not provide them at less than cost, and it is highly likely that they will make at least a small profit. If the Global Fund or the United States has newly appropriated billions to spend on AIDS, it is expected that a great deal of this money will go to the purchase of ARVs. And whatever the profit that accrues to the drug companies, it will come from a market that currently does not exist, thus it will be additive to current profit levels. For this reason, drug companies are—or ought to be—in favor of the ARVs-for-the-poor idea, as long as they can prevent the cheaper drugs that will circulate in resource-poor countries from being resold in developed countries.

There were a few lone voices at the Barcelona conference defending the need for prevention, even from the PLWHA community. In the following speech posted in summarized form by af-aids@healthdev.net calling for local and community action by a Ugandan PLWHA (July 8, 2002):

"The way this epidemic is, especially in the developing world, a lot needs to be done," says Milly Katana of People Living with AIDS in Uganda. "Government structures are wanting in many ways, not only for HIV but across the board. So people in NGOs and CBOs have a vital role to play."

We have realized that we need to do things in a more organised way. In prevention, less than 1% of the world's population is infected with HIV, so we have 99% to take care of.

But even in this statement, it seems that the real lessons of prevention were not mentioned, unless the summary filtered out any mention of the PBC that has occurred in Uganda. Indeed, there was little evidence in the entire conference that abstinence or fidelity/partner reduction plays any role in AIDS dynamics.

ISSUES SURROUNDING ARV DRUGS

Let us look more closely at the issue of treating HIV infections in Africa with expensive triple combination therapies, especially now that the prices are declining due to political pressure and the manufacture of cheaper generics drugs in some developing countries. This idea seems very appealing at first. It offers a relatively simple-sounding technological fix to a complex problem, even if it might cost $7–10 billion a year for an indefinite period. (This is the sum said by the Global Fund to be minimally necessary.) Perhaps the thinking is, Condoms didn't prevent a massive, deadly epidemic in Africa, so let's try drugs. This proposed solution, in fact, has some of the same appeal as condoms did fifteen to twenty years ago: It involves Western ("northern") technology and industry; we can export Western products; we can count the things we export and feel good about how many units we have exported and distributed; we can involve both the public and private sectors in distribution; and we can avoid the messy business of trying to change peoples' sexual behavior.

Some of the same people calling for drugs for the poor have been arguing that poverty is the root cause of AIDS. Yet even they realize that the solution called for if this is true, eradicating poverty, is an achievement that is hard to realize during anyone's lifetime. Focus on poverty can even become an excuse for inaction, for not doing the more mundane things necessary to avert HIV infections. As Halperin and Allen (2000) put it, "While well-meaning expressions like 'poverty causes AIDS' implicitly appear pro-African, they may actually do more harm than good through inadvertently encouraging a fatalistic attitude that, at least in the short run, 'nothing can be done' to prevent the continuing spread of HIV and other STDs" (p. 15).

There is even the promise of ARV's contribution to prevention: Triple combination therapy can lower viral load, which in turn should lessen the likelihood for HIV transmission. It has been estimated that if serum viral burden is reduced to less than 3,500 copies per milliliter, HIV transmission will be reduced by 81.4 percent (Quinn, Gray et al., 2000). However, ARV treatment would likely be provided mostly to those near the end stage of their disease, therefore it might have minimal impact on reducing transmission. And since ARVs prolong life, the pool of the HIV infected would grow with availability of ARV. This might lead to more opportunities for infection and possibly a net increase in HIV infection due to this factor alone, since not all viral loads will decrease. In fact, recent research has shown that even "men with excellent virological and immunological response to antiretroviral therapy may intermittently shed high levels of HIV in semen" (Gross, 2003).

On the other hand, the availability of treatment can encourage people to be tested, and this could contribute to prevention. In the words posted by the president of the Malaysian AIDS Council, "When they come forward to be tested, they can be counselled on how to prevent infection to themselves if they are still seronegative (not infected), or counselled on how to prevent infection to others if already seropositive (infected)" (Mahathir, posted on sea-aids@healthdev.net, June 19, 2002). Yet experience in Uganda in the early 1990s has shown that other incentives can also motivate people to be tested, for example, couples wishing to marry often wanted to know their sero-status.

Treatment of the poor in developing countries with ARVs is a worthwhile goal. But there are important considerations that are often overlooked. It is worth reviewing these. These issues become most apparent when considering implementing ARV programs in Africa, so this region will be the focus of discussion.

Infrastructure and Delivery

Africa lacks effective delivery systems in the form of adequate networks of health care facilities staffed by trained personnel. There is a lack of clean water and electricity not to mention health facilities and trained staff. There are problems of communications between far-flung health facilities; maintaining a constant supply of several drugs; teaching correct usage; and compliance with complex (although this has become less so) drug-taking regimens that result in irregular compliance even with literate, educated Americans. As recently observed, "The seemingly humanitarian efforts of drug companies, governments, and the UN could have explosive unintended negative consequences. Individual patients may not benefit, may become treatment resistant, and developing countries could become a veritable 'petri dish' for new, treatment-resistant HIV strains" (Popp & Fisher, 2002, p. 676).

Kevin DeCock, director of CDC's Kenya field office, recently pointed out that health practitioners in Kenya and elsewhere cannot focus on delivering ARV drugs to infected mothers when there is no mechanism for identifying HIV-positive women, basic necessities such as running water may be lacking, and infants are vulnerable to other preventable infections, such as malaria. He suggests that a reinvestment in African public health and an effort to rebuild basic infrastructure will be necessary before treatment of AIDS (or for that matter, prevention or vaccine) can make a substantial difference (DeCock, 2001).

In fact, to ensure a modicum of safety and to ensure effectiveness of ARV regimens and schedules, it would be necessary to provide various types of tests: liver and renal function, CD-4 levels (viral load tests would be required in wealthier countries), full blood counts, toxoplasma IgG, cryptococcal meningitis, and sputum analysis for TB among them. This requires significant training, the presence and availability of trained personnel, lab equipment, and, of course, considerable funding.

We cannot pass lightly over the issue of compliance. Even though there have been improvements in the direction of greater simplicity and fewer pills, the treatment regimen is still sufficiently complicated and onerous that many educated Westerners do not follow the regimens properly. Estimates of HIV medication nonadherence (sometimes called "pill fatigue") range from 50 percent to 70 percent (Chesney, 2000; Jones, 2002). It may be assumed that compliance would be much worse in remote areas of Africa where both patients and health care providers may lack much formal education. And with poor compliance comes the risk of resistance to ARVs.

Equity

Next we might ask if it is reasonable or even ethical to provide $1,000 (or $500, or $200) per year for one high profile disease in countries that currently spend $5 to $10 per person, per year, for all health care expenditures (drugs, operations, delivery of babies, immunization, and indeed all prevention programs). This becomes even harder to justify if malaria is killing more people in that country than AIDS. On what grounds could donors refuse to vastly increase treatment programs for malaria or tuberculosis if they were providing $500 per person per year for AIDS?

The quick response to questions like these might be that in a country like Botswana, where over one-third of sexually active adults are HIV infected, the answer may be yes. But in a country like Brazil or India, where less than 1 percent of the population is HIV infected, and where other diseases account for far more morbidity and mortality than AIDS, one faces legitimate issues of health priorities. Yet if the international community provides $1,000 per patient in Botswana, there will be great political pressure to do the same in India and Brazil, whatever other diseases might deserve higher priority.

In addition, organizations of African PLWHAs have pointed out that however cheap ARVs become, there will still be people who cannot afford them unless the total costs are paid for by donor organizations. Therefore, classes (if not clashes) will arise between the infected, basically between the privileged and the unprivileged. Resentment, jealousy, and perhaps conflict would follow. Ironically, problems of fairness and equity would likely plague programs begun precisely in the name of fairness and equity.

Disinhibition

Another consideration is disinhibition. There has been a return to risky sexual practices among some groups in the United States, Great Britain, and elsewhere in recent years, due apparently to the availability of ARVs. The Global AIDS conference in Durban summarized trends evident even in 2000. "In industrialized countries, there is now increasing evidence that in some populations, reductions in risk behavior over the last decade are reversing. . . . These developments may be the result of a false sense of security following the perception that HIV is now a 'normal' treatable disease" (DeLay et al., 2000). A year later, a UNAIDS report (UNAIDS, 2001) summarized overall trends in high-income countries, pointing to rising infection rates in various Western populations. Other recent studies have also measured a resurgence of STD and HIV infections, as well as higher-risk sexual behavior (e.g., recent CDC Morbidity and Mortality Weekly Reports). In a recent AJPH lead article, a scientist who is part of the gay community ponders the disturbing trends of HIV and rectal gonorrhea increasing among MSM in America. He notes that the Internet makes finding sexual partners easier, and that a rise in amphetamines and Viagra are also fueling the MSM epidemic. He notes that condoms are hardly ever used consistently; "barebacking" is on the rise (Gross, 2003). Latex is the only form of prevention mentioned in this article, although a new solution is also offered: implore the drug companies to invent an anal microbicide.

Gabriel Rotello, author of *Sexual Ecology* (Rotello, 1997) wrote to me in 2003 about disinhibition in the United States:

The lifting of the automatic death sentence here has resulted in a situation far more dire even than what I predicted in my *New York Times* op-ed during the Vancouver conference, when I compared the promise of this incomplete cure to the promise of antibiotics against standard VD in the 1950s (which ultimately caused those diseases to rise, or contributed to their rise). Who would have guessed that a proud, "out" culture of barebacking would emerge, which defiantly rejects safe sex? I didn't. And I was considered a pessimist. (Rotello, 2003)

There is a danger that risky sexual behavior could also increase in Africa if it became widely believed that there is now a cure for AIDS. Erosion of behavior in the direction of greater risk might outweigh or exceed any benefits that might result from availability of effective treatment drugs. Are we willing to take the risk of losing millions more lives than would otherwise be the case if the proposed experiment doesn't turn out quite as we hoped?

Diversion of Drugs

Another consideration is that if ARVs were distributed through the public sector, they would likely meet the same fate as any other free drugs that are actually valued in poor countries: They would not reach the poor. They would be diverted and end up being sold to those who could afford them. Indeed , this has already begun. In October 2002, the Dutch government recalled a quantity of Glaxo's Combivir and Epivir drugs after they found that "more than 35,000 packets of pills valued at some $15 million had been diverted from Africa to Holland and Germany" (Reuters Health News, October 10, 2002). During the same month, 290,000 Diflucan tablets donated to Uganda by Pfizer to treat AIDS-related infections were discovered being sold on the open market. Moreover, a bogus pill industry would likely arise since demand for the real drugs would be high and would still be too high for many or most. People would take fake pills, both as prophylaxis and treatment.

Health Complications

In addition, there are high rates of severe liver toxicity associated with ARV therapy, even in otherwise healthy, well-nourished populations with access to yet other drugs to take care of such dangerous side effects. For example, in a comprehensive retrospective review of more than 10,000 adult AIDS patients participating in twenty-one different AIDS Clinical Trials Group studies in the United States, "10% of patients developed grade 3 and 4 hepatotoxicity and 23% of them had to discontinue therapy permanently. According to the data, 2.5% of all deaths in the study period were liver related" (Reuters, 2001). Liver failure and death from this would likely be substantially higher in Africans whose immune systems may be compromised from coinfection with a variety of tropical diseases, sickle-cell anemia, anemia from malaria, parasitic loads, poor diet, and the like, and who may lack access to medical guidance, liver tests, or treatment of hepatic side effects.

A study of 659 men and 116 women in The Netherlands found that 53 percent had to switch their initial protease inhibitor-containing HAART regimen in the first year of therapy, 24 percent due to toxicity (Dieleman et al., 2002). We see from these statistics that ARVs cannot simply be given out; patient reaction to these powerful drugs needs to be monitored. This requires infrastructure and trained personnel.

Neveripine is now given to mothers and infants to prevent vertical transmission of HIV; it may also be given in cocktail combinations to HIV+ patients. It alone can also cause hepatotoxicity. According to Piliero & Purdy (2001),

The European Medicines Evaluation Agency's scientific committee issued a warning regarding the potential hepatotoxicity of nevirapine. This warning was issued because of "additional reports" of severe hepatic reactions. As a result, prescribing information has been changed to recommend biweekly monitoring of AST and ALT levels during the first 8 weeks of therapy, with specific recommendations to stop nevirapine depending on the degree of enzyme level elevation. . . . Bartlett presented the results of the FTC-302 trial, in which one group of patients received nevirapine as part of their HAART. Seventeen percent of these subjects had moderate to severe elevations in liver function test results, usually in the first 4 weeks of treatment. Two patients, including 1 with chronic hepatitis B, died of liver failure. (p.379)

There are additional problems with ARVs, even in American populations. By 2001, guidelines on how to use these were still being radically revised. Instead of starting ARVs as soon as HIV infection is suspected or confirmed, in order to hit the virus early and hit it hard, the guidelines were being changed to wait a few years until viral loads reach a certain level indicating disease. And rather than use ARVs consistently and nonstop, guidelines that were revised to suggest one week on ARVs, followed by one week off, may be optimal. Moreover, by 2001, half of Americans taking ARVs were found to have developed resistance to at least one ARV used in combination therapy (Blower, 2001). If resistance developed so quickly under optimal conditions of therapeutic administration, it would likely develop more quickly in poor countries that lack delivery and monitoring systems. This is just further evidence that ARVs ought not to be taken as a permanent or long-term solution to AIDS in Africa and other low-resource areas.

The following recent comments by a doctor treating HIV-infected patients in Zambia capture several of the problems just mentioned:

Zambia's population needs to be educated about HIV and AIDS and how HIV spreads. They do not need to hear about "cures" from the industrialised world that they cannot afford. For viral load testing, CD4 counts, and even liver function tests, the patients from this region need to travel 500 km to the capital, Lusaka. The cheapest bus fare is roughly equivalent to a nurse's weekly wage. However, zidovudine can be bought in a private chemist in the local town (80 km away). Currently only very wealthy patients can afford even a few weeks of this drug. This is how some patients spend all of their meager savings in the few weeks before they die. If the population is not educated about HIV, and antiretroviral drugs are made cheaper in Zambia, then a greater proportion of the young adults dying from AIDS related diseases will have no money to leave their families after they have died. . . . Patients need education and very basic medicines before they need these very expensive drugs made just about affordable. (Elphick, 2002, p. 895)

Even if ARV proponents get funding for the mass ARV programs they call for, it will still take years before ARVs are actually available to the masses in Africa and other resource-poor populations. In the meantime, the shift of funds and attention to treatment could have the effect of increasing the numbers of infection that could have been prevented through effective prevention programs. Interest in ARV programs also diverts attention from what can be done now in resource-poor countries in the form of low-cost, home-based care and support programs. We should not assume that all the solutions to the problems of the Third World poor lie outside those communities and countries, and that they can be found only in the donor organizations, corporations, and universities of the developed world.

LOW-COST, HOME-BASED CARE

Meanwhile there are low-cost, home-based care and support programs in Africa that are available now and that could usefully be supported while the many problems just outlined are being resolved. It must be admitted that resolution of these problems will likely take years. During this time, many people will die. What can be done for infected Africans right now? There are some community-based programs that provide information and advice on improved nutrition, therapeutic use of locally produced and available herbal medicines (several of which have been proven effective against opportunistic infections of HIV, if not for HIV/AIDS itself), psychosocial and spiritual issues, participation support groups, prevention and treatment of standard diseases and opportunistic infections, stress avoidance, promotion of good general immune system health, cessation of smoking and alcohol consumption, development of positive attitude, and the like. Considering only the role of improved nutrition, it has been established that concentrations of HIV in the genital tract are increased by vitamin A deficiency (Mostad et al., 1997), thus supplementation of this vitamin alone might play a role in prevention of HIV as well as treatment.

In April 1993, I conducted interviews and made observations in two indigenous healer clinics in Dar es Salaam that specialized in the treatment of STDs and AIDS. Both emphasized diet, nutrition, exercise, and other elements of relatively low-cost, holistic treatment. One clinic was run by a nurse who said she worked as a hospital nurse for fourteen years before she returned to her earlier calling as an herbalist. Some of her activities are as follows:

She presently uses only medicines derived from herbs or minerals. Mrs. N. sees about 150 patients a week, of whom roughly half are STD and HIV/AIDS patients; in fact she specializes in the latter. For her HIV/AIDS patients, she recommends a high protein diet along with plenty of vegetables, especially wild greens. She also recommends seafoods, and eating a lot of fruit and spices, believing that spices are good for the nerves and stimulate the appetite. There should be no smoking or alcohol consumption. She also recommends exercise, especially social-type hobbies or sports such as netball and dancing. Mrs. N. said that such activities are in part to help patients overcome depression and morbid thoughts. She emphasized the importance of "encouraging" AIDS patients. (Green, 1994, p. 250)

Even in the absence of evidence that the herbal medicines in use are effective against opportunistic infections, or against HIV infection itself, we can see there is value in such treatment and advice to PLWHAs. Indeed, programs have arisen in Africa that do not necessarily involve traditional healers but they promote positive behaviors and lifestyles. One such program is Positive Living, which arose in South Africa and is now spreading to neighboring countries.

Vida Positiva, as the same program is called in Mozambique, is a program of empowering people infected or affected by HIV in order to improve the quality of lives. From brief interviews I conducted in Mozambique in 2002, this program appeared to be low-cost, low-tech, sustainable, and apparently well accepted wherever it is introduced. There is a booklet written for PLWHA and their families which provides detailed advice for handling the physical, mental, social and spiritual problems faced by PLWHA. The program also focused on advocacy, awareness raising, and prevention.

One strength of the Positive Living approach appeared to be that it gave hope to those who are, or suspect they might be, HIV positive. The message is that infected persons can live longer, more productive lives if certain steps of self-care are taken. This approach and message contradicts the belief widespread in Mozambique that AIDS is little more than a death sentence. This belief leads to PLWHA hiding their HIV status (indeed, not being tested), abandoning hope, weakening their immune system health with fear and anxiety, and, of course, not becoming involved in AIDS education roles as in Uganda. The Positive Living approach seemed likely to increase VCT, which itself has been shown in some studies to contribute to positive behavior change and therefore to AIDS prevention. Another effect may be that PLWHA will become involved in community- and school-based IEC. According to stakeholders I consulted, PLWHA in Mozambique would sometimes attend certain workshops sponsored by NGOs or the Ministry of Health, but they did not participate at the community level due to fear, social stigma, and defeatist thinking.

There is obvious potential to save and improve the lives of millions if ways can be found to pay for the drugs and to overcome the many problems of cost, distribution, monitoring, and the like just reviewed. This will not happen quickly. Yet money from donors, such as USAID and some pharmaceutical companies, is already starting to become available for ARV programs in Africa and elsewhere. And countries such as Brazil and India are making relatively inexpensive ARVs. Since the problems outlined have not yet been adequately considered, programs of ARV provision in poor countries should begin only as small-scale pilot programs and they ought to be carefully monitored and assessed in a number of ways before they are scaled up to national programs. The possibility that ARV availability might lead to increased risk behavior should give particular pause, especially since this has already been documented in the United States and parts of Europe. After one recent modeling exercise in Botswana to examine the effects of ARV and of behavioral change, it was concluded, "Programs that provide HIV medication have been noted to make behavioral change more difficult to achieve, resulting in fewer AIDS deaths in a short period and more AIDS deaths later. . . . The solution for the HIV/AIDS epidemic lies in prevention programs that promote behavior change" (Sanderson, 2001, p. 12).

Uganda once again provides guidance in the area of what many call palliative care of the HIV infected. The role of THETA and its relationship with the Ugandan Ministry of Health is described in Chapter 6 on Uganda. Instead of taking the position that people should stay away from traditional healers and only seek any sort of treatment from biomedically trained practitioners, the Ministry of Health recognizes that most people in Uganda, as elsewhere in Africa, consult traditional healers for STDs and virtually everything else, including AIDS. It recognized the role of healers in palliative care and it collaborated with THETA in research that could identify locally available herbal medicines that could treat at least the opportunistic infections associated with HIV. Early research showed that a local mixture of plant-based medicines were as effective in the treatment of herpes zoster as expensive, imported drugs (Homsy et al., 1999). Herbal medicines for diarrhea were also identified and used with HIV/AIDS patients. The National Strategic Framework for HIV/AIDS Activities in Uganda 2001–2006 affirms the government's continuing relationship with THETA and the reliance on traditional healers and their local medicines in treatment of PLWHAs. It mentions the objective of "increasing accessibility to traditional medicines that work" (p. 16). This is in spite of Uganda being among the first, if not the first, country in Africa to pilot programs of treating HIV patients with ARVs, showing that the latter does not exclude the former.

Even before the AIDS scourge, critics sometimes charged that those who show any sympathy for indigenous medicine and healing are really advocating a "double standard of health care, [with] second class medicine for the rural masses" while Western medicine is reserved for urban elite (Green, 1994, p. 34; Velimirovic, 1984). This has long been one of the arguments used against collaboration between biomedical and indigenous health practitioners in Africa (cf. Green, 1996). It doesn't seem fair on the face of it: Why not insist on expensive medicines for the poor as well? The answer to this is certainly yes, if we can find a way to pay for it, let's also give expensive medicines to the poor. But keep in mind all the cautions and considerations when the medicines are ARVs and we may be talking about poor countries that spend less than $10 per year per person on all health care. Moreover, we ought not devalue and dismiss locally available therapies out of hand without unbiased consideration of available evidence relating to efficacy. Evidence of this sort exists. With powerful medical databases available online and ever-improving search engines, it is no longer difficult to find.

Better medicine (food, manufactured goods, etc.) is already more available to the urban elite than the rural poor, and always has been. And until a better, more equitable system is in place regarding ARVs—and the various problems mentioned are addressed—it makes sense to use whatever is currently available that contributes to improved lives for the HIV infected.

In treatment, care, and support, as in prevention, we need to never forget that conditions in Africa and other resource-poor areas are not the same as they are in the West. Schemes developed in Washington (e.g., at USAID, World Bank) or Geneva (e.g., at UNAIDS, WHO) may seem workable and humane, but they may not be suited to the realities of the less-developed world. What about more design input from Africans themselves? The problem, of course, is that this is too often only cosmetic involvement. The donors call the tune with their earmarked funds: Africans may make recommendations about plans for community-based distribution of condoms. But not, for example, for involvement of FBOs. These influential, resourceful groups are not part of the Washington–Geneva scheme. Very few faith-based organizations in Africa are nowadays directly supported by major donors in AIDS prevention efforts.

NOTE

1. Posted on intaids@healthdev.net, August 1, 2002.

Part III

INDIGENOUS APPROACHES TO AIDS PREVENTION IN DEVELOPING COUNTRIES

There have been some genuine success stories in Africa and elsewhere, despite nonrecognition by Western experts. The problem is that in these countries, Africans did not change behavior in the expected, predicted, and dictated way. In order for HIV prevalence to decline, we nearly all believed, high proportions of Africans would have to be using condoms, "every time." They would have to have their STDs treated, which meant "appropriate health-seeking behavior" (I have often used phrases like this myself). They would learn the dangers of not using health facilities, as well as unprotected sex.

But as we have already seen, the African countries that most followed this model are the ones with high infection rates and little or no sign of infection decline. Those few countries that did something that is not supposed to work are the ones among whom infection rates have declined. It is a very awkward situation for Western experts who have invested hundreds of millions of dollars and as well as their professional reputations.

This section highlights findings from several countries that have much to teach the West and the rest of the world. I begin with the country which has experienced the greatest decline in HIV prevalence, which is also the country for which I have the most information. I also present findings from Senegal, Zambia, and Kagera district in Tanzania. Programs and HIV prevalence levels may have changed recently for the better in Kenya, and so there is a brief update of a story that is otherwise typical for most of Africa. Following this, I provide details of a relative success story in the Caribbean: Jamaica. U.S. assistance to Jamaica has been atypical in the way it has been channeled since 1995. Instead of going through a U.S. organization, the money has gone to the Jamaican government. This has provided an unusual degree of national autonomy in the development and implementation of an AIDS control program in a developing country.

Finally, I provide the example of Thailand, which has a different epidemic pattern than that characteristic of Africa or the Caribbean. Thailand is often held up as the best example of how 100 percent condom policy (sometime said to be 100% condom use) can reduce national HIV prevalence. In fact, there is more to Thailand's story than condoms.

I hope the Western reader will come away with a new sense of humility from reading this section, because in fact some of the countries of the developing world have much to teach the West. The fair-minded reader will probably also wonder why, if these findings are true, they are not better known, or known at all. This was discussed in Chapter 3. But the short answer is bias. In fact, Africans and others have been telling survey researchers that they have been having fewer sexual partners, and delaying sexual debut, for years. As we will see, in some populations there seems to have been enough behavioral change of this sort to help bring down HIV infection rates.

What Can We Learn from Uganda?

As noted earlier, the best evidence for primary behavior change and the best links between PBC, program interventions, and impact on national levels of HIV infection, come from Uganda. This chapter is long and detailed, but earlier versions of this chapter that I have summarized in a few unpublished papers have set off a firestorm of debate, and so I want to present as much evidence as I have been able to amass with my limited resources.

EPIDEMIOLOGICAL DATA

Uganda seems to have experienced the most significant decline in HIV rates of any country in Africa or elsewhere. Surveillance data based on pregnant women seeking antenatal care at fifteen sentinel sites show a significant downward trend. The national average prevalence rates among pregnant women declined from 20.6 percent in 1991 to 6.1 percent in 2000. The decline has been most pronounced among younger age cohorts (15–19 and 20–24 years). See Figures 6.1 and 6.2.

As noted in the 2001 sentinel surveillance report, "Desegregation of the data by age group in both the rural and urban surveillance sites reveals continuing declines in the young age 15–19 and 20–24, but this time this trend of decline seems to get more expressed in the older age group 25–29" (Uganda ACP, 2001, p. 6).

Studies from 1986–1990 suggested that infection rates in youth ages fifteen to nineteen were driving the national epidemic; many surveys showed that the highest infection rates were found in just this age group

Figure 6.1
Uganda Poster

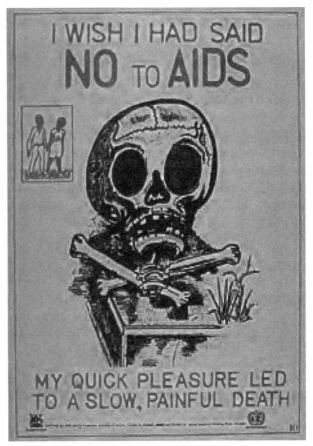

Source: Courtesy of Uganda Ministry of Health.

(Konde-Lule, 1995). An analysis of trends found that HIV prevalence rates declined 75 percent in fifteen to nineteen-year-olds (from 20.9% to 5.2%) and 59 percent in twenty to twenty-four-year-olds (from 24.9% to 10.2%) between 1991 and 1998, compared to about 50 percent for all age groups (Stoneburner & Low-Beer, 2002a).

There have always been skeptics concerning declines in Uganda's sentinel surveillance rates. The most recent may be a paper by Parkhurst (2001) charging that analysts tend to seize upon "a few pieces of data" from single Ugandan districts and then treat them as representative of national trends. The critic continues, "This is reflected in

Figure 6.2
Decline in National HIV Seroprevalence in Uganda, Based on Fifteen Sentinel Surveillance Sites

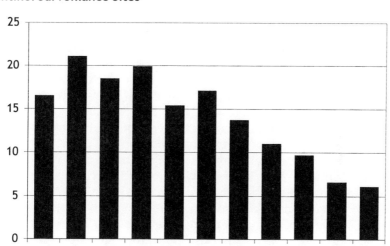

statements that discuss how Uganda has seen HIV rates decline from '30 to 10 per cent', for example, when these data, in fact, reflect the reality seen in only one surveillance site" (pp. 4–5).

However, the 21.1 percent to 6.1 percent prevalence decline represents national data, derived by the Uganda Ministry of Health, based on calculating averages from all sentinel surveillance sites. In the following words of the 2000 surveillance report:

Sentinel surveillance prevalence rates have continued to decline in the different surveillance sites in the different parts of the country both urban and rural. The weighted overall antenatal prevalence rate was 6.1% in 2000, down from 6.8% in 1999. The rates were skewed towards the urban sites where the weighted average dropped from 10.9% in 1999 to 8.7% in 2000 as compared to weighted averages of 4.3% and 4.2% prevalence in rural sites for 1999 and 2000 respectively. (Uganda ACP, 2001, p. 3)

It is a valid caution to point out that there were only seven sentinel surveillance sites in 1991, when rates peaked nationally, while there were fifteen sites in 2000. If we only compare the seven Ugandan districts for which we have surveillance data in 1992 with the same surveillance sites in 2000, average prevalence for those seven sites has fallen from 20.64 percent to 7.88 percent in eight years, still a dramatic decline.

According to estimates of UNAIDS and the U.S. Census Bureau data, national prevalence in Uganda peaked at around 15 percent in 1991 and has fallen to 5 percent as of 2001. The two rates are lower than the rates used by the Ugandan government because of weighting that reflects the proportion of the population living in rural areas. There has still been a significant decline in HIV prevalence by this estimate.

Focus on national trends can obscure the dynamics of local epidemics among different populations who may exhibit different risk factors. There are districts in Uganda where HIV prevalence among the sexually active population reached only relatively low rates. According to the current HIV/AIDS surveillance report (Ministry of Health, 2000), seroprevalence in Moyo district fell from 5.0 percent in 1993 to 2.7 percent in 2000; in Pallisa district it fell from 7.6 percent to 3.8 percent between 1992–2000; in Soroti it fell from 9.1 percent to 5.0 percent; and in Matany it fell from 2.8 percent to 1.9 percent between 1993–2000. Consideration of these data in districts of relatively low seroprevalence weakens the argument that Uganda's HIV seroprevalence decline might have been caused by either the saturation stage of the epidemic or firsthand experience with dying and dead family members, rather than behavior change or possibly better STD treatment.

CAN WE BELIEVE DATA FROM UGANDA ANC SURVEILLANCE SITES?

First of all, there are non-ANC data that show parallel trends. According to local studies compiled by the U.S. Census Bureau, HIV prevalence among Ugandan blood donors fell from roughly 25 percent to 2 percent between 1989–1996; and from 62 percent to 23.0 percent among STD patients between 1989–1999, even though there is considerable variation in results with the same year.

Sentinel surveillance data from Ugandan ANCs were accepted when that country seemed to have the highest HIV infection rates in the world, but when they began to decline, many experts thought something was wrong with the data (e.g., Zaba & Gregson, 1998). As a result, ANC data from Uganda have been scrutinized more than comparable data from most African countries (Bunnell, 2001).

Moreover, sentinel surveillance among women attending ANCs is the standard used by major agencies for trend analysis and for comparison between countries and regions. A UNAIDS/World Bank committee recently focused on the usefulness of sentinel surveillance and concluded that for all its shortcomings,

Several studies have shown that HIV prevalence among antenatal clinic attendees still gives a reasonable overall estimate of HIV prevalence in the general adult population, although they tended to underestimate HIV prevalence among women and overestimate HIV prevalence among men. As a result of these concerns, there is a continuing interest in research comparing HIV infection in pregnant women and in the majority population. (UNAIDS/MAP, 2000, p. 15)

It sometimes suits the fund-raising or political agendas of some players in international AIDS to minimize or deny evidence of falling HIV or STD infection rates, to present worst-case scenarios and perhaps even to exaggerate HIV prevalence rates. Such a position is believed to maximize donor interest and funding levels for a given country. I have encountered the pessimistic posture in both Uganda and Jamaica, and the stated reason for worst-case depictions is, We cannot rest on our laurels; we cannot become complacent; infection rates may begin to rise again. However, officials have also told me privately that the publication of findings pointing to success might result in HIV/AIDS donor funds being shifted to a country in greater need. My response was always that success stories in AIDS prevention are so few and so greatly needed to point the way that it is highly unlikely that a successful country would lose funds—it is more likely that they would receive higher funding levels. Nor have I seen any evidence of a country receiving less donor funding following reduction in HIV infection rates. Probably the opposite is true. In fact, as this is written, USAID will focus its AIDS expanded response to only fourteen high-priority countries. Despite its success—or because of it—Uganda is one of the fourteen.

Those somewhat pessimistic about ANC data may note that HIV infection reduces fertility, suggesting that sentinel surveillance data from antenatal clinics in Africa may in fact underestimate the true prevalence of HIV infection (e.g., Glynn et al., 2000; Zaba et al., 2002). On the other hand, it was observed in a careful review and comparison of ANC and population-based study trends that women with low education were overrepresented in the ANC sentinel surveys, compared to women in the majority population, because of their higher fertility, and lower education correlated with higher HIV infection levels, at least after 1996 (Fylkesnes et al., 2001). This would mean that ANC women might have higher HIV infection levels than women in the majority population.

There are other ways in which ANC data might overestimate infection levels in the broader population. Males tend to be infected less than females in the late stages of Pattern II infection. Recall that in early epidemic stages in sub-Saharan Africa, male-to-female infection is about 5:1. Later it becomes about 1:1 and finally about 1:2. The UNAIDS Multicentre study (Carael & Holmes, 2001) tested blood of randomly selected men and women and found in sites in Kenya, Cameroon, and

Zambia that prevalence of women was 50 to 100 percent higher than that of men, meaning that ANC surveillance data on women only would significantly overestimate national seroprevalence in these late-stage epidemics. Moreover, prevalence is calculated from only the sexually active, therefore it will not pick up rises in age of sexual debut or decreases in levels of premarital sex (Grulich & Kaldor, 2002).

Kwesigabo and his colleagues (2000) conducted population-based sero studies and incidence studies in Kagera region, Tanzania, which borders southwest Uganda and has a similar epidemiologic and socioeconomic profile as adjacent districts of Uganda. They found as follows that their population-based surveys validate the accuracy of ANC sentinel surveillance:

Our findings show that in this high prevalence area, monitoring the epidemic through a sentinel surveillance system involving pregnant women who are attenders at ANCs can be informative of the actual situation as it exists in the majority population. This recommendation is perhaps valid only for situations in which the epidemic is approaching a peak, stabilizing, or declining. (pp. 415–416)

There is also the issue of whether changes in HIV prevalence really tell us anything about changes in incidence, about the rate of new cases of HIV each year. It has been suggested that changes in prevalence in Uganda might have been due to alterations in the base population resulting from migration and mortality (Serwadda et al., 1996). However migration can also confound incidence studies. And mortality would have the least effect on prevalence in the fifteen to nineteen age group, followed by the fifteen to twenty-four age group.

Prevalence among Kampala females ages fifteen to nineteen declined from 22 percent in 1990 to 10 percent in 1996. As Sittitrai (2001) notes, "The steady drop for the youngest women suggests a real fall, not just of prevalence but also in incidence" (p. 7). In fact, prevalence in women ages fifteen to twenty-four has come to serve as a proxy for incidence among epidemiologists. By tracking infection rates among women ages fifteen to twenty-four, one can approximate incidence, for at least two reasons. There are fewer biases associated with HIV-related loss of fertility in younger women who have been infected for a shorter time. And because women in this cohort are closer to the age of sexual debut, HIV prevalence more closely reflects HIV incidence (Grulich & Kaldor, 2002). On the other hand, if there is a trend toward later sexual debut among women, such as we find in Uganda and Zambia, an increasing proportion of virgins will result in declines in prevalence even in the absence of changes in incidence among the sexually active

(Grulich & Kaldor, 2002). This means we still need to be cautious in interpreting trends in HIV prevalence among even the youngest.

Still, incidence is considered more useful than prevalence in measure of the spread of HIV. The problem is that such data rarely exist in developing countries as seen in the following:

Collecting incidence data, which involves testing the blood of the same group of people repeatedly over time or testing large numbers of people to detect a relatively small number of infections, is too costly and difficult for most national HIV/AIDS programs. Instead, these programs gather information on prevalence—the percentage of people in a population who are infected with HIV at a given time. This prevalence data is usually derived from testing blood samples taken for other reasons. (Henry, 1998, pp. 12–13)

In fact, Uganda has some incidence data. A cohort 17,000 people in 5,000 households were followed over an eleven-year period. Overall incidence has fallen from 7.6 per thousand per year in 1990 to 3.2 per thousand per year by 1998. As with prevalence, decline is more pronounced among younger age groups (Okware et al., 2001). It is a pity that the incidence study in Uganda begins in 1990, since there must have been incidence decline in the late 1980s prior to the 1991 peak year of HIV prevalence.

HIV prevalence data represent a combination of new infections and those that could be years old. As a result, there are many possible explanations for any changes in HIV prevalence. Still, significant changes in prevalence in specific age groups can suggest such things as change in patterns of risk behavior. STD prevalence is another biological measure; however, the quality of STD data in most developing countries is poor. Due to these weaknesses, one tries to triangulate findings, namely, to look for compatible trends between HIV, STD, and behavioral data derived from both qualitative and quantitative research (Pisani et al., 1998).

Before looking at the evidence for behavior change, we need to consider some other factors that might account for HIV prevalence decline.

OTHER FACTORS THAT MIGHT EXPLAIN PREVALENCE DECLINE

Some researchers believe, or once believed, that saturation accounts for almost all the HIV infection recorded in Uganda, at least in certain districts with especially high infections rates (e.g., Rakai and Masaka). Saturation refers to a stage of an epidemic where most of those who might be infected are already infected, and so incidence must begin to decline. In other words, high mortality among the infected decimates the ranks of those susceptible to infection, leaving those of less risk. Thus high mortality can in itself lead to lower incidence for a time, until new cohorts reach sexually active age and bring rates up again with high-risk behavior.

One argument against the effects of mortality explaining HIV decline in Uganda is that HIV prevalence fell first and to a greatest degree among the youngest cohort tracked, those ages fifteen to nineteen, among whom mortality would have the least effect. Even more compelling, rates have continued to fall to the greatest degree in this cohort between 1991–2001.

There is also the possibility that fear of AIDS independent of any interventions might account for behavior change. By the early 1990s, Uganda had the highest known HIV seroprevalence rate in the world, about 15 percent nationally, to use the figure weighted to reflect rural/urban proportions. Virtually every Ugandan knew people that had died of AIDS or were sick with the disease. This is a powerful incentive to change behavior. It is probable that a certain amount of behavioral change was in fact motivated by fear of death by AIDS, independent of any interventions. Yet there is a demonstrable relationship in Uganda between the types of behavior targeted in behavior change interventions in this time period, and the types of behavior change that have in fact resulted and been measured.

Let us consider further the spontaneous behavior change factor. Fear of AIDS caused by knowing someone sick with AIDS, or who has died of AIDS, ought to be a powerful motivator of behavioral change. Researchers examined DHS data from three countries, Uganda (1995), Zambia (1996), and Kenya (1998), specifically to understand determinants of behavioral change and to analyze the relative importance of knowing someone who has died of AIDS, comparing this with other factors, such as age, education level, knowledge of HIV/AIDS, economic status, and marital status. They concluded that "personal experience of AIDS is a significant predictor of behavior change in Uganda and Zambia, and is marginally significant in Kenya" (Macintyre, Brown, & Sosler, 2001, p. 160).

Knowing someone with AIDS, or who has died from AIDS, is clearly related to the social and political climate for even discussing AIDS. Stoneburner and Low-Beer (2000) have tried to pin this variable down, operationally defining "open personal networks" as situations when someone can discuss HIV status with 20 to 30 percent of contacts. In a country like Uganda, people have long known people with AIDS because it is possible to identify such people without much fear of reprisal. In countries like South Africa or Swaziland, few people know someone with AIDS because infected or sick people go to great lengths to conceal their status and illness. In South Africa, a woman named Dlamini (an ethnic Swazi) was killed by her neighbors after she revealed her HIV positive sero-status. On a tragic personal note, my closest friend in Swaziland, a man I had worked with closely for over twenty years, fell ill and died of AIDS in 2000 without telling me what was wrong with him. So powerful was the stigma and shame associated with AIDS that he forewent the possibility of obtaining ARV drugs through his friendship with me and died in silence.

We can conclude that, other things being equal (such as HIV infection rates), people are much more likely to report knowing someone with AIDS when there is an open social and political climate for discussing AIDS, and stigma associated with AIDS has been reduced. It certainly helps create an open climate and reduce stigma when PLWHAs become involved in these processes, such as has happened in Uganda. PLWHAs there visited schools, churches, and local communities, teaching about the disease and speaking candidly about their personal experiences. A study in Uganda shows that school-based AIDS education conducted by PWLHAs can lead to positive behavior change. "Young people in schools can be accessed with HIV/AIDS messages to influence them to adopt forms of safe sexual behaviour that do not expose them to the risk of HIV/STD infection and early unwanted pregnancies" (Sekirevu & Lukenge, 1998).

Personal experience with AIDS no doubt motivates some degree of behavioral change. But if fear from personal experience were sufficient to change behavior that impacts national HIV seroprevalence levels, why did this not have such impact in the dozen or so countries whose HIV infection rates became higher than Uganda's ever were? Other countries either remained in denial about AIDS for many years (and may still be in denial as I write), or they never used a deliberate-fear–personal-risk perception approach in AIDS education, at least to the same extent that Uganda did (discussed later).

Another argument against attributing HIV reduction to high mortality is that other countries in Africa have achieved higher infection rates than Uganda had in the early 1990s, and yet while there may be signs of plateauing in an increasing number of these, there has not yet been a clear reduction of incidence or prevalence, with the exception of youthful cohorts in Zambia. This suggests that behavior change may have had at least as great an influence as saturation in reducing HIV infection.

In addition, there are districts in Uganda where HIV prevalence among the sexually active population reached only relatively low rates.

According to the HIV/AIDS surveillance report (Uganda Ministry of Health, 2001), HIV prevalence in Kotido peaked at around 3 to 4 percent and then fell to 1.9 percent. In Moyo, it peaked at 5 percent and then fell to 2.7 percent. These two districts now have the lowest prevalence rates in Uganda. Evidence from especially these two districts weakens the argument that saturation and firsthand experience with dying and dead family members accounted for HIV declines (although it is true that some rural people may have had relatives in urban areas whose deaths influenced behavior change).

In sum, it is unlikely that either saturation or fear of AIDS unrelated to program interventions account for the dramatic decline in HIV experienced in Uganda, even though these may have contributed to part of the decline. This conclusion is supported by evidence that behavior change interventions were focused on youth, and both incidence and prevalence have declined more among Ugandans ages fifteen to nineteen and twenty to twenty-four than among other groups. These were the groups primarily targeted in AIDS education. A growing number of epidemiologists and others who work in international AIDS now attribute Uganda's HIV decline to behavioral change. Unfortunately, there is far less consensus about which behaviors changed.

BEHAVIOR CHANGE OVERVIEW

It is useful to look at knowledge before behavior, since the former is often regarded as the precursor to the latter in behavior change theories. By 1989, around the time HIV incidence probably peaked, we have findings from a WHO/GPA survey that point to high levels of knowledge about AIDS prevention. Remember that this was a time when most of Africa was still in denial about the epidemic. The (unpublished) survey shows that 92.7 percent had heard of AIDS; 93 percent believed that sex with many partners caused AIDS; 85.8 percent believed AIDS can be prevented by changing one's behavior; and 61.9 percent said some of their friends' behavior has changed because of AIDS.

It is clear that behavior changed in Uganda, although not necessarily the behaviors anticipated. By 1995, according to the DHS, 95 percent of men and women ages fifteen to forty-nine were reporting either having one partner (or no partner outside a polygynous marriage) or abstaining during the past six months.[1] By 2000, there was a slight decrease in the percentage reporting monogamy or fidelity, to 93 percent (discussed later). About 11 percent of those who reported any sexual activity, or 8 percent of all Ugandans ages fifteen to forty-nine, reported condom use during last intercourse with any partner (DHS/Uganda, 2000). This figure seems to be the best measure of regular use, although we don't really know about regularity and we certainly do not know about how correct condom use is.

In addition to the changes reflected in these broad measures, the proportion of men reporting three or more nonregular partners fell from 15 percent to 3 percent between 1989 and 1995. These figures come from the WHO/GPA survey (Bessinger & Akwara, 2003). Thus we see a significant decline in multipartner sex among men who can be considered core transmitters.

It is difficult to conclude that a risk reduction behavior reported by 8 percent of the population is contributing more to HIV infection aversion than two risk avoidance behaviors reported by 93 percent of the population, even in 2000 when reported condom use is highest. The case was even stronger in 1995, when the proportions were even more polarized.

The greatest degree of all major types of behavior change promoted (partner reduction, abstinence or delay, condom use, seeking appropriate STD treatment) has been found among those ages fifteen to twenty-four, paralleling the greatest decline in HIV infection rates, and therefore suggesting causal linkage between interventions and declining infection rates. Analysis of data on behavior change shows that there has also been more positive change among females than among males, and generally more change among urban and better educated than among rural and less educated. HIV ANC prevalence decline among age group fifteen to nineteen was more dramatic than that of older Ugandan women, on the order of 75 percent rather than around 50 percent by 1998. If HIV decline can be attributed at least in part to changes in behavior, then it seems there was more of this among younger people.

THE MUSEVENI APPROACH

AIDS prevention interventions found in Uganda, especially those of the early period, need to be looked at carefully. It is useful epidemiologically to define the early period as between the beginning of a national response to AIDS (1986) until the year HIV prevalence peaked (1991). As bold an activist as he was when it came to AIDS, President Museveni of Uganda did not have much faith in condoms during at least this period. He had his own approach to AIDS prevention that was at odds with the donor community and international experts. He put it as follows in a 1991 speech:

Sex is not a manifestation of a biological drive; it is socially directed. . . . I have been emphasizing a return to our time-tested cultural practices that emphasized fidelity and condemned premarital and extramarital sex. I believe that the best response to the threat of AIDS and other STDs is to reaffirm publicly and forthrightly the respect and responsibility every person owes to his or her neighbor. (Museveni, 2000, p. 251)

In the context of AIDS and STDs, respect is often a Ugandan or broader African code word referring to fidelity to one's spouse or partner. For example, a group of Zimbabwean chiefs commented to some local traditional healers, "To solve the problem (of AIDS) we would like things to be the way they were yesterday and not today. Wives and husbands must respect each other as they used to do before" (Musara, 1991, p. 32). In my own fieldwork in South Africa with indigenous healers, "respect" in this context means respecting marriage and therefore practicing fidelity.

A Ugandan government booklet entitled *Control of AIDS*, published in 1989, stated unambiguously: "The government does not recommend using condoms as a way to fight AIDS." The booklet expressed the view that condoms were not readily available, they were unreliable, they were likely to be used incorrectly, and they gave users "a false impression that they were safe from AIDS" (Kaleeba, Namulondo, Kalinki, & Williams, 2000, p. 17). In fact, when President Museveni gave the keynote address at the International AIDS Conference in Florence, Italy, in May 1991, he surprised the audience by denouncing condoms as an AIDS prevention strategy (Kaleeba et al., 2000, p. 17).

Incidentally, President Museveni has been mischaracterized about his position on condoms. The *Washington Post* gave the following account of a summit that twelve African leaders had with the World Bank president and the IMF managing director in Dar es Salaam, February 22–24 (AIDS was high on the list of discussion topics):

"Malawian President Bakili Muluzi wanted to know about the role of church and religious leaders. Simple, (Uganda Pres.) Museveni responded: he said he invited church leaders in, discussed with them how to carry out their awareness drives and gave them condoms to distribute." (March 14, 2001)

This account has nice shock appeal, and it suggests that Museveni's views on condoms changed over time. But at least during the early epidemic period, Museveni was opposed to the single-minded emphasis on condoms that he found on the part of the international community, meaning donors and health experts. In the following extract from a 1991 speech to the First AIDS Congress in East and Central Africa (in Kampala, November 20, 1991), he made himself quite clear:

Just as we were offered the "magic bullet" in the early 1940s, we are now being offered the condom for "safe sex." We are being told that only a thin piece of rubber stands between us and the death of our continent. I feel that condoms have a role to play as a means of protection, especially in couples who are HIV-positive, but they cannot become the main means of stemming the tide of AIDS. . . . In countries like ours, where a mother often has to walk twenty miles to get an aspirin for her sick child or five miles to get any water at all, the question of getting a constant supply of condoms may never be resolved. (Museveni, 2000, p. 252)

Since polygamy exists in Uganda and elsewhere in Africa, admonishing people to stick to one partner was problematic. Ugandan programs began to use the term "zero grazing" or "graze at home" to take care of this issue. The term meant that both monogamists and polygamists (polygynists, strictly speaking) should remain faithful to their married partner(s). It was recognized early in the epidemic that if polygamous spouses were uninfected, then it was far safer for a man to have sex with his two or three wives than to have occasional sex with a CSW (Sabatier, 1988).

To continue with Museveni's distinctive approach, Museveni launched a national awareness campaign that involved a great deal of face-to-face discussion and learning (and desensitizing and "destigmatizing" of a highly sensitive topic), involving opinion leaders at all levels of society, both urban and rural, such as religious leaders, political leaders (including chiefs), school teachers, heads of women's and youth organizations, traditional healers, and many others. More on this will be found in sections to follow. But it is important to note that was not and is not the usual approach to AIDS prevention in Africa: Use mass media to raise awareness, promote condoms, and close the condom gap between knowledge and behavior. In this scenario, interpersonal education is usually focused on community-based distribution of condoms.

It was only in 1992 that President Museveni began to yield to the entreaties of the international AIDS community and agreed, reluctantly, to add condom promotion to Uganda's approach that emphasized fidelity and delaying sexual debut. By that year, HIV infection rates had already started to decline, strongly suggesting that the earlier approach had worked. Before 1992, national condom user rates (ever-use) were in the single digits nationally. In fact, significant condom distribution did not begin until the mid-1990s (Kaleeba, Namulondo, Kalinki, & Williams, 2000).

Another distinctive characteristic of Uganda's program is that the risks of the C option were not dismissed or glossed over. In the words of one Ugandan health official, "First, abstain from sex. If you cannot abstain, stick to one partner. If you can't stick to one partner then you have to use a condom. *But be sure that condoms are not 100 percent effective"* (Tayebwa Katureebe, quoted in Torres, 2000). The last part of this statement provides important information that is usually not mentioned in prevention messages, especially in Africa. Its inclusion by a Ugandan shows both insight into transmission dynamics and honesty in conveying this to the public. And it may provide us with insight into how and why Uganda was able to promote the A and B of the prevention ABCs so successfully. That is, the public was warned not to put more trust into condoms than they deserve.

My Ugandan colleague, Vinand Nantulya, who was an early advisor to President Museveni, explained to a skeptical, largely American audience in Febuary 2003 that the message in Uganda was phrased something like, Practice A or B. If you fail, then be sure you fail with a condom.

In 1998 I examined district workplans of the Ugandan Ministry of Health and was able to measure in a rough way the relative number of persons trained or sensitized under Option A (safer sex, or partner reduction, abstinence/delay) and option B (condom promotion). There seemed to be at least four times as many persons trained under Option A. This may again help explain why A and B options have been reported more than condom adoption when we look at actual studies of behavior change. It may also demonstrate the relative national impact of public sector AIDS programs at the district levels compared to better-known national NGO or government programs—at least better known to the international AIDS community. The major bilateral donor in AIDS, USAID, has only funded NGO programs.

With increasing foreign donor funding and program priorities since the early 1990s, AIDS prevention in Uganda has begun to look like AIDS prevention elsewhere in the world. Emphasis on PBC has diminished, while emphasis on condoms, VCT (which increasingly urges adoption of the condom option upon those tested), and to a lesser extent treatment of STDs has increased. More and more funds have been channeled through NGOs, whose activities reflect foreign donor priorities. Indeed, the majority of these NGOs developed precisely because money was available from donors like USAID. By 2001, there were over 1,000 NGOs and community-based organizations working in AIDS in Uganda.

The major player in the early years was the Ministry of Health, and support came from WHO/GPA. Fortunately for the continuation of the ABC approach and emphasis on PBC, the World Bank funded public sector AIDS prevention through the STI project, beginning in 1994. The Museveni approach seems to have continued because the Uganda government had a great deal of control over how these project funds were spent. In fact, the project's requirement of decentralized planning and implementation meant that the prevention strategy had considerable input from district health officials. It appears that these officials had a better idea—certainly than foreign donors—of what was needed, what was feasible, and what had worked to date in prevention.

This remains true today. In spite of foreign donor spending priorities, the National Strategic Framework for HIV/AIDS Activities in Uganda 2001–2006 describes sensitizing the public about the dangers of early sex, infidelity, unprotected sex, and substance and alcohol abuse in relation to HIV/AIDS as a key activity to support IEC for sexual behavior change. Religious organizations continue to be listed among other NGOs under key sectors involved, sometimes being listed first, covering the broad range of activities relating to prevention, care and support, treatment, stigma and discrimination reduction, orphans and vulnerable children, and policy development. Five risk factors are mentioned, including high number of reported lifetime sexual partners and sexual intercourse before sexual organs are mature.

Before looking further at Uganda's response to AIDS, let us consider more evidence for behavioral change.

FIDELITY AND ABSTINENCE

There was substantial reduction in the proportion of Ugandans reporting casual sex between the late 1980s and the mid-1990s. Before looking at the statistics, it is useful to look at the following snapshot of Uganda in 1986, the year AIDS prevention began:

John Kiwanuka remembers what it was like as a medical student at Makerere University in Kampala, Uganda, in 1986. The nightmare years of dictators Milton Obote and Idi Amin were over. Yoweri Museveni had won the civil war, and Uganda had entered a time of relative peace.

"My friends and I wanted to party and celebrate. We had girlfriends," said Dr. Kiwanuka, a public health physician at the Africa-America Institute in New York responsible for HIV/AIDS policy.

Then the Ugandan president began to speak out.

"There was a dramatic change among students in 1987 and 1988. I took precautions. My friends changed their behavior. The ones that didn't succumbed to the disease," Dr. Kiwanuka said. (Carter, 2003, p. A13, http://www.washingtontimes.com/world/20030313-21315566.htm)

By 1995, according to the DHS, 95 percent of unmarried men and women ages fifteen to forty-nine were reporting either one or zero partners during the past six months. As seen in Table 6.1, women were more likely than men to abstain or report one partner. Comparing those in union and single, abstinence was the main behavior reported by the unmarried, while monogamy was the main behavior reported by the married, as might be expected. Otherwise, for combined "abstinence-monogamy" levels, there was little overall difference.

It is useful to consider the sexual behaviors recorded before HIV prevalence levels peaked in 1991, knowing that sero-incidence peaked somewhat earlier. First, we must acknowledge that multidistrict surveys from the 1980s are not directly comparable with the DHS of 1995 and 2000, which are national surveys. Thus, any exercise in assessing degree of behavior change using the former must be highly qualified. On the other hand, it does not seem heuristic to ignore random sample surveys that cover five or six districts and have sample sizes of between 2,000 and 4,500, especially since it is crucial to know something about sexual behavior prior to 1989. In fact, comparisons between the Uganda DHS 2000 and Ministry of Health sample surveys of southern districts from 2000 and 2001 produce rather similar data on casual sex. Comparisons between the DHS and the WHO/GPA surveys conducted in 1995 likewise show similarities in findings about casual sexual behavior. These similarities suggest it is permissible to make at least general comparisons between the DHS and both earlier and later surveys in southern districts only, at least on measures such as casual sex.

Still, the most cautious way to handle these early data is to make essentially qualitative rather than quantitative comparisons between them and later DHS data. That is, we may conclude that there was significantly more multipartner behavior in the late 1980s, compared with the mid- or late 1990s, but we cannot know the precise magnitude of change.

An Adolescent Fertility Survey was conducted in six districts (Jinja, Kampala, Masaka, Kabale, Hoima, and Mbale) between 1988 and 1990. A multistage, random sample of 4,510 respondents ages fifteen to twenty-four were chosen on the basis of age, regardless of marital status (there were 594 men and 1,009 women from rural areas, and 951 men and 1,956 women from urban areas).

Among the findings was the following:

Approximately 82% of male and 80% of female respondents in both rural and urban areas had had a sexual partner in the last three years. Two-thirds of the males had had more than one sexual partner; of these males, more than half had had four or more partners. Most young women had had only one sexual partner; only one-third had had more than one, and of these young women, fewer than half had had more than two partners. Distributions were almost equal for urban and rural respondents. (Turner, 1993, p. 76)

Table 6.1
Percentage Distribution of Men and Women by Number of Sexual Partners (Excluding Spouse or Cohabiting Partner) in the Six Months (1995) or Twelve Months (2000) before the Survey

	Marital status	Number of partners				Percent with 1 partner, or abstaining*
1995		0	1	2	3+	
Male	Not currently in union	80.4	12.0	4.0	2.6	91.1
15-54	Currently in union	90.3	6.3	1.4	0.3	90.3
Female	Not currently in union	94.7	4.2	0.6	0.2	98.6
15-49	Currently in union	98.5	1.0	0.2	0.0	98.5
2000						
Male	Not currently in union	65.4	23.4	8.7	2.4	88.3
15-54	Currently in union	88.0	9.7	1.4	0.8	88.0
Female	Not currently in union	71.9	26.0	2.0	0.0	97.6
15-49	Currently in union	97.4	2.4	0.1	0.0	97.4

Source: Macro International (2001) and Macro International (1995).

*Missing data or "don't know" not included, so values do not add up to 100 percent.

Meanwhile, reported condom use in urban areas was higher than might be expected at that time: 18 percent for urban males (5% for rural males). Use was less than 1 percent of females in both urban and rural areas (Turner, 1993). Twenty-one percent of men and 8 percent of women reported they had had one or more STIs.

In another published version of these study findings (that specify use of only 1988–1989 data), we see that risk of STDs among those not reporting (ever) use of condoms was 46 percent higher than that of those who did report condom use. Moreover, 32.5 percent of respondents had four or more sexual partners during the past three years (Agyei & Epema, 1992).

In 1988, a national sample survey was done with support from the Ford and Rockefeller foundations. It was known as the AIDS and Reproductive Health Network (ARHN) study. The survey was described as a randomized sample of 3,160 respondents, 44 percent men, drawn from ninety-one rural and urban clusters in eight districts (Ankrah, Asingwiire, & Wangalwa, 1990). Some data from this survey have been presented at global and regional AIDS conferences. Some of the findings were that there was "already evidence of decline" of commercial and extramarital sex, and that use of condoms seemed to have little acceptance among the males in this 1988 sample of Ugandan men (Ankrah et al., 1990). A paper showing partial findings from eastern Uganda reported the following:

First sexual experience for both males and females commenced at an early age. While extramarital sex was supposedly declining, reported numbers of current partners revealed that 69% of the participants at the time of the study had more than one. Admission of multiple sex partners was most common by men in cities and towns. (Ankrah et al., 1990, from abstract)

A 1989 baseline survey conducted by WHO/GPA in eight districts found that 39.2 percent of men and 18.4 percent of women (28.8% combined) reported "at least one sex partner other than a regular sex partner in the past year" (UNAIDS/Uganda, 2000, p. 9). By 1995, only 16 percent of all men, or 20 percent of sexually active men, were reporting nonregular partners in a second WHO/GPA survey. A seemingly significant decline in commercial sex can also be seen by comparing the 1989 WHO/GPA survey and the Uganda DHS 2000. In 1989, 33 percent of men ages fifteen to twenty-four reported commercial sex in the past year. In 2000, 2 percent of men reported paying for sex in the previous year (Ankrah, 1993; Macro International, 2001). We should keep in mind that there are differences in sampling between the 1989 GPA and later DHS surveys.

The WHO/GPA survey asked open-ended questions on behavioral change (e.g., Did you change your sexual behavior because of AIDS? If so, how?). Of the 69 percent who reported change, virtually everyone reported something other than condoms; only a fraction of 1 percent reported condoms, even though that is the only behavior change specified in the report. Another sample survey of three southern districts conducted by the Uganda Ministry of Health AIDS Control Programme in 1991 asked the same questions about change. The behavior change overwhelmingly reported was reducing the number of partners; 1 to 2 percent mentioned condoms (Moodie et al., 1991). The Moodie and colleagues (1991) study also sought behavioral data based on three-year recall, as well as data on current and recent behavior. Forty-three percent of a random sample of respondents reported two or more sexual contacts per year for the three years prior to the 1991 survey, compared to 17 percent who did so in 1991 (Moodie et al., 1991).

Moodie and colleagues (1991) conclude that the numbers of partners reported for the earlier period "suggest that either a definite change has occurred or perhaps that respondents are more willing to report numbers of sexual contacts they have had in the distant past rather than in the present" (p. 41) or more recent past.

At the end of this study report, the authors conclude the following:

There is good evidence that some changes in sexual behaviour have occurred. As discussed previously, questions can be raised about the validity of self-reported behaviour change. However, the 45% of the sample who reported a reduction of sexual partners can be combined with other indices to gauge behavioural change. These other indices are the 14% of respondents who volunteered a change in the sexual behaviour of family members, and the more than 20% who spontaneously reported changes both in social behaviour and in concomitant sexual behaviour in their communities.

Taken together, these markers suggest that a reduction in sexual partners has occurred, albeit not uniformly across our sample. It should be noted that reduction of sexual partners does not always mean reduction to only one partner or contact, although this was the most commonly reported number. (Moodie et al., 1991, p. 52)

In addition to the 1989 GPA and the 1988 national survey, studies by Konde-Lule and his colleagues (Konde-Lule, 1993; Konde-Lule, Berkley, & Downing, 1989) found that between 1987 and 1992, those who reported two or more concurrent partners fell from 43 percent to 12 percent among men, and from 13 percent to 1 percent for women. "Concurrent" was defined as partners in the past six months. Condom ever-use was 3 percent in 1987, and 20 percent of the entire sample reported an STD (defined as "purulent genital discharge or sore") in the five years prior to the survey (Konde-Lule et al., 1989, pp. 515–516). These data come from random (multistage, cluster) sample surveys in two semirural communities not far from Kampala. The sample was 3,928 in 1989, 54 percent of whom were women.

Data from these foregoing early surveys are summarized in Table 6.2. Averaging findings from these five surveys, it seems that about 40 to 45 percent of Ugandans reported a casual partner or more than one partner in the previous year.

Additional studies show that by the mid-1990s, Ugandans were reporting fewer multiple partners than some earlier baseline studies suggest. For example, Wierzba and Tumushabe (1994) reported 8 percent; Clarke (1994) reported 1 percent; and Musinguzi and colleagues (1997) reported between 5 percent and 11 percent all cited in Barton (1997). This partner reduction among core transmitters must have had considerable impact on national prevalence rates.

From all these studies, it is clear that there has been considerable reported partner reduction between the late 1980s and the mid-1990s, as well as a reduction of men reporting using commercial sex, even if the exact degree of change cannot be known.

If we only want to look at the least debatable statistics, we can compare results of the two WHO/GPA surveys: Looking at all age groups, 39 percent of males had more than one sex partner in 1989. This declined to 21 percent by 1995. For females, the decline was from 18 percent to 9 percent. Furthermore, the proportion of males reporting three or more sex partners fell from 15 percent to 3 percent between 1989 and 1995 (Bessinger & Akwara, 2003). These in fact are the figures I used in congressional testimony on March 20, 2003, just to avoid debates over methodological differences between surveys. The magnitude of actual behavioral change was undoubtedly greater than these WHO data show, especially considering that there must have been behavioral change before 1989. But even with these figures there has still been significant change, and no one can dismiss the data on the grounds of methodological differences.

Incidentally, a period of special risk for African men is during wives' pregnancy and the postpartum abstinence period. Several studies show that men are more likely to engage in extramarital sex during these periods. Yet Uganda DHS data show that the postpartum abstinence period was shortened from 4.1 to 2.1 months, reducing the period of risk. This might suggest that men are resuming sex with their wives earlier, instead of engaging in extramarital casual sex, as a strategy to avoid HIV infection.[2] This may be further evidence of PBC in Uganda.

For the record, during my first trip to Uganda in 1993, there was already evidence available that STD infection rates were starting to decline, although no foreign expert that I met at the time believed it (some Ugandans did). I wrote the following in my consultant report to USAID:

There is anecdotal evidence that STD incidence has significantly decreased in Uganda in the last year or two. While this may reflect wishful or politically motivated thinking, it would be extremely significant if this were true. If a high AIDS-prevalence country like Uganda shows a significant decline in STDs (presumably a harbinger of a later decline in HIV seroprevalence) *in the absence of a male condom prevalence rate of over 5%*, it might suggest that *other* types of behavior change (premarital chastity, "zero grazing," marital fidelity, abstinence, non-penetrative and other safer sexual practices) can significantly affect STD incidence if not HIV incidence. (Green, 1993b, p. 4)

USE OF CONDOMS

The proportion of surveyed males who had ever used a condom was about 3 percent in 1987 and rose to between 5 and 13 percent by

Table 6.2
Respondents Reporting Casual Partner or Two or More Partners in the Previous Year

Data year	Name of study	Male (%)	Female (%)	Both (%)
1988-1990	AFS (age 15-24)	66	33	53
1988	ARHN			69
1989	WHO/GPA	39	18	29
1988	Moodie et al. 1991, based on 3-yr recall			43
1987	Konde-Lule	43	13	26
1995	WHO/GPA	21	9	
1995	DHS	In Union: 8 Single: 6.6	In Union: 0.9 Single: 2.5	

Source: Early behavioral surveys in Uganda.

1991, the year HIV infection rates reached peak level (UNAIDS/Barton, 1997). Probably a fair national average of condom ever-use in 1991 among men would be 5 percent. In fact, condoms were not widely available in Uganda until after 1993 (Stoneburner & Carballo, 1997). It therefore seems unlikely that condom use contributed much to initial stabilization and decline in HIV incidence and prevalence, whatever its later contribution.

Ever-use of condoms does not tell us much. By 1995, about 6 percent of sexually active Ugandans used a condom with some regularity, measured as condom use during last intercourse with any type of partner. By 2000, this had risen to 11 percent of those sexually active (14.7% of men and 6.9% of women), or about 8 percent of all Ugandans ages fifteen to forty-nine, factoring in those who report abstinence (DHS/Uganda, 2000). Since only consistent use of condoms is likely to have significant effect on HIV prevalence at the population level (Hearst & Chen, 2003a), levels of 6 to 8 percent (condom use, last sex, any type of partner) in the latter 1990s are not likely to have had nearly as much impact on prevalence as delay of debut and partner reduction.

For recent measures of inconsistent and more regular condom use in Rakai, a largely rural area, we can look at the results of a project of promoting condoms and providing them free of charge to discordant couples. In spite of the known risk and the efforts of this project, 6.3 percent reported occasional condom use, and only 1.2 percent reported consistent use (Gray et al., 2001). The authors observe, "This finding is consistent with previous Rakai studies that showed low condom use within marriage. In contrast, European, U.S., and Thai investigations found frequent condom use among HIV-1 discordant couples" (p. 1149).

Another random sample survey (N = 1,627) in Rakai found that "only 10% reported consistent condom use with every non-spousal partner. Condom use with spouses is negligible" (Morris, Wawer, Makumbi, Zavisca, & Sewankambo, 2000, p. 736).

Focus group findings about condoms are also available from Rakai. For example, a study by Konde-Lule (1993) sheds light on other be-havior changes as well as condom KABP in the early 1990s as seen in the following:

In rural areas a marked sexual behavior change was reported. In all rural groups there was a strong consensus that promiscuity had sharply declined or even disappeared from the rural communities. . . . Most of the focus group partici-pants had heard about condoms and many had seen them but hardly anyone trusted or used them. There is a widespread fear that they are not effective barriers. "They may contain small holes through which the disease may pass," was a statement made by several groups. . . . Among groups other than those of barmaids, there was an added fear that condoms may increase promiscuity. Relevant statements were "Condoms will ruin society," and "Condoms will make the youth less careful and AIDS will spread even more than now." These arguments were particularly common among the rural groups. . . . Many groups saw no need for using condoms and recurring statements in many rural groups went as follows: "if you are happily married then what is the condom for?"; "they are not effective anyway and they can tear during intercourse"; "condoms are only used by a few young people." (Konde-Lule, Musagara, & Musgrave, 1993, p. 681)

In spite of low condom use in the majority population, user rates are fairly high among those who need them most. Condom use has been found to most likely occur among younger, unmarried men and women, and with a noncohabiting or nonregular partner (DHS, 2001; Ministry of Health/Uganda, 2000, 2001). Condom use has also risen significantly among female sex workers. A survey in Kampala sug-gests that 98.9 percent of female sex workers used a condom during last intercourse (Ministry of Health, 2001), up from rates of around 42 to 70 percent three years earlier (Kasirye et al., 1998, p. 1133). A USAID–supported program of IEC through peer education in the Uganda People's Defense Forces was formally started in 1994, although the interventions began earlier. By 1996, Ugandan soldiers had distrib-uted over 4 million condoms supplied by USAID. HIV prevalence among soldiers had declined from more than 45 percent in the early 1990s to 26 percent in 1996 (USAID/Uganda, 2000).

DELAYED AGE AT FIRST SEX

In Uganda there seems to have been significant changes in the delay of age at first sex during the early period under consideration. Asiimwe-Okiror and colleagues (1997) reported a two-year delay in the onset of sexual intercourse among youths ages fifteen to twenty-four. From analysis of DHS data, Bessinger and colleagues (2002) found between 1989 and 2000, median age at first sex increased by 1.2 years for girls and 1.7 years for boys.

Comparisons of average age of debut are not the best measure of change of this sort. Males (never married, ages 15–24) reporting premarital sex decreased from 60 percent in 1989 to 23 percent in 1995, according to the WHO/GPA surveys from those years. The 1995 DHS found that 33 percent reported premartial sex in 1995, still a significant decline from 1989. For females, the decline was from 53 percent to 16 percent between 1989 and 1995 (Bessinger & Akwara, 2003). Since we know HIV incidence peaked in the late 1980s (Low-Beer, 2002), it is highly likely that there was PBC before 1989, so that the magnitude of behavioral change between 1986, when the national response started, and 1995 would have been even greater than the figures just cited suggest.

The section on *AIDS Education in the Schools*, which will be presented later, has more data on increases in abstinence and delay.

MODELING STUDIES

If sizable numbers of men and women reduce their number of sexual partners, can this have significant impact on HIV infection rates? Studies that have modeled the impact of different interventions on HIV infection rates in East Africa suggest that reduction in number of partners can indeed have great impact on averting HIV infections, in fact greater than either condom use or treatment of STDs (Auvert, Buonamico, Lagarde, & Williams, 2000; Auvert & Ferry, 2002; Bernstein et al., 1998; Robinson, Mulder, Auvert, & Hayes, 1995).

Robinson, Mulder, Auvert, and Hayes (1995) developed a simulation model for the transmission dynamics of HIV infection, drawing on data from a rural population cohort in Southwest Uganda (Rakai). They found the following:

39% of all adult HIV infections were averted, in the 10 years from 1990, when condoms were used consistently and effectively by 50% of men in their contacts with one-off sexual partners (such as bar girls and commercial sex workers). Reducing by 50% the frequency of men's sexual contacts with one-off partners averted 68% of infections. Reducing by 50% the duration of all STD episodes averted 43% of infections. (p. 1263)

In other words, partner reduction has a powerful effect on averting infections, more than consistent condom use, as seen in Table 6.3 based on the preceding data.

The authors concluded that "a substantial proportion of HIV infections may be averted in majority populations through interventions targeted only on less regular sexual partnerships" (p. 1263). Of course, impact of partner reduction on HIV infection rates would be especially strong where there is relatively high HIV seroprevalence among potential partners, such as in Uganda.

Kretzschmar and Morris (1996; also Morris & Kretzschmar, 1997) have also done modeling exercises which suggest that the number of concurrent sexual partners increases both the intensity and the variability of the intensity of an HIV epidemic and that the final size of the epidemic increases exponentially as this number increases. These results are independent of changes in HIV transmissibility over time, due to changes in viral load (Carael et al., 2001). The UNAIDS Multicentre study seemed to challenge this hypothesis, however, as noted previously, when researchers later reanalyzed the data from this study and concluded that lifetime number of sexual partners was a crucial determining factor in explaining differences in HIV prevalence rates between African cities (Auvert & Ferry, 2002).

The effect of abstinence or delay, which might be as great as partner reduction—or greater among youth—was not measured by Robinson, Mulder, Auvert, and Hayes (1995), nor am I aware of other modeling studies that have modeled abstinence. But the reported delay in onset of sexual activity in youth in particular (and especially female youth) ought to be contributing to HIV declines at the national level, and even more immediately and substantially to HIV declines among Ugandan youth. Laga, Schwartlander, Pisani, Sow, and Carael (2001), citing Asiimwe-Okiror and colleagues (1997), comment, "Although scientific evidence that would help quantify this effect is lacking, a delay of a few years in first sexual activity has been associated with a reduction of HIV prevalence among young people in Uganda."

Stoneburner and Low-Beer (2002b) also conclude that partner reduction was the single most important factor, or behavioral change, that accounts for HIV reduction in Uganda. They observe the following:

This suggests that the extent and connectedness of sexual networks may impart a mathematical relationship to epidemic dynamics that may not be adequately expressed in classic epidemic theory and its application to modeling HIV and effects of interventions. Although interventions that reduce HIV risk at the individual exposure level should not be considered ineffective, our comparative analysis emphasizes the greater importance of partnership reduction. (p. 10)

"Interventions that reduce HIV risk at the individual exposure level" refers to condom programs.

SHOULD WE BELIEVE THE DATA?

It is true that partner reduction and abstinence/delay could be exaggerated by survey respondents, as can happen with any type of survey question. Certainly the same can be said of self-reported condom use. And, as Busulwa (1995) has cautioned, local Ugandan definitions of abstinence might differ, and might sometimes include potentially dangerous practices, such as coitus interruptus. These definitional problems can occur anywhere; a reliability study in Switzerland found that 12.5 percent of the men and 1.9 percent of women included nonpenetrative sex in their definitions of sexual intercourse (Jeannin, Konings, Dubois-Arber, Landert, & Van Melle, 1998).

There are also methodological issues surrounding measures of faithfulness, as Barton (1997) points out in the following:

Terminology has been somewhat flexible in the various AIDS prevention campaigns, leading to lack of clarity in various related concepts such as "sticking with one partner", "faithfulness", and "zero-grazing". For example, in one multi-district study (results presented only by district and not totaled), the researchers found different proportions of persons reporting sticking with one

Table 6.3
Estimated Proportion of Infections Averted

Intervention	HIV Reduction Rate
Condom use	39%
STD reduction	43%
Partner reduction*	68%

Source: Robinson, Mulder, Auvert, and Hayes (1995).

*Reduction in frequency of contact with nonregular partner.

partner (range 26–68%), faithfulness (range 13–45%), and zero-grazing (range 1–21%) [Musinguzi et al., 1996]. There was a general failure to clarify faithful polygamy, or faithfulness to multiple regular partners where persons had more than one partner. These variations in interpretation lead to difficulties in comparing studies that have not specified which of these terms or not used a mixture of all of them in seeking information about faithfulness. (p. 29)

Many of these definitional problems disappear if the measure is simply the number of partners within a specified time, namely, the last twelve months. We can say with minimal ambiguity from the 1995 DHS that about 95 percent of Ugandans ages fifteen to forty-nine reported one or zero partners in the past six months. And behavioral research findings in Uganda are in the rather unusual position of being corroborated or triangulated by biological data, both by HIV and STD prevalence as well as by limited incidence data. And there have been numerous surveys conducted by diverse public and private groups, funded by several countries that point to the same trends.

THE DEVELOPMENT OF THE UGANDA APPROACH

In late 1998, I was asked by the World Bank to evaluate the impact of preventive interventions, especially IEC, on behavioral change and, if possible, on declining HIV infection rates. For this effort, I reviewed all available statistics and qualitative studies, reviewed district work plans between 1995 and 1998, conducted in-depth interviews with relevant informants, and facilitated group discussions. I also made site visits to observe how various prevention (and a few care and support) programs were implemented. Through this assignment, and two earlier ones in Uganda, I began to piece together the following information about Uganda's distinctive response to AIDS. It has been aided by subsequent research including follow-up visits to Uganda in 2001, 2002, and 2003.

High Level of Government Commitment

A necessary, but not by itself sufficient, cause of behavior change and HIV decline in Uganda seems to be a high level of government commitment. Every informant I spoke with from every organization, Ugandan and expatriate, gave credit to the Ugandan government—especially President Museveni—for its high level commitment to discussing AIDS openly and dealing with it strongly. There was consensus that none of Uganda's success with AIDS could have been possible without this level and degree of government support. One effect of this was to reduce stigma, make open discussion of AIDS, and set the stage for sexual behavior change.

Other results can be seen to have followed from this high level of openness and support. For one, an open and accepting attitude began to develop that made AIDS education easier to implement, that helped attract Ugandans to VCT programs, that also reduced fear and stigma associated with AIDS, and that helped people go public about their HIV status. This helped involve PLWHAs in AIDS prevention, which seems to have played an important role in both raising awareness and changing behavior (see *The Role of Fear* in IEC later). For another, Uganda attracted donor funds for AIDS prevention earlier than most other African countries. More money and programs soon followed earlier programs, especially given the supportive role of the Ugandan government and positive results that began to be evident after 1993.

By 1988, two other African national leaders had joined Museveni in speaking openly and frankly about AIDS and becoming involved personally in national AIDS efforts: Abdou Diouf of Senegal and Kenneth Kaunda of Zambia. Diouf's role is discussed in Chapter 7. Kaunda became involved after his son died of AIDS. Like Museveni, he did much to simply raise awareness about the threat of AIDS at a time when the rest of Africa's leaders—soon to include Nelson Mandela—were largely in a state of denial.

How important is it to have a national leader raise awareness about AIDS and put the topic on the national agenda? In fact, Uganda, Senegal, and Zambia may all be regarded as AIDS success stories, as sections to follow document. Leadership at the level of prime minister in AIDS also helped Thailand become the first AIDS success story in Asia, as the section on Thailand shows. As we will see in the section on Jamaica, that country had strong leadership in the ministry of health, but not at the level of prime minister, and it was able to have a relatively successful national AIDS prevention program.

Leadership at the highest level seems to allow prevention programs to have maximum impact. It is probable that one of the factors inhibiting such a government response elsewhere in Africa and beyond is fear of negative reaction from religious authorities. This only strengthens the argument for involving religious leaders and FBOs as early as possible. In each of the first five countries that stabilized or reduced national HIV seroprevalence—Uganda, Senegal, Thailand, Jamaica, and Dominican Republic—the government made efforts to involve major religious groups early in the local epidemic.

It was not just a high level of openness and commitment on the part of Uganda's president that was crucial to Uganda's success. President

Museveni and his advisors developed a model that was suited to the economic and sociocultural realities of Uganda. And it differed quite considerably from the model being urged by well-meaning foreign experts, not only concerning the role of condoms. Part of the Ugandan model involved fighting stigma and empowering women and youth.

Reducing Stigma

AIDS-associated stigma prevents open discussion and therefore awareness of the problem, let alone its solution. It undermines community action and blocks access to services. As I write this, there is still a great deal of stigma and shame in two of the African countries I know best, Swaziland and South Africa. Effective AIDS prevention is still hampered by these. A nurse in South Africa (Ndwedwe) told me that it is difficult implementing home-based care because people seem more worried about their neighbors suspecting who might be infected than they are about receiving treatment.

In Uganda, popular singer Philly Lutaya became the first well-known Ugandan living with HIV/AIDS. He traveled all over Uganda educating people about AIDS, and he was soon followed by other PLWHAs.

It is difficult to quantify degree of stigma by means of survey research, or perhaps even to prove its existence in a population. Qualitative research seems a more appropriate set of tools. Focus group research was conducted in the early 1990s in rural and urban Rakai district, where infection rates soared early and reached high levels, and where there was a great deal of preventive education and open discussion about AIDS. The study found, "In all the focus group discussions there was a striking positive attitude towards people with AIDS. There is no noticeable stigma or fear of contact with persons with AIDS. Virtually everyone in all the groups expressed the feeling of sympathy for the people with AIDS" (Konde-Lule, Musagara, & Musgrave, 1993, p. 681).

It appears that government support and proactivism in AIDS prevention helped reduce shame and stigma, initially by speaking out openly about AIDS and sexual behavior. The IEC message was that everyone could become infected, not just certain groups, therefore we are all in this together. A widely-used metaphor was that of a hungry lion that has entered a village; people must act together to protect the village and the nation. This openness and call to action helped encourage the participation of PLWHAs in prevention, and this participation in turn helped greatly in spreading awareness and assisting in prevention. Even so, it took great courage for the first PLWHAs to reveal their sero-status in the early years of the epidemic.

Stigma is to some extent a relative concept. Ugandan PLWHAs may still feel there is considerable stigma and discrimination in their country. Several groups of PLWHA groups (NGEN+: National Guidance and Empowerment Network of People Living with HIV/AIDS; NACWOLA: National Community of Women Living with HIV/AIDS) posted complaints on the internet in 2001 under the title, "Discrimination Of People Living With HIV/AIDS in Uganda." I can only comment that stigma seems worse in other African countries.

Advancement of Women and Youth

President Museveni took concrete steps to advance the status of women and youth. I am not using the term empowerment because President Museveni saw this as a Western term that grew out of the feminist movement. He thought the term implied a zero-sum game and he thought it might therefore threaten Ugandan men, or at least wound their pride. So he used "advancement" instead. The crucial fact is that he did something positive for women and youth that among other things, seems to have provided an enabling environment for PBC and declining HIV infection rates.

Today there are representatives from both women and youth groups in parliament, one from from each district. There are also more women in higher educational institutions, due in part to affirmative action measures such as adding points to female admission test scores. There have additionally been legal reforms pertaining to rape and seduction of minors (Nantulya, 2002). A recent editorial summarizes aspects of women's advancement as follows:

Critical elements of Uganda's national AIDS strategy are political and economic empowerment of women and girls through universal education, women's political leadership, and economic opportunity. Moreover, appointment of women to key Cabinet posts, including vice president, and a law that says women must comprise one-third of the Parliament have reinforced national gender equity policy, which includes efforts to increase boys' respect for girls' rights.

President Yoweri Museveni mobilized religious leaders, youth, women, journalists, artists, and—perhaps most important—Ugandans living with HIV/AIDS to repeat explicit, well-targeted messages about the need to change sexual behavior. (Diarrah & Rielly, 2002, p. A19)

These authors (the first one being Mali's current ambassador to the United States) recommend, in a memorable turn of phrase, a "democratic triple therapy" consisting of public participation, poverty reduction, and women's rights, in order to "turn the corner on HIV/ AIDS." It appears that Uganda has gone a considerable distance in achieving the first and last of these three remedies.

There is also a defilement law against seduction and rape of minors. Apparently this law had been around for years with little enforcement, but then began to be enforced in the mid-1990s. Rape of a minor can be punishable by death or life in prison. A teacher who impregnates a high school girl can get seven years in prison. At this writing, a domestic law that would give wives the right to refuse sex with their husbands under certain circumstances is being considered and debated in parliament.

But how much improvement in the position of women has there actually been in Uganda? In reproductive health circles, certain indicators have been used to measure this. Indicators include increase in educational attainment, increase in the proportion of women in the labor force, increase in age of marriage, and increase in use of modern contraceptives. Regarding employment, DHS data reveal an interesting finding: There has been a great rise in employment of women in Uganda, something that went unnoticed until a colleague of mine reported on this. She found that the rise in rate of women's employment may be unprecedented in Africa (Murphy, 2003). She produced Table 6.4, showing the degree to which (self-described) employment has risen, and comparing it with Zimbabwe, a country with very high HIV prevalence and that began with higher female empowerment indicators— including high contraceptive user rates—than almost any other African country.

In rural Africa, it is hard to think of a single indicator of independence more important than employment. Remember that this is self-defined, so that whatever the weakness of the measure, it would be more or less the same across national boundaries. Most Ugandan women are rural and have little formal education. This rapid rise of women's employment may well be spurred by AIDS deaths among traditional male breadwinners, but then, of course, women's employment ought to rise in other countries with high mortality from AIDS, especially countries with even higher mortality like Zimbabwe. On the other hand, Uganda's epidemic is older than those of southern Africa.

In any case, there is other evidence of women's empowerment in Uganda. The Uganda DHS 2000 asked women and men whether women have the ability to negotiate safer sex. The numerator was defined, "The number of respondents who believe that, if her husband has an STI, the woman could refuse to have sex with him or propose condom use." The denominator is total number of respondents. Looking at the data available for Africa, Uganda has the highest percentage

Table 6.4
Percentage of Women Working

	Time Period		
	Early	**Middle**	**Late**
Uganda	9	61	73
Zimbabwe	34	51	49

Source: DHS data from three time periods (Murphy, 2003).

of women able to negotiate safer sex, by this definition: 91 percent. This compares with 73 percent in Malawi, 87 percent in Rwanda, 55 percent in Tanzania, and 71 percent in Zimbabwe (from DHS/Measure data on Web site).

Government efforts to raise the status of women and youth might have had the effect of making both feel that they themselves could do something to protect themselves against AIDS. This may have assisted positive behavior change among women and youth, the groups in which change has been most pronounced. In a recent keynote address written by President Museveni, and delivered by Crispus Kiyonga, chairman of the Working Group to establish the Global AIDS and Health Fund (October 13, 2001, New York Hilton Hotel), Museveni wrote the following:

Permit me to tell you the obvious. In the fight against HIV/AIDS, women must be brought on board. In sub-Saharan Africa most women have not yet been empowered and men dominate sexual relations. To fight this epidemic, the women must be empowered to take decisions about their sexual lives and women in Uganda have been empowered and participate, today at all levels of governance. This has made them more assertive of their rights than ever before. To fight AIDS effectively, we must empower women. (Kiyonga, 2001)

Changes in A and B behaviors can involve the exercise of some degree of power. We often hear that women throughout Africa and other resource-poor parts of the world are too subordinate to negotiate condom use. The low status of African women is often cited as a barrier to condom use and to AIDS prevention efforts in general. A typical recent study in South Africa found that women believe their partners have a right to multiple partners and to not use condoms; yet women have no right to refuse sex with their partners or to insist on condom use. The authors conclude that women cannot reduce their risk of HIV because of their "lack of a right to safer sex, lack of skills to adopt safer sex practices, financial dependence on their sex partners, and the threat of violence" (Karim, 2001, p. 193).

Sophia Mukasa Monico, a Ugandan AIDS expert, credits the ABC approach with changing Ugandans, especially women: "Women had to take responsibility for their own lives. Wives told their husbands to be faithful, use a condom, even in marriage, or there would be no sex. Many women in Uganda had celibate marriages or moved out on their own" (Carter, 2003, p. A13). The high level of self-defined women's employment now found in Uganda support this statement.

Thus, something seems to have occurred in Uganda to alter the status of women, including their power to negotiate sex, unless it can be demonstrated that the status of women in Uganda already differed substantially from the rest of Africa in the 1980s. By the mid-1990s, Ugandan women were not only negotiating sex, they seem to have also been negotiating non-sex, not having intercourse. This is an area of research crying out for more attention, since Uganda's experience suggests there may be something governments can do to empower women, and this in turn might somehow assist a process of sexual behavior change and HIV prevalence decline.

The Early Role of USAID in Uganda

One of several reasons Uganda developed a distinctive and different response to AIDS prevention is that President Museveni and his advisors developed a program before outside experts showed up in significant numbers. As veteran researcher Dr. Norman Hearst said in a recent press interview, "I've had people tell me that the only reason they were successful in Uganda is that there were no European or American experts there" (Carter, 2003, p. A13).We will encounter evidence in other chapters and sections of this book that successful programs were developed in a handful of other countries, often in spite of, rather than because of, foreign expert advice.

Another factor in Uganda's success may be that the U.S. organization that implemented the first major U.S.–funded AIDS program there had relatively little experience in AIDS and was therefore not committed to the condom solution. Nor was the implementing organization one that makes its living by promoting contraceptives. World Learning Inc., a U.S.–based private voluntary organization formerly known as the Experiment in International Living, implemented the AIDS Prevention and Control Project (APCP) in Uganda between 1989 and 1995.

World Learning Inc. was not one of the major contractors or grant-ees in AIDS prevention, thus its APCP team did not arrive in Uganda as experts who thought they already knew exactly what was needed. The chief of party of the APCP happened to be a Protestant minister (although I never knew this when I consulted for this project in 1993), and it is possible that this made him more open-minded to the type of PBC program President Museveni favored. In any case, the ACPC team had the wisdom and cultural sensitivity to engage in listening and learning during the early months and years of its project implementa-tion. They were thus able to learn from Ugandans who were already carrying out AIDS prevention lessons with surprising effectiveness, as we now know.

Relatively early in the project, the ACPC commissioned an evalua-tion to assess the impact of prevention efforts to date. The evaluation found clear evidence that PBC was already well underway by 1991 (Moodie et al., 1991). Perhaps because World Learning was not an or-ganization with great expertise in HIV/AIDS, the evidence of PBC that emerged in the evaluation was not filtered out by risk reduction biases or preconceived notions about how behavior was supposed to change. This evaluation study provided World Learning with empiri-cal justification to continue with programs that promoted PBC through such novel groups (for the donors) as Christian and Muslim organiza-tions and primary schools.

The AIDS technical expert at USAID during this time, Dr. Elizabeth Marum, was also open-minded and allowed the first USAID–funded bilateral AIDS project to be implemented as it was, without undue insistence on business-as-usual interventions. Indeed, these latter were also funded, and as noted elsewhere, Uganda in some ways had the same kind of prevention programs as other countries. After all, donor-funded interventions are usually designed by outsiders and funds are earmarked to the programs and projects they favor. But enough of what some call the Museveni approach was supported by USAID in the early days, and by the World Bank even later, that Uganda ended up with more PBC than other countries.

Uganda's IEC Strategy

Uganda's IEC strategy has been to use multiple channels (electronic, print, interpersonal), recognizing that each has both advantages and disadvantages, and believing that synergy and maximum exposure can be achieved if all channels are used, especially in complementary and mutually reinforcing ways. Research has in fact demonstrated that synergy can be achieved when multiple channels are used (e.g.,

Kanyesigye et al., 1998). USAID and other donors have financed social marketing and other mass media IEC efforts (e.g., through the DISH project, the SOMARC project, and more recently, Commercial Marketing Strategies). In 1999, local NGO Straight Talk began broadcasting AIDS education and life skills content aimed at youth ages fifteen to twenty-four through seven FM stations. Several local languages were used and the target audience was youth.

Indeed most countries follow some version of a multiple channel IEC strategy. Uganda stands out among most countries in (1) where it has put its behavior change emphasis; (2) its emphasis on interpersonal (or face-to-face), community-based, culturally-tailored IEC. A great amount of training and sensitization of various community leaders occurred. This seems to have resulted in the awareness and subsequent involvement in AIDS education of not only health personnel and traditional healers as well as traditional birth attendants, but influential people normally not involved in health issues, such as political and religious leaders, teachers, traders, leaders of women's and youth associations, and the like. Methods of training and sensitization often use drama, song, dance, music, poetry, and other indigenous cultural forms of expression.

An evaluation of responses to IEC in local communities in Masaka and Ssembabule districts (the population was 62% literate) found that interviewees felt that AIDS dramas were more interesting and applicable to their daily lives than videos or pamphlets (Kamali, Nakamanya, Mitchell, & Whitworth, 2001). I suspect that this traditional or culturally tailored interpersonal approach has had significant impact. Research-based evaluations (and improved monitoring) will probably be able to prove (or disprove) this hypothesis.

There is already some evidence of the impact of interpersonal IEC. DHS evidence has shown that the main sources of information about HIV/AIDS among Ugandans have been family members and friends, as distinct from radio or print media. In fact, Uganda seems atypical in this regard; in countries like Kenya and Zambia, sources of AIDS knowledge tend not to primarily be interpersonal (Low-Beer, Stoneburner, Barnett, & Whiteside, 2000). Zambia and Kenya have not had Uganda's success in declining infection rates or behavior change. As Low-Beer and colleagues (2000) note, "Integration of mass AIDS knowledge into personal/friendship networks is important in the adoption of new behaviours, and for AIDS integration of mass AIDS knowledge into personal/friendship, networks (are) important in the adoption of new behaviours and for AIDS" (p. 5).

In a later paper, Low-Beer and Stoneburner (2002) describe their comparative findings more precisely as follows and in Figure 6.3:

Personal channels were dominant in Uganda in 1995 among women (82%), men (70%), in urban and rural areas. Personal knowledge of someone with AIDS was also higher in Uganda (91.5% of men and 86.4% of women). These communication elements were related to behaviour changes in Uganda, with risk ratios for reducing partners (1.65), condom use with last intercourse (2.19), and starting condom use (4.6) Conclusions: The results suggest there are unique communication elements which affected behaviour changes and enhanced HIV prevention in Uganda. (Low-Beer, 2002, from abstract)

In fact, diffusion of innovation theorists Rogers and Shoemaker (1971) hypothesize that mass media channels are more important in spreading knowledge, while interpersonal channels are more important "at the persuasion function," or actually motivating new or modified behaviors (p. 255). And among "peasants" in less-developed countries, mass media are found to be far more effective when coupled with interpersonal communication in "media forums" (p. 263). This refers to groups in which new ideas (innovations) are openly discussed.

The decentralization of the Ministry of Health (and all ministries) required by the World Bank under its loan to Uganda for AIDS prevention may have led to even more reliance on interpersonal education. For example, Moyo district reported in its 1998 work plan: "One important aspect of this plan is to move to interpersonal communication as a drive to behavior change, departing a little from the mass communication strategies that were being employed previously" (Green, 1998, p. 21). This may be due to the relative costs between training local leaders compared to developing and running radio spots. There is also less technical expertise at the district level for the latter. Moreover, good quality, culturally appropriate print and film materials may not exist at the district and lower levels. It may also be because interpersonal IEC has simply been found by district and lower AIDS committees to be effective at the local level. Some Ugandan NGOs feel strongly that this is the case, as I found out during interviews in December 2001.

In fact, one or more important hypotheses arise from the foregoing that almost beg for testing in Africa and other parts of the resource-poor world: (1) When health ministries decentralize, there is a tendency to invest or engage less in more technologically sophisticated IEC (i.e., mass electronic media) and more toward community-based, lower-tech interpersonal IEC; (2) Such interpersonal IEC may be more sustainable, more tailored to sociocultural realities, and (therefore) more effective than mass media intended for a country as a whole.

My review of district workplans and district-level activities between 1995 and 1998 confirmed that a great deal of training and face-to-face

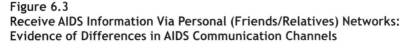

Figure 6.3
Receive AIDS Information Via Personal (Friends/Relatives) Networks:
Evidence of Differences in AIDS Communication Channels

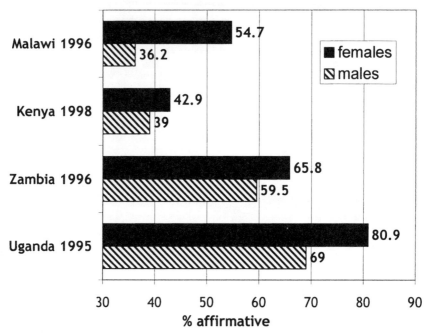

Source: Stoneburner and Low-Beer, 2002.

Note: Ugandans are more likely to receive AIDS information through personal friendship networks. Women cite this source more than men.

AIDS education occurred at the district and lower levels during those
years. There are variations in the number and type of local people
trained and sensitized, but they seem to always include school personnel, youth and women's leaders, religious leaders, and local council members (the national Draft IEC Strategy, which was finalized
during my 1998 consultancy, advised "Sensitization of local councils
and religious leaders" at all subcountry levels). District workplans often include traditional healers and midwives, local political figures,
and other local opinion leaders. They also often include groups at special risk, such as military and police, disco and bar or restaurant owners, forest workers, plantation workers, fishermen, and refugees.

What level of intervention are we talking about? If there are roughly
150 religious leaders trained per district (a roughly average number
found in district workplans), then with forty-five districts (as there

were in 1998), there would be 6,750 per year. Or assuming only 100 religious leaders per year, then only 4,500 would be trained. But even then, in two years, there would be 9,000 trained. There are equal or even greater numbers of women and youth opinion leaders trained annually through the district health education units of the Ministry of Health. These are substantial numbers of trained or sensitized community educators.

Stoneburner (2000) worked with model simulations and suggested that knowledge can diffuse rapidly early in an AIDS epidemic, and that the openness of personal networks is more important than the stage or level of the epidemic in determining levels of infection. They provide the following three scenarios of diffusions:

1. Knowledge networks are highly multiplicative and can lead to a high percentage of the population knowing someone with AIDS at an early stage of the epidemic. Knowledge diffusion is very sensitive to conditions of openness.
2. AIDS status is hidden from friends.
3. Segregation of people with AIDS socially, and uprooting of knowledge networks through migration.

The first scenario is found in Uganda, where there was a relatively open political and social atmosphere for discussing AIDS from an early stage of its epidemic. I would suggest at least two ingredients that led to diffusion of AIDS knowledge and highly multiplicative interpersonal networks. One is the widespread sensitization of local leaders of all sorts. Another is the bold enlistment of PLWHAs in AIDS preventive education quite early in the epidemic, including the education which occurred in the schools. This PLWHA involvement helped reduce stigma and furthered the openness in scenario one.

Print Materials

In 1998 at least, print IEC appeared to be relatively weak compared to interpersonal IEC. This was particularly true at the district level where not much print material appeared to be available. District health education units appeared not to fully understand that, with decentralization, they were now expected to design and produce much of their own IEC materials—in fact, electronic as well as print IEC.

In view of the apparent success of IEC in Uganda, it is interesting that printed materials related to AIDS seem only average in quality and quantity. From the IEC materials I saw, there seemed to be a disproportionate number promoting condoms, no doubt reflecting the interests and beliefs of foreign organizations and consultants. Some relied too much on language, in a country with high illiteracy rates, and some of the language was too technical for all but a handful of more educated Ugandans to understand.

Some of the earlier materials employed what today might be called negative imagery or fear arousal. Let us look at this more closely.

The Role of Fear Arousal

In the early years of AIDS prevention in Uganda and several other countries of Africa, governments used images and messages intended to frighten people about the serious nature of the new STD for which there was no cure. In Uganda, there were somber radio messages accompanied by the slow beating of a drum and a stern, raspy voice of an old man talking about AIDS in the manner of announcing funerals. Posters used imagery of human skulls, coffins, and Grim Reapers harvesting humans. A recent paper by an educator in the Uganda Ministry of Health depicts the IEC approach during Uganda's early stage of national response (making allowances in the use of English): "General awareness was comprised of alert messages, ghostly pictures, drums that culturally symbolize danger. The immediate output was instillation of fear and negative reaction as the messages were related to death" (Byangire, 2002). Sam Okware, the first director of the National AIDS Control Programme, recounted, "At first, we focused on instilling fear in the population" after which options for avoidance of risk were promoted, starting with "avoidance of sexual contacts" (Okware et al., 2001, p. 1114.) In a recent interview, Okware told me, "The first approach was that we drove fear into people." He further explained that the ABC message was often phrased "ABC or D." In other words practice A, B, or C, or choose D for death (Okware, 2003).

Considerable involvement by PLWHAs in face-to-face AIDS education, such as in primary schools and villages, led to people taking AIDS more seriously, and even to being more fearful of becoming infected. As some Ugandan AIDS educators told me, when people saw PLWHAs looking sick and emaciated, it scared people into behavior change. But when healthy, normal looking PLWHAs visited schools and communities, there was another kind of powerful impact. It put a human face on the disease; it showed that people can live positively even if they test positive, and so it reduced stigma and marginalization of PLWHAs and it motivated people to be tested.

Members of the European gay community and those sympathetic to them seem to have been the first to reject the fear-based approach to

AIDS prevention. An American observer condemned this in the following article in *Mother Jones*:

In most parts of the world, AIDS propaganda is controlled by the state and the educational model is highly authoritarian. Official AIDS information campaigns tend to address the citizenry as misbehaving children and employ either fear or moral exhortation—what the British writer and gay activist Simon Watney refers to as the "terrorist" or "missionary" strategies. (Talbot, 1990, p. 41)

This author praises the approach some Scandinavian health ministries had begun to develop to educate gay men about AIDS, stressing "hope, eroticism, and humor." This was the opposite of a missionary approach; indeed ads conveyed the message that men could "stay hard" and keep it up!" (Talbot, 1990, p. 41). This laissez-fair, erotic, and at times humorous approach to AIDS prevention seems to have become the norm in American as well as European gay communities. In the *Mother Jones* article, Talbot heaps scorn upon chastity crusaders and asserts that the conservative morality campaigns of the U.S. government aimed at the general ("straight") population "had virtually no impact on the nation's high rates of adolescent sexual activity" (Talbot, 1990, p. 42). In fact, he criticized the U.S. government for not promoting condoms enough to the American population. As an example of a "terrorist, missionary" message from Africa, he cites "One man, one woman" for life, used by the Zambian health ministry, and he claims this to be "a typical skull-and-crossbones poster" (Talbot, 1990, p. 44).

Talbot quotes the head of the first USAID global AIDS communication project, AIDSCOM, who likewise rejected fear-based approaches: "These campaigns may temporarily discourage sexual activity, but then there is a boomerang effect as people react against the scare tactics." Another AIDSCOM program officer likewise believed that Africans and West Indians, like gay Americans, respond better to a "more lighthearted, upbeat approach" (Talbot, 1990, p. 44).

I am quoting at some length to provide some history and information about the clash of values between governments like those of Uganda or Zambia, which were and are authoritarian, conservative, and influenced by religious groups; and gay Westerners, who were and tend now to be laissez-faire, sexually hedonistic, and antimoralizing about sexuality. One of the men just quoted later died of AIDS himself, raising question about the effectiveness of the erotic, lighthearted approach to AIDS prevention. Meanwhile, HIV prevalence fell in Uganda and among Zambian youth. Yet fear-associated approaches initially favored and indeed developed by African governments were eventually replaced by the softer, gentler approach favored by Western AIDS experts. Donor assistance, especially American, comes with Western technical experts such as those who design IEC programs and behavior change campaigns. It is hard to mount serious challenge to foreign experts who come with millions of dollars and advanced degrees. Few if any resource-poor African governments asked the simple question, How can you foreigners know more about influencing African behavior than we Africans? They needed the assistance and so they accepted the experts and the advice.

This happened everywhere. Talbot (1990) approvingly quotes a Brazilian AIDS educator who learned to educate in the preferred manner: "We don't terrorize the kids and we don't get preoccupied with moral habits" (p. 44). Yet, how well has softer, gentler AIDS education worked in the United States? Infection rates among gay men and IDUs is on the rise at this writing. A gay actor recently admitted in a *New York Times* op-ed that something is not working with the messages to which the gay community is exposed; in fact, they might even be contributing to higher infection rates:

In our effort to remove the stigma of having AIDS, have we created a culture of disease? We all see the advertisements for HIV drugs. They illustrate hot muscular men living life to the fullest thanks to modern science. Other advertisements show couples holding hands, sending the message that the road to true love and happiness is being HIV positive. Is that message You're going to be okay? (which is terrific), or is it You want to be special? Get AIDS. HIV equals popularity and acceptance (which would be tragic) (Fierstein, 2003).

A member of the Uganda AIDS Committee told me in 2001 that messages that employed fear may not be pleasant to receive, but he believed they helped change behavior when Uganda used this approach prior to the early 1990s. Indeed, there was enough behavior change in the latter 1980s that the HIV epidemic was turned around. This Ugandan official commented that Western experts might have been misguided when they condemned the way Uganda educated its people about the dangers of AIDS. After all, it worked, and the same cannot be said for the Western approach, even in the West. He made these comments before we knew that levels of abstinence and fidelity were eroding in Uganda, and national HIV prevalence was about to rise slightly for the first time in a decade.

In Uganda, in surveys that ask why, in a general way, people changed their sexual behavior, the most common response, even most recently, is simply fear of AIDS, followed by the perception that so many people are dying from AIDS (Uganda Ministry of Health, 2000, 2001). Stoneburner and Low-Beer (2002b), who have carefully analyzed Uganda's AIDS prevention program, likewise conclude this program used "health education messages that presented a clear warning of the health risks and behavioral options for avoidance" (p. 11). Thus it seems that even though AIDS education messages may have become more positive and lighthearted, the earlier messages are still remembered, and still have some influence on behavior.

The DHS asks a question designed to measure perception of risk of AIDS (What are your chances of getting AIDS?). Senegal, in spite of having the lowest HIV prevalence in continental sub-Sarahan Africa, shows the highest percent of (female) respondents who report their chances of getting AIDS as great, 38.2 percent. This finding might prove to be a measure of an effective AIDS education effort, one that has instilled a perception of risk, even in a country where actual risk is perhaps the smallest in Africa.

President Museveni was interviewed about Uganda's success in AIDS prevention by the BBC in August 2002. According to the following BBC summary,

President Museveni said he has tried to boost public awareness of the disease since first coming to power in 1986. "I could not take chances with a disease which we had no knowledge of," he told the BBC World Service.

"It had no vaccine but it was easily prevented. That is why we went for the prevention and awareness solution."

The president used political rallies and public broadcasts to educate people on Aids. "When I had a chance, I would shout at them," he said. "[I used to say] 'you are going to die if you don't stop this. You are going to die'." (Posted on af-aids@healthdev.net August 12, 2002)

He does not specify what "stopping this" means, but it probably refers to casual sex. An early advisor to Museveni agrees: "Yes, it was to stop the business of casual sex with several partners which was at the time considered the in thing!" (V. Nantulya, personal communication, August 2002). And clearly he was not soft-peddling the message that AIDS kills, that if risky behavior does not change, there can be severe consequences. It is interesting that Museveni speaks in the past tense, perhaps suggesting recognition that his approach to prevention has fallen out of international favor.

What do we know empirically about the role of fear in behavioral change? Fear may be a powerful motivator of behavior change, although it is more accurate to describe the process as internalizing or personalizing risk. American campaigns against smoking and use of illicit recreational drugs have used disturbing images of bodily harm to provoke personalization of risk on the part of the target audience. It also appears that if fear is overused, the credibility of the message suffers and behavior change is less likely to follow. A classic example in America is the 1950s film *Reefer Madness* that exaggerated the dangers of marijuana smoking.

In 2000, a meta-analysis was published on fear appeals or fear arousal and behavioral responses, in the context of public health. The researchers found, "The meta-analysis suggests that strong fear appeals produce high levels of perceived severity and susceptibility, and are more persuasive than low or weak fear appeals. . . . It appears that strong fear appeals and high-efficacy messages produce the greatest behavior change, whereas strong fear appeals with low-efficacy messages produce the greatest levels of defensive responses" (Witte & Allen, 2000, p. 608). Kim Witte and others have suggested that how people respond to fear appeals depends on their assessment of the threat and their perceived efficacy in avoiding or reducing the personal threat. These terms are defined as the following:

Total perceived threat
= *Perceived severity* (Is this a serious health risk? If I get HIV will I die?)
    + *Perceived susceptibility* (Can this happen to me? Am I at-risk for contract-
        ing HIV? What are the chances that I will contract HIV?)

Total perceived efficacy
= *Response efficacy* (Is the recommended action really going to avert the danger?)
    + *Self-efficacy* (Am I capable of taking the recommended action? Am I able
        to use condoms to prevent HIV transmission?) Witte, 1992, quoted in
        Thesenvitz, 2000, pp. 6–7; cf. Witte, Girma, & Girgre, in press).[3]

Ugandans were made to fear AIDS, to feel personally at risk of infection. Yet they also knew what to do to avoid AIDS; they heard the message loud and clear, including from their president and from leaders and peers in their local communities. Thus there was a high level of self-efficacy, which, paired with fear arousal, created optimal conditions for behavioral change.

Perhaps paradoxically, the Talbot (1990) article I have quoted at length concludes with a comment with which I could not agree more: "This global plague will not be stopped by medical ingenuity alone. It will require a deeper sense of reason and compassion, a respect for human diversity, and a commitment to the free flow of information" (p. 47). I am sure I interpret this in a way quite different from Talbot, since I take this to mean we ought not to rely only on condoms or drugs. Nor should we develop the same programs for African primary school children as for gay American men. We must indeed respect diversity and realize that people, cultures, and indeed AIDS epidemics are different, therefore different approaches are needed to accomplish something as complex as changing—or delaying—sexual behavior.

AIDS EDUCATION IN THE SCHOOLS

In early 2002, an article circulated on the Internet saying the following:

"Uganda to Introduce Sex Education in Schools to Fight AIDS" (Xinhua News Service, January 17, 2002). On Thursday, local media reported that Uganda's Health Minister Jim Muhwezi said that President Yoweri Museveni had directed the head teachers of primary and secondary schools to address their students on HIV/AIDS issues every two weeks. During a visit by a delegation of Japanese legislators, Muhwezi said that this was one of the new measures the government employed to combat AIDS. "Abstinence is the answer for children," he said, adding that teachers will have to take responsibility for talking about sex.

The implication is that something new is being initiated in Ugandan schools, implying that there was no sex education in Ugandan schools earlier. This is untrue. As noted, IEC has always focused primarily on youth. HIV/AIDS sensitization and preventive education have been in the primary school curriculum and syllabus since 1987 through the School Health Education Program (SHEP) of the Ministry of Education. SHEP has required and involved significant cooperation between the Ministries of Education and Health, as well as between countless health educators and local schools. The main donor was the Swedish AID agency (SIDA). Danish AID (DANIDA) and UNICEF also contributed to SHEP. The first director of Uganda's National AIDS Control Programme commented in an interview that SHEP must have contributed to prevalence decline among youth in the early years. He said this program brought "AIDS education into the classroom and into the school syllabus. There were end-of-year exams on AIDS that students needed to pass" (Okware, 2003). Okware stated that SHEP got AIDS information into the minds of youth in schools.

The aim of this program was to reach youth with AIDS prevention information before they become sexually active. It was also known that dropout rates after primary school were high. AIDS was not the only component of SHEP, but it was an important one. The behavior change emphasis was on delay of debut, but condoms were also promoted. In fact, SHEP was very bold in this regard, for Africa in the 1980s, or for primary schools anywhere, anytime. I have seen a 1987 book used in this program; it shows an erect penis and shows how a condom should be worn.

I have corresponded with one of the UNICEF officials involved in the design and initial implementation of SHEP. He told me there was a sense of urgency about getting this program started. Instead of taking all the steps necessary to develop and fine-tune the SHEP curriculum, he and his colleagues just jumped in and learned by doing. That is, they got the program started using common sense and accumulated experience. The formal curriculum continued to be designed while the program was being implemented.

Master trainers were trained at the highest level, and they in turn trained district trainers, who then trained subdistrict level teachers. Students themselves were trained as peer educators; they were expected to teach their parents and peers about AIDS. This was all done in a relatively short time. The basic facts about AIDS and how to prevent it were taught. A version of Life Skills was also introduced (as will be discussed later).

SHEP has been implemented in primary schools, but similar NGO-run programs, such as Straight Talk, have also been implemented in secondary schools as well in private schools (Kaleeba, Namulondo, Kalinki, & Williams, 2000, p. 78). Most private schools are run by religious groups. A useful if not crucial side benefit of involving religious organizations early in the epidemic and in significant ways seems to have been that AIDS prevention, including the use of condoms, can usually be taught in schools run by religious groups.

Universal primary education and the integration of HIV/AIDS education into the science curriculum also appears to have contributed substantially to AIDS-related knowledge, if not behavior change, among youth. It may be, however, that public sector efforts aimed at AIDS education in schools has become weaker in recent years. The current recommitment may be due to recognition that A and B behaviors have started to erode, and HIV prevalence may no longer be declining as of 2002.

Life Skills education has been taught in schools for a number of years, beginning with SHEP. Life Skills refers to training youth in such skills as interpersonal relationships, self-awareness and self-esteem, problem solving, effective communication, decision making, negotiating sex or lack thereof, resisting peer pressure, critical thinking, formation of friendships, and empathy. These are referred to as cognitive skills and the idea is to empower youth through such training. The idea is also to help youth sustain life- and health-promotive decisions and behavior. It would seem that these programs motivate behavior change and help sustain it. Indeed, they were developed specifically to bridge the gap between high HIV knowledge and awareness levels and lagging behavior change. It was recognized that young people, particularly females, needed certain social and other skills to change behavior and sustain this over time. Related youth-oriented programs, such as Straight Talk, Young Talk, and the like, also seem to have had positive impact on promoting and sustaining youthful behavior change, using approaches very similar to Life Skills. These two programs were reaching well over a million young people by 2000, mostly through primary and secondary school programs (Kaleeba, Namulondo, Kalinki, & Williams, 2000, p. 78).

Straight Talk has recognized the need to address male as well as female adolescent sexual issues. Female issues have been more widely recognized and addressed to date, in Uganda and perhaps elsewhere in Africa. Yet young males face pressures to have sex early and often to prove manhood. Straight Talk developed IEC approaches designed to change adolescent male norms to make it more acceptable to not initiate sex until a later age.

The Sara Communication Initiative initially developed under UNICEF also promotes a Life Skills type of intervention. Straight Talk and some other youth programs target out-of-school as well as in-school youths. In the regular work of the Ministry of Health we can see a large number of trainings and sensitizations aimed at youth and women's leaders in the district work plans.

In sum, public and private sector programs in Uganda have targeted exactly the groups in which HIV prevalence has declined the most. Recall that HIV infection rates among Ugandans ages fifteen to nineteen fell more dramatically than the roughly 50 percent for all age groups—more on the order of a 75 percent decline between 1991 and 2000. Moreover, behavior has changed the most in the age group fifteen to nineteen: delay of debut, abstinence, fidelity, and condom use. A recent analysis by UNAIDS researchers reaches the following similar conclusion:

A delay of a few years in first sexual activity has been associated with a reduction of HIV prevalence among young people in Uganda. Efforts to reduce early exposure to sex include promoting abstinence throughout adolescence as a "cool" behaviour for young people, and teaching negotiation skills and alternatives to penetrative sex. (Laga, Schwartlander, Pisani, Sow, & Carael, 2001, p. 933)

The relationship between programs targeting youth and behavioral change is illustrated in the experience of a program of AMREF, an East

African NGO. AMREF recently evaluated the impact of a school-based project to strengthen AIDS IEC in schools in Soroti and Katakwi districts (AMREF/Uganda, 2001). Project objectives were as follows: (1) to strengthen and sustain school health education in 90 percent of primary schools in the Katakwi/Soroti district to incorporate effective change strategies; and (2) to demonstrate a 50 percent decrease in sexually risky behavior in upper-level primary students.

Multistage cluster random sampling was used to select schools in nine subcounties representing each of the counties in the project districts. A baseline KABP survey was conducted in 1994 and the same instrument was used in a postintervention survey conducted seven years later in 2001. Respondents were Primary 7 pupils (ages thirteen to sixteen) who themselves were randomly selected. Respondents' mean age was 13.9–14.0, and boys and girls were more or less equally represented.

Self-reported sexual activity among boys dropped from the preintervention 61.2 percent for the class of 1994 to 5.2 percent for the class of 2001, while in girls the change was of similar magnitude, from 23.6 percent in 1994 to 1.9 percent in 2001. The data suggest increasing delay of sexual debut by the pupils from the baseline of 38.8 percent in boys to 94.8 percent and from 66.4 percent to 98.1 percent among girls. Since questions about personal sexual activity always have the potential for distortion, the children were also asked about sexual activity among friends. The results of "other reporting" confirm self-reported data that the pupils were increasingly abstaining from early sex. While among boys 58 percent were reported to be sexually active in the 1994 class, this figure dropped to 2.7 percent among the 2001 class, representing a delay in sexual debut from the baseline of 42 percent to 97.3 percent. The proportion of girls reported to be sexually active dropped from 60 percent for the class of 1994 to 1.6 percent for that of 2001, representing delay in sexual debut from the baseline of 40 percent to 98.4 percent among girls. The increasing number of children choosing to delay involvement in sex is a much more significant result than the often-cited reference to the age at which children first got involved in sexual activity. For instance, the mean age at first intercourse in this study was 11.3 years in 1994 and 11.4 for 2001, obscuring these very significant results ($p < 0.0005$) (AMREF/Uganda, 2001). See Figure 6.4.

Incidentally, one of the recommendations of the AMREF study was that the "Science Teacher should continue to co-ordinate health matters and ensure that budgetary provisions are made to sustain Health Activities in the school" (AMREF/Uganda, 2001, p. 32). This is evidence of where responsibility lies for AIDS-related IEC in Ugandan schools.

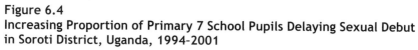

Figure 6.4
Increasing Proportion of Primary 7 School Pupils Delaying Sexual Debut in Soroti District, Uganda, 1994-2001

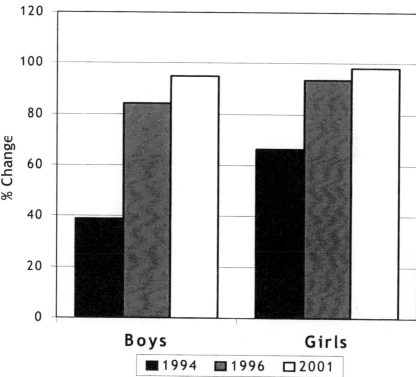

Source: AMREF, 2001.

An assessment of this project admitted that there were objections to teaching sex education in primary schools in Soroti and Katakwi districts and elsewhere from tradition-minded parents as well as cultural and religious leaders. Objections were largely overcome by sensitizing local community leaders, including religious leaders, headmasters, and local political figures. Pupils were very embarrassed to talk about sex openly at first; the ice had to be broken slowly over time (Kaleeba, Namulondo, Kalinki, & Williams, 2000).

A student from Soroti was quoted at length in the chapter in Kaleeba, Namulondo, Kalinki, and Williams (2000) about school-based AIDS programs. This fourteen-year-old girl had experienced AIDS deaths in her immediate family. She was exposed to the intensive AMREF program in Soroti just described. She had read about AIDS in *Straight Talk* and *Young Talk* newspapers, and heard about it on Straight Talk radio and a program called "Capital Doctor." She and her school friends openly discuss AIDS. Is it any wonder that she is postponing sexual debut, abstaining? Western AIDS experts need to overcome their skepticism about abstinence and put themselves in the position of this Ugandan girl. Clearly Uganda's strategy of reaching young people early, before they have initiated sex, is an important element of its youth strategy.

But when it comes down to it, how does one actually promote abstinence to teenagers? What are the exact messages, and who delivers them, in what way? I observed an abstinence education session in December 2002 in Kampala. The setting was an elite Christian school for girls. The following is directly from the notes I took that day:

Demonstration of Abstinence Education, December 9, 2002

The educational session was held at a very old girls school—religious but somehow also government. Apparently many of the elite women of Uganda including the current ambassador to the United States went to this school. The abstinence educator was a self-described born-again Christian, Dr. Luboga. Most of the 200 or so girls present appeared to be quite enthusiastic Christians themselves, judging by their "Amens," etc. Therefore it should not be assumed that this school audience would resemble the mixed, secular audience one would find at a U.S. public school.

Dr. Luboga (Dr. L.) described his wife as a desirable role model for the girls present, especially since she attended this same school. He described his wife's achievements and wonderful attributes, including being the mother of seven children.

Dr. L. began with the basic ABCs of AIDS. He said that Uganda has begun to increasingly emphasize "C" because a lot of people make money on the condom intervention. He then explained the vulnerability of young girls to HIV and STD infection. He talked about the stages of growth of the pelvic bones, the delicacy of the immature womb, etc.

Dr. L. had seven children himself and he seemed to appeal to pronatalist attitudes, e.g., work hard, abstain, be like me and you can have many babies in the future. Do not abstain and you will end up getting pregnant, not finishing your education, and quite possibly undergoing a terrible abortion experience. At this point, Dr. L. went into graphic detail about girls who try to self-abort with knitting needles, etc. (my American colleague began to whisper to me that this was really horrible, this was totally uncalled for, this is religious indoctrination, etc. I said yes, maybe, but regarding the last, this is a religious school and they have already been "indoctrinated").

On the other hand, Dr. L. was definitely trying to empower these girls. He kept telling them they could finish their education, make something out of their lives, become an ambassador, a parliament member, a doctor, a lawyer, even a vice president (such as Uganda currently has). He urged, "Don't just become an appendage to some man, even if he's your husband!"

Dr. L. then became quite animated as he lampooned teenage boys appealing to their girlfriends that if they didn't have sex with them, they would "explode and die" (many giggles over this from the audience). He said girls that fall for this line will get pregnant or infected with HIV, and then where will these boyfriends be? At best, the girl will be at home taking care of a baby and dropped out of school. At worst, she will also be HIV infected.

He again told the girls that they could graduate from university, perhaps get an M.A. like his wife: "Don't be a pregnant school dropout. Be the next vice president of Uganda!" Dr. L. used the word "self-esteem" often.

He then took questions from the audience. One girl asked, "If condoms are not 100 percent protective, why are they promoted in Uganda?" The doctor said that condoms reduce the frequency of infection, but they do not eliminate the risk. He said the only device that doesn't tear, slip, or break is delay of first sex. Condoms in fact prevent the ability to delay. "Virginity can only be lost once. When that happens, you lose the option to decide your destiny yourself." (Author's field notes, Uganda, December 9, 2002)

It must be remembered that this is only one example, and one model, and a religious one at that. I know that some other approaches to abstinence used in Uganda are less fear based and more focused on developing self-efficacy. But before we reject either the general "abstinence" intervention or this particular example of preventive education, we must remember that Uganda has somehow managed to reduce significantly the proportion of youth sexually active before marriage.

THE ROLE OF FBOs

The strategy of the Ugandan government was to involve religious or faith-based leaders and organizations from the beginning of the struggle against AIDS. The Uganda Ministry of Health, through its ACP, began to work with the major religious organizations in Uganda (Catholic, Anglican, Muslim) in AIDS prevention as early as 1987, with support from the WHO. A book on global AIDS published in 1988 explained that Uganda used its religious organizations to reach people in the way other countries might have used its mass media. Illiteracy was widespread and much of the country's infrastructure had been crippled by years of brutal dictatorship and poverty. Few people had radios or read newspapers. Yet it was estimated that 92 percent of the population attended Anglican or Roman Catholic services regularly. The Ministry of Health decided that leaders of these churches, as well as Muslim leaders, could play a major role in spreading awareness about AIDS. The leaders of these three religious organizations were more than willing to cooperate (Sabatier, 1988).

About 60 percent of all health facilities in Uganda are private, the great majority run by FBOs. According to a 2001 survey, about 44 percent of private health care is Catholic, 34 percent is Protestant, 8 percent is Muslim, and 14 percent is "other." This underscores the importance of the role of FBOs in AIDS prevention and mitigation.

According to Anglican informants I interviewed, the government took steps to educate religious leaders as AIDS educators from late 1986 or 1987. Trainers from Makarere University were asked to do some of the early training, which was centered in Kampala. The government at first promoted the slogan "Love Carefully," which might in fact have been suggested by foreign advisors. Whoever coined it, religious leaders thought this message was ambiguous. They preferred "Love Faithfully" and so this is what they used in AIDS eduction. It was meant to convey restricting sex to marriage. A 1991 external evaluation of this ACP in fact found that "Love Faithfully" was remembered more often than Love Carefully, zero grazing, or any other slogan (Moodie et al., 1991). Zero grazing seems to have become better known somewhat later.

Condom promotion was a component of the awareness and prevention programs of these religious groups, except for the Catholics. Yet from the beginning, the FBOs explained that they wished to emphasize "fidelity" and "abstinence" rather than condoms. As noted previously, President Museveni was skeptical about the value of condoms and favored the fidelity/delay approach of the religious groups. Yet foreign AIDS experts were urging the ACP to promote condoms. In response, the ACP and the Uganda AIDS Commission (whose original and current chairmen were Anglican or Catholic bishops) were "not very forceful in promoting (condoms) in the beginning" (Kirungi, 2001, p. 27). In the words of the Uganda AIDS Commission's Director of Research and Policy Development Dr. John Rwomushana, "We adopted a policy of inclusiveness that avoids confrontation with the different social and religious groups. . . . We encourage groups that preach morality to promote means to HIV avoidance they are comfortable with, without, however, undermining other agencies that may be promoting methods less acceptable to them" (Kirungi, 2001, p. 27).

The ACP's first evaluation, based on survey and qualitative research (Moodie et al., 1991), documented positive behavior by 1991, some of which appeared attributable to FBOs. The CDC technical advisor in AIDS assigned to USAID, Dr. Elizabeth Marum, commissioned a consultancy in 1991 to assess the potential and actual response of the religious community to AIDS and to make recommendations for their greater involvement if warranted. The resulting seventeen-page report, submitted to the CDC and USAID, found some resistance to the religious leaders themselves emphasizing condom use (but not to low-key condom promotion or to other groups promoting them). The rest of the report mostly uses language like "willingness and openness." There were no reported findings pertaining to religious leaders condemning PLWHAs or to anything else promoting stigma.

USAID/Uganda began to support Ugandan FBOs in 1992. But at that time there was still an impasse over the contentious issue of condoms between FBOs and donors such as USAID. But for this issue, USAID might have funded what were later to be called FBIs even earlier than 1992. By that year, HIV infections rates were so high—the highest in the world then—that USAID decided to allocate funds for religious groups to work in prevention, even if this had to be on the FBO's own terms. The FBOs had said from the beginning that they wished to promote fidelity and abstinence rather than condoms. Of course, many foreign experts working in HIV/AIDS prevention thought that fidelity and abstinence promotion would have few if any measurable results. Indeed, most AIDS experts still seem to believe that.

Has involvement of FBOs impacted behavior in Uganda? As already noted, the behavior changes that the FBOs—and the government—emphasized are the very ones that changed the most. Moreover, there is some direct evidence from studies of the impact of FBO projects. The Anglican Church CHUSA program was funded by USAID through World Learning's project, ACPC. It began in 1992 and was implemented in 10 districts (Uganda had 40 or less districts at the time, so this was relatively large coverage.) Clergy and laity were trained in AIDS prevention, using peer education, although perhaps the approach was based more on Diffusion of Innovation theory (see below). AIDS messages were delivered from the pulpit in sermons on days of worship, as well as at funerals, weddings, and other occasions. This project cost $370,000, a modest sum as donor-supported AIDS prevention projects go.

Baseline and follow-up surveys of sexual behavior among CHUSA clients in two widely separated districts between 1992 and late 1994 found that those reporting two or more sexual partners declined from 86 percent to 29 percent for men, and from 75 percent to 7 percent for women (Ruteikara et al., 1995, pp. 24–25; cf. Lyons, 1996, pp. 8–9). Ever-use of condoms rose from 9 percent to 12 percent in the same period. There were also focus group discussions involving community leaders and youth. Evidence of behavior change emerged to corroborate surveys' findings, for example,

Before the onset of AIDS, one could have five sexual partners, or even have sex on a chain basis, but these days you realize that there is a lot of self-constraint. Burials, people falling sick from AIDS, and religious leaders have awakened people.

People in the area have made a recognizable behavioural change in light of the AIDS scourge. People realized that AIDS is here to stay and they had to change or else perish." (Ruteikara et al., 1995, p. 21)

Comments about condoms were not very favorable:

God meant us to have sex without using condoms.

Condoms may minimize the transmission of AIDS but on a very small scale.

Condoms are always contaminated with AIDS-virus before they are sold out. (Ruteikara et al., 1995, p. 22)

Interviews with CHUSA and other Anglican AIDS educators in 2003 shed some light on religious—or at least Anglican—views regarding condoms. I was told in three separate interviews that the government and donor-supported AIDS programs promote condoms as if they were 100 percent effective. Meanwhile Catholic groups were said to dismiss condoms as largely ineffective. Anglicans saw themselves as occupying a middle, reasonable ground. They said they teach that condoms are 85 percent or 90 percent effective if used consistently. Two informants went into highly accurate detail about why condoms fail between 10 and 15 percent of the time in Africa. In one interview, an Anglican informant commented spontaneously that so many groups "medicalize the problem of AIDS," and think that condoms are the solution. "But AIDS has nothing to do with medicine. They forget about the community and behavior" (Author's interviews with Dantes Kashangirwe and Medard Muhwezi in Kampala, July 22, 2003).

Another project that began in 1992 with USAID funding has been written up as a UNAIDS "Best Practices" project. The Islamic Medical Association of Uganda (IMAU) project (Kagimu et al., 1998) shows that AIDS prevention activities carried out through Muslim religious leaders and laity had significant direct impact on particular populations targeted.

As PBC has increased and HIV infection has continued to decline, the number of religious leaders and groups involved in AIDS prevention has expanded under district Ministry of Health AIDS prevention activities (funded by the World Bank STI Project). As a result, there is now a high level of involvement on the part of religious organizations and leaders.

How high? By 1995, over 2,745 trainers and peer educators, as well as 5,629 community volunteers in the Muslim IMAU project, had reached 193,955 households and had counseled or sensitized 1,059,439 sexually active people, according to the external evaluation of the

USAID–funded project that supported the first FBOs (Lyons, 1996). In the Anglican CHUSA project, the project trained ninety-six diocesan trainers and 5,702 community health educators and had sensitized 736,218 members of the community, also by 1995 (Lyons, 1996; Ruteikara et al., 1995).

By 1998, I estimated that an average of 150 religious leaders (ministers, imams, deacons, elders, etc.) were being trained in each of Uganda's then forty-five districts per year, resulting in some 6,750 religious leaders trained in HIV/AIDS per year. In case there might have been overreporting of training numbers, we can reduce figures by a third and there would still be 4,500 trained per year since 1995 (Green, 1998). "Training" here refers to religious leaders being educated or sensitized about AIDS and what they could do to help prevent it, usually in brief workshops. Those trained in this way then function as peer educators and group discussants, talking to others in their denomination or religious group about AIDS and how to prevent it.

Taken altogether, there is at least suggestive evidence that religious organizations and perhaps other more conservative opinion leaders in Uganda (e.g., school authorities, traditional healers, and political leaders, such as chiefs) that have advocated abstinence and fidelity have had a significant impact on overall infection rate decline.

One reason USAID took a chance on funding FBOs in Uganda in 1992 was because it believed that religious leaders would not openly criticize condom programs once they were working with AIDS prevention funds (Marum, 1993). Indeed this is what happened for the most part. The experience of working in AIDS prevention and having contact with public health partners helped desensitize the issue of condoms to the point that some pastors, priests, and imams would often quietly direct those asking for condoms to the appropriate place to obtain them. In fact, some FBOs became rather open and active in condom promotion and even provision. For example, the Anglican CHUSA project was implemented in five of its twenty-seven dioceses using the church's community network and church leaders' pastoral home visits. Sample sermons and other awareness materials were distributed—along with free condoms. In its first eighteen months, CHUSA distributed 2 million condoms (Ruteikara et al., 1996).

In spite of this example, experience in Uganda and elsewhere has shown that FBOs should not be forced to promote condoms. This component of HIV/AIDS prevention already receives the lion's share of AIDS prevention resources. FBOs ought to be given support in doing what they themselves prefer to do, and what they do best, namely, promoting fidelity and abstinence. This is discussed further in the section that follows.

How Do FBOs Change Behavior?

What still needs to be empirically researched is exactly how FBOs have changed behavior. I conducted a focus group discussion on this topic with religious leaders in Mbale in December 1998 and one approach became apparent. Discussants from the (Anglican) Church of Uganda described AIDS sensitization workshops in which people "confessed their misbehavior with tears in their eyes." Some of those providing such testimonials were PLWHAs, whom discussants felt were particularly effective in motivating behavior change. Some discussants described this process as a public confession, namely, one in which people confess, I have sinned and misbehaved, and now I see how I endangered my life and that of others ("others" often referring to wives). They then make a public commitment to a new way of life.

Clearly this approach to behavior change is not for everyone, but it may be highly effective with Christian believers and quite possibly with adherents to other religions. It resembles the approach of Alcoholics Anonymous (AA) in which drinkers in effect confess their dysfunctional behavior (I am an alcoholic, my life became unmanageable, I could not stop drinking on my own) and make a public commitment to a new way of life, a life of sobriety. Again, this may not be an approach that works with everyone; in fact it is abundantly clear that no single approach to alcoholism works with everyone. But AA has a better record of changing alcoholic behavior than any other approach. This record, and Uganda's overall success in combating AIDS, would seem to suggest that the approach described by religious leaders in Mbale should not be dismissed out of hand as moralistic. If the AA or Mbale approach to changing behavior works and saves lives, it should be taken seriously. Uganda's FBO approaches to behavior change certainly merit empirical investigation.

Other observations from my Mbale focus group notes include the following:

It was clear that the emphasis in AIDS prevention from this group was on "morality and faithfulness." One leader said that it is only if the person is "not serious" about changing behavior that "we tell him to use a condom so you don't go killing people." He said that not all religious leaders will promote condoms, but most will.

A Catholic leader said that speaking very directly about a sensitive subject, such as is seen in Straight Talk, "is offensive to our culture. So we develop an indirect way of getting the message across."

One elder mentioned that an early reaction on the part of women first hearing about AIDS was a lamentation like, "We women will die due to our husbands' behavior!"

The Church of Uganda initially opposed condoms, "but then we began to see it as a life and death issue. . . . But still we emphasize abstinence and fidelity." All the religious leaders agreed with that statement. Others made comments like "upholding upright behavior" and "upholding biblical standards." Several leaders commented that they have counselors in their local church counseling young people. Sometimes there is a parenting program, a couples program, and an outreach program to single mothers and widows.

The Church of Uganda spokeswoman commented that they have mobilized many volunteers. It seems that virtually the whole religious mobilization from whatever group is entirely based on volunteerism. She also mentioned that in her church, they deal with the "whole human being: physical, mental, and spiritual."

One of the religious elders is a retired headmaster and former schoolteacher. He thanked the government for instituting universal primary education, which among other things helps spread the AIDS message to all in primary school.

The IMAU Muslim representative said he wanted to thank the Ministry of Health and the United Nations Development Program (USAID was also a major funder of IMAU) for support of its AIDS prevention program. His group has sensitized eighty mosque imams. These imams in turn have trained others, such as Family AIDS Workers (FAWs). FAWs have been motivated and enabled in their work by providing them bicycles. The representative said that their project had recently come to an end, but they are continuing anyway. They take advantage of large crowds which even include non-muslims who show up at funerals, to get across the AIDS message. They also use the Friday summons to prayer to conduct AIDS education. He said that the use of condoms was controversial, but IMAU has worked through this issue. Local religious leaders managed to reconcile condoms with the teachings of the Prophet.

I asked about the influence of radio: Is it a help or a hindrance, given the moral approach used by the religious leaders? One elder said that not too many people hear the radio, but another elder disagreed and said that it is widely listened to. There was general agreement that the radio focuses too much on condom promotion, and not on the options of abstinence or fidelity. One elder said he hadn't heard these options even mentioned. Another said that they may be mentioned, but they are certainly not emphasized. One elder said that the radio is only interested in the sale of condoms. (Author's field notes, Uganda, November 27, 1998)

There seem to be many clues in these notes about how FBOs approach behavior change in the context of AIDS. It is astonishing to me that there has not been more systematic investigation of the role of Ugandan FBOs in AIDS prevention in general, and in behavior change in particular. But then there is little discussion at all nowadays about changing sexual behavior, even though we are dealing with a pandemic driven by risky sexual behavior. These notes also provide clues as to how a great deal of AIDS education probably occurs in schools, remembering that a high proportion of Ugandan schools are run by religious organizations.

We might pause to ask why the role of FBOs in behavior change in that country is not better known outside of Uganda. Part of the answer is that it is very difficult and costly to measure separately the independent effects of various programs operating simultaneously and aimed at the same behavioral responses. There may also be an unconscious bias against reporting or even noticing findings that do not fit the usual expectations of Western public health professionals. Countless millions of dollars have gone into condom promotion. In 1998 I examined the returned questionnaires of a national survey that sought to measure the impact of an AIDS education program aimed at Ugandan youth. In a number of responses, interviewers had checked the "other" (miscellaneous) response category, but had written explanatory comments like, "The respondent says he has been 'Saved.'" Respondents had in fact made a number of references to the role of religion in influencing their sexual behavior, or abstinence. Yet no reference to any sort of religious response was made in the report of this research. One could read the research report and have no idea that religion played any role whatsoever.

A more recent analysis of behavior change in Uganda mentioned "turning to God" as one of the behavioral changes reported by informants, along with condom use, abstinence, and sticking to one partner (Ntozi et al., 2001, p. 9). Perhaps this was recognized in this paper because an African is the senior author. In fact, being "saved" is currently one of the recognized response categories used by the Ministry of Health in its KABP surveys related to HIV/AIDS.

Recent Marginalization of FBOs

I was part of a delegation to Uganda during December 7–13, 2002, the purpose of which was to investigate trends in behavioral change and HIV prevalence, which latter had started to rise again (albeit very slightly) in 2001. We met with several leaders of FBOs, and we asked them how they saw their contribution to AIDS prevention. One pastor was quite outspoken. He told us that the chair of the Uganda AIDS Commission admits that ABC is official prevention policy, yet no funds are actually allocated to A or B these days. He believed strongly that Uganda should return to the approach that worked in earlier years, emphasizing abstinence and fidelity. Others from the FBO community agreed with him. Several were so bold as to say it was the United States and other foreign donors who came to Uganda with their own funding priorities, and this changed the program that Uganda developed for itself.

The outspoken pastor asked us if we would tell the minister of health and the First Lady (with whom we were about to confer) to stand up to the donors. His message to the minister was the following: "Don't just accept any donor materials for AIDS education, for example, We should bring in our cultural, traditional, and local leaders together and make sure they have a voice in selecting what is distributed and implemented in Uganda." That, and bring the FBOs back into the mainstream of AIDS prevention. In fact, I spoke with the Anglican minister who administered the highly successful CHUSA project in the 1990s. I asked him why the USAID part of the project ended. He said he was told the funding cycle just came to an end. He also told me that the Anglican church stands ready to work with USAID or any other donor in AIDS prevention, and that the Anglican network of clergy, volunteers, and the like can be mobilized at any time.

VOLUNTARY TESTING AND COUNSELING

Voluntary counseling and testing (VCT) is one way to get patients into treatment, whether palliative or ARV. What I want to discuss here is the possible role of VCT in behavioral change and prevention. There is some empirical evidence that VCT has had the effect of promoting positive behavior change of all types. By 1993, studies in Uganda seemed to show that VCT led to safer sexual behavior, whether the person tested and counseled (both were found necessary) HIV positive or negative. Later studies in East Africa also suggested that VCT could result in less risky practices among sero-discordant couples, although not necessarily with casual partners (Coates et al., 1998; UNAIDS, 1999b). However a more recent study in Uganda seemed to cast doubt on the effectiveness of the intervention for behavior change. In Kigoyera Parish, western Uganda, 495 persons were selected and interviewed about their sexual behavior, out of 2,267 people in the parish. The conclusion was as follows:

Persons who were HIV tested showed no difference in sexual behavior compared to those who were not tested (condom use, 4.3% vs. 5.5%; mean number of sexual partners in the past 3 months, 1.8 vs. 2.0). The conclusion is that only knowing the HIV serostatus is not enough to reduce high-risk behavior. The study results also showed that there is a demand for HIV counseling services without being HIV tested. (Kipp, Kabagambe, & Konde-Lule, 2001, p. 279)

Knowing how low condom user rates are among married or in-union couples, even if they know one partner is HIV infected, I wonder how much condom use there really is after VCT. In one much-studied district in Rakai, only 6.3 percent of discordant couples reported occasional condom use, and only 1.2 percent reported consistent use, in spite of condom promotion by a U.S.–funded project (Gray et al., 2001).

A summary by Wolitski, MacGowan, Higgins, and Jorgensen (1997) showed that VCT can motivate positive behavior change in some people, but not always, and there are differences between populations and situations. The following summarizes a study in rural Uganda:

A study in rural Uganda compared risk behaviors over 20 months follow up for four groups: (a) HIV+ subjects who received VCT (N = 370); (b) HIV− subjects who received VCT (N = 2,304); (c) HIV+ (N = 562); and (d) HIV− subjects (N = 2,860) who did not receive VCT. For all subjects, there were no statistically significant difference in most risk behaviors between those who had participated in VCT and those who had not, regardless of HIV status, although there was a slight increase in condom use. (Nyblade et al., 2000)

VCT programs have been developed in Uganda perhaps more than anywhere else in Africa. Because of Uganda's success in destigmitizing discussion of AIDS and indeed PLWHAs themselves, and because of high-quality programs, such as AIC, TASO (The AIDS Support Organization [Uganda]), and many others, Uganda may lead Africa in the sheer amount of VCT accomplished. Moreover, the quality of VCT appears to be quite good. However, it must never be forgotten that neither VCT, condom social marketing, mass treatment of STDs, nor prevention of mother-to-child transmission were in existence in Uganda when prevalence began to decline. Nor are these programs available even today in remote districts like Kotido and Moyo, yet there has been a 50 percent decline in prevalence in these areas. As evidence accumulates showing that condom promotion has not lived up to expectations, many American and other experts now want to see VCT as the next magic bullet. It is not. To the extent that VCT may have a preventive function, many programs are aimed at persuading people to use condoms. Thus VCT may be a more complicated and expensive way to promote condoms.

On the other hand, VCT can lead people to treatment, care, and support. The AIC, supported by USAID and other donors, is the Ugandan NGO that pioneered VCT. In addition to testing people and providing results the same day, AIC provides counseling and a variety of other services including preventive education. It also provides face-to-face IEC during the counseling it conducts in local communities.

Why might VCT lead to positive behavior change? Knowing serostatus is thought to empower people to change behavior, to enhance self-efficacy. As one Ugandan informant told me in 2001, "It's like the person thinks, 'I am negative! I have been lucky up to now. But now I had better change my ways if I am to remain healthy.'"

There may be other, indirect contributions of VCT to prevention. Uganda developed care and support programs relatively early in its epidemic, once again being something of a pioneer in Africa in this area. The availability of some sort of care and support for those infected served to motivate people to come forward to be tested and counseled, even though there were few resources for care and support as we think of it today. Care, support, and VCT all helped destigmatize AIDS and discussing sexual behavior, and this helped prevention efforts (Marum, 2002).

The main reason AIC clients give for seeking sero-status is marriage or planning to marry. It seems that religious leaders have joined the AIC in promoting the idea that VCT or knowing one's sero-status is a necessary foundation for a happy marriage, planning families, being honest, protecting lives, and reducing the number of AIDS orphans.

The following shows that the AIC has also become an exception to the emphasis on individual counseling by VCT programs in most of Africa:

While the AIC's principal focus has been one of providing VCT to individual clients, the Centre's clientele has changed. The number of persons requesting VCT as couples has steadily increased from 8% of all clients in 1992 to nearly a third currently. Nearly 80% of these couples request HIV testing as a kind of premarital screening process, described as "planning for marriage." (Baryarama et al., 1996; Turyagyenda, 2000; quoted in Painter, 2001, p. 1399)

In addition, it appears that AIC, along with TASO, have contributed substantially to reducing stigma associated with AIDS. Both NGOs have helped people go public about their HIV status, and they encouraged PLWHAs to become involved in AIDS sensitization and prevention.

However, some analysts have gone too far in crediting VCT as the major intervention that should be credited for Uganda's overall success. As will be discussed, there have been no VCT programs in the two districts (Kotido and Moyo) where HIV prevalence peaked at the lowest levels, that have the lowest seroprevalence currently, and where there has also been significant behavior change along with prevalence decline. Moreover, a good deal of behavior change and prevalence decline occurred prior to 1991–1992, when VCT and other high-profile programs began, as seen in the following:

It appears that the process of behavior change in Uganda resulting in reduced HIV risk was well in effect prior to 1991–1992 (the apparent crest of HIV prevalence in youth). This excludes a clear, direct causal association with many proposed intervention strategies, e.g., voluntary testing and counseling, enhanced treatment of sexually transmitted diseases, widespread use of condoms or other strategies. (Stoneburner & Low-Beer, 2002b, p. 10)

MASS MEDIA AND CAMPAIGNS

There have also been mass media, particularly radio, campaigns that have reached a great many people. There is evidence that these have helped raise at least awareness and knowledge levels. The USAID–funded DISH project in the latter 1990s feels that its radio campaign has also been able to directly motivate behavior change, especially condom adoption. Others feel that the strength of radio is to promote general awareness and to reinforce and remind about messages that are presented through other channels. Kanyunyuzi-Asaba and Mwesigye (1998) researched broadcast media in AIDS prevention and concluded as follows: "Audio-visual communication has a significant positive impact on reducing HIV spread. Broadcast media is particularly effective among populations with low literacy. It should however be used with sensitivity to prevailing cultural, religious, and moral norms" (online abstract).

According to a 1998 interview with the general manager of Radio One, Uganda's leading newspaper sells about 32,000 copies a day. Television had about 12 percent national penetration in 1995, and therefore reaches only urban, better-off Ugandans. Radio has 90 percent national penetration.

There has been a great deal of attention given to mass electronic media in the AIDS prevention literature, and so implementers in Uganda, such as Johns Hopkins University, have many reports and publications available to the interested reader. My purpose is to shed light on the less well-known interventions, especially the ones that occurred earlier in the epidemic prior to the peaking of HIV prevalence in 1991. And as we will see later, there are districts in northern Uganda where radio listenership is very low, yet there has still been prevalence decline on the order of 50 percent. This of course is not to say that electronic mass media did not help in spreading awareness about AIDS.

ROLE OF NGOs

There are over 1,100 NGOs and CBOs assisting in AIDS-related activities in Uganda. This represents an unusually vigorous nongovernment sector by African standards, and there are reasons to attribute some of the declining HIV and STD infection rates to the efforts of this sector. A body of evaluation and other research data exist that demonstrates the impact of various well-known NGOs, such as AIC, TASO, and numerous others. CBOs are appropriate (although not exclusive) vehicles for the involvement of various religious groups, people living with HIV, traditional healers, and many others who wish to contribute to the mitigation of AIDS.

I will focus on the role of one of the less well-known NGOs, one consisting of traditional healers.

Involving Ugandan Traditional Healers

As noted previously, Uganda sensitized or trained many types of community leaders. To use a classic definition suggested by the sociologist Merton (1957, quoted in Rogers, 1962, p. 236), opinion leaders may be "monomorphic," meaning they exert influence in a narrowly defined area, or "polymorphic," meaning they exert influence in several areas. Many of the local leaders sensitized in Uganda do not necessarily have any influence in health matters. However, their support (and lack of opposition) was necessary to provide a climate in which school sex education programs, faith-based AIDS programs, and the like could be implemented successfully. Moreover, AIDS is a behavioral as well as a health or medical issue, and sexual behavior is arguably a moral or at least normative issue, however uncomfortable medical professionals feel about this. This makes the support of local leaders extremely useful.

African traditional healers are monomorphic in the sense that they are highly influential in health matters. They are also polymorphic because their influence often extends to spiritual/religious, family, social, and broader normative domains. In many ways they are ideal AIDS educators and behavior change agents, if they can be enlisted in such efforts (see Chapter 10).

The first significant effort to engage Ugandan healers in AIDS prevention began in 1992 through an NGO called THETA. Professor John Rwomushana, a member of the Uganda AIDS Commission, summarized recently as follows:

Traditional Healers (TH) in Uganda came out openly to contribute to the national struggle against HIV/AIDS. This was made possible by the Government's policy of openness about the epidemic. Through mutual education and training, Traditional Healers have been successfully involved in HIV/AIDS prevention through community mobilization, care, counseling, social support and research. They are encouraged to use their own traditional approaches and methods. Collaboration, rather than integration, strategies are applied in joint interventions. (Rwomushana, 2000, from abstract)

By 1998, THETA had trained 125 healers in HIV/AIDS prevention over a five-year period. But these very modest numbers provide an incomplete picture because they overlook THETA's multiplier effect. Shortly after a UNAIDS evaluation was completed in 1998, I was asked by the World Bank to assess the impact of education and communication programs on HIV decline in Uganda. I have already mentioned that traditional healers were among the local community leaders trained or sensitized in AIDS in short workshops. It appeared that the THETA program was often the stimulus or inspiration for including healers in local-level training, yet these thousands of healers sensitized by district-level AIDS educators were not among the healers counted in the UNAIDS evaluation.

At least three districts—Moyo, Mbarara, and Mbale—were training and involving traditional healers in promotion of STD early health seeking behavior. Given the reality throughout Africa that many or most STD cases are brought to traditional healers (cf. a review of evidence of this in Green, 1994), it makes good sense to involve healers in referral and in treatment itself, as well as in promotion of behavior change. Other districts (e.g., Mubende) were involving healers in promotion of safer sexual behavior, which refers to encouragement of fidelity and monogamy among couples and delay of sexual debut among youth.

From my review of district workplans in 1998, I was able to estimate that about one-third of districts trained traditional healers, meaning that over 1,800 healers were trained every year for four years under the public sector STI project. Of course, this estimate is based on written records. These and other numbers might be exaggerated by district officials. But even allowing for considerable inflation of figures, this still amounts to a greater number of indigenous healers officially involved in HIV/AIDS prevention than most—perhaps any—other country in Africa that I am aware of. And that does not include programs in the private sector. Of the hundreds of local NGOs that work in AIDS education or care and support, some involve traditional healers. In fact, district-level public sector programs involving healers often worked through local level NGOs and CBOs; they may be classified as public sector because funding comes through the Ministry of Health. These NGO and CBO efforts have also led to the development of low-cost treatments, or what is now called community-based or home-based care and support of PLWHAs.

None of this amounts to hard evidence that Uganda's impressive decline in HIV infection rates is due even in part to the influence of traditional healers working in AIDS prevention. Such evidence would require more rigorous evaluation research than I was able to carry out in late 1998, due to time restrictions. Yet we can say that involvement of local opinion leaders, such as traditional healers and religious leaders, in HIV/AIDS prevention has occurred on a scale uncommon in Africa and the world; and Uganda leads the world in magnitude of HIV decline. It is therefore reasonable to hypothesize that involvement of healers and clergy has made some contribution to HIV decline.

As AIDS commissioner John Rwomushana mentioned in his Durban conference paper, the open attitude of the Uganda government and— I would add—a recognition of the important role healers in community-based health care, has led to a *sustained* national effort of cooperation in AIDS prevention. I emphasize the word "sustained" because many programs involving traditional healers are fragile and short-lived (Green, 1994).

There is every indication that the Ugandan government and NGO sectors plan to continue this collaboration. The National Strategic Framework for HIV/AIDS Activities in Uganda (2001) affirms the government's continuing relationship with THETA and reliance on traditional healers and their local medicines in treatment of PLWHAs. It mentions the objective of "increasing accessibility to traditional medicines that work" for the opportunistic infections of AIDS (p. 16). The framework acknowledges that clinical trials have in fact confirmed the efficacy of such locally available herbal medicines for herpes zoster and AIDS-related diarrhea (Homsy et al., 1999).

During an assignment in Uganda for USAID in late 2001, I found that particular USAID mission unusually interested in building upon accomplishments to date and supporting AIDS prevention interventions that involve traditional healers. Actually, global USAID has probably supported more traditional healer, collaborative public health programs than any other donor organization, starting in the 1970s in Ghana, so they are to be commended (Green, 1994).

TARGETING HIGH-RISK GROUPS

We have focused on interventions as well as behavior and prevalence changes in the majority population of Uganda. What about high-risk groups? In Uganda, these groups include (but are not limited to) sex workers, truck drivers, soldiers, police, refugees, out-of-school youth and street children, forest workers, plantation workers, and owners or workers in bars, discos, and restaurants, and perhaps some types of migrants.

The Ministry of Health strategy has been to reach these groups in ways that do not contribute to the stigmatization of such groups, nor lead the general public to think that AIDS is mostly a problem of special groups. Such efforts have been low profile and low key, for example, avoiding use of mass media. Instead, the kind of peer education and sensitization of leaders that is being done by some NGOs and by many districts at local levels seems appropriate and often effective. Some groups, such as CSWs, require special informal approaches and methods to educate. Programs targeting CSWs have been successful in promoting condoms.

There has been some dramatic impact on at least one other special group of people at special risk, namely, soldiers. It is said that President Museveni came to realize the extent of the AIDS epidemic in Uganda after he received a telephone call in the mid-1980s from Cuban military authorities informing him that many of the Ugandan military personnel training in Cuba were HIV positive. By the early 1990s, it was estimated that more than 45 percent of the Ugandan military was infected. Because of restrictions prohibiting direct USAID funding to the military, USAID provided funds to WLI through its APCP to support HIV prevention activities in the Ugandan military (USAID/Uganda, 1996). In fact, WLI supported the pioneer FBO projects described in this chapter, as well as many other high-impact programs. The following is from a USAID summary fact sheet:

AIDS prevention interventions in the army have included HIV testing and counseling, health education, STD treatment and prevention, condom promotion and distribution, and post test clubs. Through an arrangement in the WLI project, army personnel on temporary leave assumed staff positions on the UPDF's HIV/AIDS prevention project. This UPDF project began in April 1994 with the objective of reducing HIV transmission among target UPDF personnel in four army divisions together with their civilian dependents and surrounding communities. Ugandan soldiers volunteered to become AIDS "peer educators". After a three-day training course, these volunteers provided education to fellow soldiers, particularly to motivate fellow soldiers to use condoms. These volunteers also serve as condom distributors. As a result of the project, over 2000 soldiers were trained as peer educators and over 53,000 soldiers and their dependents received HIV/AIDS sensitization. In addition, Ugandan soldiers distributed over 4 million condoms supplied by USAID. (USAID/Uganda, 2000)

The implication here is that condom adoption was the sole or at least major change in behavior in the military. And it may well be that, at least with soldiers, as with CSWs, it is appropriate to emphasize condom use over, say, abstinence. A cartoon appeared in a Ugandan paper while I was in Kampala in 1998. It depicted the situation of the developing civil war in eastern Zaire and it showed prostitutes rushing to pick up Ugandan soldiers, while ignoring soldiers from Rwanda, Burundi, Zaire, and other countries that had troops in eastern Zaire. Why? Because it had recently been reported that Ugandans were the only soldiers in the area who actually used condoms.

But were someone to conduct the research, it may be that many soldiers (also) limited their contacts with women, such as CSWs, that would have been at increased risk of HIV infection, or remained faithful to one partner, whether they were married or not.

It should also be emphasized that condom use reported by Ugandan sex workers rose to nearly 100 percent (one always has to take such figures with a grain or two of salt) by the late 1990s. In fact, reported condom use among CSWs and men reporting two or more sexual partners in the past year are among the highest in Africa. It's just that the denominators here are small. For example, only 1.6 percent of men reported engaging in commercial sex in the past year by 2000, according to the Uganda DHS 2000.

WHICH THEORIES OF BEHAVIOR CHANGE WERE EMPLOYED?

There is interest in theories of behavior change in the context of AIDS among a number of analysts. Many or most prevention programs are said to be based implicitly if not explicitly on such a theory, even if "most intervention reports . . . do not explicitly state the theoretical framework of the project" (UNAIDS, 1999c, p. 5). This was true especially outside the United States until recently (Denison, 1996). Earlier AIDS-related theories were individual centered and included the health belief model, social cognitive (or learning) theory, theory of reasoned action, stages of change model, and AIDS risk reduction model. These theories focus for the most part on the individual's perceived susceptibility to infection and benefits that would result from changing behavior, as well as on constraints to such change. They assume that people are rational and will do the right thing once they are provided adequate information and see that change is in their personal self-interest (UNAIDS, 1999c).

The following health belief model (UNAIDS, 1999b) that was developed in the 1950s is typical of this type of theoretical model:

1. Perceived susceptibility to a particular health problem (Am I at risk for HIV?)

2. Perceived seriousness of the condition (How serious is AIDS; how hard would my life be if I got it?)

3. Belief in effectiveness of the new behavior (Condoms are effective against HIV transmission.)

4. Cues to action (Witnessing the death or illness of a close friend or relative due to AIDS.)

5. Perceived benefits of preventive action (If I start using condoms, I can avoid HIV infection.)

6. Barriers to taking action (I don't like using condoms.)

The stages of change model was introduced in 1982 for smoking cessation but it was also used in international health programs to promote oral rehydration for child diarrhea (UNAIDS, 1999b). The stages are as follows:

1. Has not considered using condoms (precontemplation)
2. Recognizes the need to use condoms (contemplation)
3. Thinking about using condoms in the next months (preparation)
4. Using condoms consistently for less than 6 months (action)
5. Using condoms consistently for 6 months or more (maintenance)
6. Slipping-up with respect to condom use (relapse)

I use these examples from UNAIDS in part to illustrate (once again) the widespread belief in international AIDS that condoms are the best, or only, intervention for AIDS prevention.

Behavioral researchers came to realize that complex health behaviors, such as those involving sexual intercourse, take place in a social and cultural context. Therefore social and cultural factors surrounding the individual must be considered in designing preventive interventions (Sweat & Denison, 1995). Sweat and Denison in fact maintain that prevention has to operate at four levels: superstructural, structural, environmental, and individual (FHI/UNAIDS, 2001).

A second group of theories, known as Social Theories and Models, is distinguished by taking these factors into account. This group includes diffusion of innovation theory, social influence or social inoculation model, social network theory, and theory of gender and power.

In the first, "There are four essential elements: the innovation, its communication, the social system and time. . . . The theory posits that people are most likely to adopt new behaviours based on favorable evaluations of the idea communicated to them by other members whom they respect. [Further,] behavioural changes can be initiated when enough key opinion leaders adopt and endorse behavioural changes, influence others to do the same and eventually diffuse the new norm widely within peer networks" (UNAIDS, 1999b, p. 9). Everett Rogers developed these ideas as early as the 1950s and applied them to family planning and contraception. One idea that is fundamental to the peer education approach used in Uganda and many other countries is homophily (its opposite is heterophily). This refers to "the degree to which pairs of individuals who interact are similar in certain attributes such as beliefs, values, education, social status, and the like." Not surprising, "more effective communication occurs when source and receiver are homophilous" (Rogers & Shoemaker, 1971, p. 14).

In practice, AIDS prevention interventions are often based on hybrids, or combinations of models, rather than individual models. For example, the peer education approach seems closely related to the diffusion of innovation theory model, but it is not the same. Opinion leaders are not really peers to those whom they influence, even though in Africa, for example, they tend to be quite homophilous in ways other than social status. My own work in collaborative AIDS prevention programs involving African indigenous healers is classified as peer education by UNAIDS (1999c), even though healers should be considered opinion leaders rather than peers.

It may be difficult to fairly characterize the dominant theoretical model in AIDS prevention programs at the country level, since there are typically a great many programs implemented by a large number of independent agencies and organizations. However, from what we have reviewed in Uganda, clearly there has been a lot of peer education, considered as a type of diffusion of innovation theory. Stoneburner and Low-Beer (2002b) seem to concur. In their comparison between Uganda and neighboring countries, they conclude the following:

The findings of heightened levels of knowledge of persons with AIDS and communications about AIDS within personal social networks, which dominate in Uganda, may reflect a contextual response to a more open and community-oriented public health strategy to address AIDS and behavioral risks. This is similar to what was observed in populations of homosexual males in the mid-1980s and consistent with social theory on behavior change and diffusion of innovation. (p. 11)

An evaluation of the successful USAID–funded APCP commented that the approach of this project most resembled the stages of change theory (Lyons, 1996).

Another apparently successful national AIDS prevention program is found in Jamaica. A recent evaluation found the following:

The BCC program uses a hybrid BCC approach based on a theoretical foundation that includes: Theory of Reasoned Action, Stages of Change Model, AIDS Risk Reduction Model, and Everett Rogers' Diffusion of Innovation Theory. The peer education model is linked to the last model, and in Jamaica, as in other countries, it is based on use of opinion leaders within particular groups as well as on true peers of the target audiences. (Amarasingham, Green, & Royes, 2000, p. 18)

I was one of these evaluators and we found that Jamaica's BCC program resembled Uganda's in its reliance on peer education (especially among in-school and out-of-school youth) and reliance on community-based opinion leaders, such as religious and school authorities.

In 2003, I interviewed a number of Ugandans who had been involved in Uganda's first interventions to address AIDS. One senior official explained that the government may have more or less been following the health belief model, although neither President Museveni nor most others in government had really ever heard of this. He said they just used common sense in approaching the problem. But now that this official has studied health education models, he was able to identify two elements which were emphasized from the beginning: internalized risk perception and self-efficacy (Kagimba, 2003). In fact, a growing body of evidence suggests that both of these are needed to achieve behavioral change (Rimal, 2001; Witte, 1998).

DOES UGANDA HAVE SPECIAL FAMILY AND SOCIAL COHESION?

If interpersonal communication and community mobilization have been key ingredients in Uganda's success, is this part of a model for AIDS prevention that could be exported to other countries in at least Africa? Some have suggested that there may be unusual family or social cohesion in rural Uganda, and that this may have facilitated Uganda's relatively quick, rational, and effective response to the threat of AIDS (Nantulya, 2002). However, Uganda has multiple ethnic groups and religions, and at the time of its first national response to AIDS, its citizens had just suffered years of repression and violence under three regimes of dictatorship. It would seem that a peaceful country like Swaziland, which is comprised of essentially a single ethnic group and major religion (Christianity), ought to have the kind of social and family cohesion that would provide fertile ground for the kind of community-based, organized response Uganda in fact had. However, it may be that male absenteeism from the family due to labor migration to South Africa has weakened the family and community in Swaziland and neighboring southern African countries. Moreover, this labor pattern leads to separation of spouses and probably to higher levels of casual sex. On the other hand, we now have evidence from Zambia that A and B behaviors have increased and prevalence has declined, at least among youth (see chapter 7).

Science journalist Helen Epstein has thought about the special social capital that may have helped Uganda in its effective response to AIDS. She points out possible additional factors in the following e-mail:

Uganda was never really colonized, and there are fewer large commercial farms there than in most other East and southern African countries. This means more people can survive on their own plots of land, there is less migrant labor (in fact very little), there are fewer street children, fewer prostitutes, and so on. As a Tanzanian AIDS worker told me recently, "wherever there are mines and big farms, there is a big HIV problem." Since Uganda has fewer of these, HIV rates might be expected to be lower, at least when the country is at peace.

The fact that Uganda is very fertile, and land ownership is more equitable, may also help explain why Uganda benefited more than other countries from the World Bank's Structural Adjustment programs, and may partly account for the country's high growth and declining poverty rates in the past few years—trends that are almost unique on the continent. Growing prosperity may also have helped the country control HIV, because wealthier families don't need to send their daughters to the city to become prostitutes (as is common in Kenya, for example), people can stay on their farms and don't have to migrate for work and so on. (Epstein, personal communication, March 20, 2002)

In fact, Sam Okware, original director of Uganda's AIDS Control Programme, believes most of Uganda does have high social cohesion. He commented in an interview, "We live closely together in groups and so we see with our own eyes the problems that people are having, including deaths in the family. Ugandans have a lot of social cohesion" (2003). Robert Thornton (2003) believes that Uganda's burial practices are atypical for Africa: relatives are buried right in the homestead, meaning that every villager knows when there has been a death.

Although these may all be contributing factors, it may be difficult to demonstrate that rural Uganda (and Senegal, another AIDS success story) have a degree of family and social cohesion not found anywhere else in Africa and that, especially in the case of Uganda, this is found throughout the country. Uganda has areas of great instability and insecurity, as well as internally displaced people living in temporary settlements. There are also African countries in states of great conflict, such as Somalia, Sudan, the Democratic Republic of Congo and Liberia, that do not have particularly high HIV prevalence rates by African standards. Still, it might be argued that a certain degree of cohesion is one of several necessary conditions that combine with national leadership, stigma reduction, community mobilization, emphasis on PBC, and empowerment of women and youth, among others, to produce an effective prevention program.

WHAT HAPPENED IN LOW-PREVALENCE AREAS OF UGANDA?

To help understand which interventions are associated with behavior change and presumably to HIV infection rates, it is instructive to look at some areas of northern Uganda where few AIDS interventions have reached. I warn the reader: This section will be an exercise in humility for those of us who work in donor organizations.

Karamoja

At one ANC site (Matany) in a northeastern district, Moroto, HIV seroprevalence has declined from 2.8 percent in 1993 (and higher in 1994, but probably not as high as the 7.6 percent reported) to 1.7 percent in 2001. We note at once that Matany peaked much lower than any other sentinel sites, where seroprevalence in some cases peaked at over 30 percent. In fact infection rates peaked at over 38 percent in Rakai district (Tarantola & Schwartlander, 1997). Unfortunately, there seem to have been no behavioral surveys in Moroto, but there was a standard (and therefore comparable) KABP survey conducted by the Ministry of Health in the adjacent district of Kotido in 1997. Matany is the nearest surveillance site to Kotido, and the two districts are homogeneous culturally, economically, and geographically. The combined area is known as Karamoja, from the Karamajong, a Nilo-Hamitic, pastoral, cattle keeping people who predominate in both districts.

For an additional biological measure from Kotido itself, reported incidence of urethritis among men was 1.1 percent, compared to 11.7 percent, 12.7 percent, 15.5 percent, and 18.7 percent for Jinja, Lira, Soroti, and Kampala, respectively.

What might account for the low HIV infection rates of Karamoja? The Karamajong are not Muslim nor do they practice male circumcision. And what might have caused a significant decline in HIV seroprevalence among the Karamajong? Ever-use of condoms was reported to be 3.3 percent in 1997, although when asked to report types of behavior change, only 1 percent of men and 0.7 percent of women cited condom use as a behavior change option adopted in the five years prior to the survey (Ministry of Health/Uganda AIDS Commission, 1997). Whether we use either figure, we must look beyond condom use for explanations.

Meanwhile, only 1.9 percent reported having had intercourse with a nonregular partner in the preceding twelve months, compared to 2.9 percent who reported a nonregular partner in the preceding five years (Musinguzi et al., 1997, p. 14). Both figures are significantly lower than the proportion found in other Ugandan districts, which themselves are low by African standards. Moroever, in questions about behavior change in the past five years, the proportion reporting faithfulness or sticking to one partner or "zero-grazing" is 94.7 percent, the apparent highest of any surveyed Ugandan districts. An additional 2.5 percent reported abstinence.

Rounding out the picture of low-risk sexual behavior patterns, "the mean age for first time sexual intercourse was 18.13 which was higher than any of the previously surveyed districts" (Musinguzi et al., 1997, p. 3). For Karamajong women, the interval between first sex and first marriage—the period when one tends to have multiple partners in most societies—is only 1.53 years.

All this may explain why HIV prevalence is relatively low in Karamoja, but we don't really know why it has declined in recent years. Of those surveyed, 74.5 percent had no formal education, 74 percent had never listened to a radio, and 88.6 percent had never seen television. Only about 16 percent had read a newspaper at least once a week. Few of the higher-profile AIDS prevention interventions often credited with impacting HIV rates are found in either adjacent district, with the exception of some faith-based programs.

Yet, AIDS awareness was found to be higher than might be expected: 87.8 percent had heard of AIDS and 65 percent were able to cite at least two correct means of prevention (Musinguzi et al., 1997, p. 19). Unfortunately, respondents were not asked from which source they had learned about AIDS, but it is possible from the foregoing to eliminate the usual candidates as significant sources: radio, TV, schools, and well-known programs such as TASO and AIC. The statistician who has been involved in the Ministry of Health KABP surveys since 1996 thinks the people in these two districts learned about AIDS primarily from local community leaders. This might include local and traditional political leaders, religious leaders, and traditional healers. Indeed, there seem to be few other possible sources of AIDS information, except perhaps from agents of the formal health care system.

One additional explanation emerged in a recent interview. There were many Karamajong men in the army during the time of Idi Amin. Soldiers away from home are at higher risk of HIV infection. These ex-soldiers probably came back to Karamoja and infected their women. But after Amin's time, few men from that area have served in the army, so there were few new infections from this source. This exposure from soldiers during one period might account for some of the prevalence decline (Okware, 2003).

Yet overall, these findings from Karamoja can be taken as further evidence that the emphasis found in Uganda on community-based, interpersonal IEC through sensitizing and educating many categories of local leaders has been important in spreading awareness and probably motivating behavior change. It also seems clear that sexual behavior was and is more conservative by standard measures than elsewhere in Uganda, and this probably accounts for the low infection rates found among these Karamajong throughout the surveillance period. There are said to be strong cultural norms regarding sexual behavior and relatively strict enforcement of these by local leaders. A reported late age of first menstruation might also be a factor.

Still, it would be most useful to conduct qualitative and survey research in Moroto itself, in the district of the sentinel site for Karamoja, to better understand the dynamics of HIV prevalence decline, behavior change, and the motivators of behavior change.

Moyo District

Much can be learned from another northern district, Moyo, which lies in Uganda's extreme northwest. There are no sizeable towns in this district, but it has population concentrations in camps for refugees and internally displaced peoples. In 1991, a Harvard researcher conducted a population-based random sample survey of 1,486 men and women, the sample divided evenly between men and women. This researcher was also interested in epidemiologic modeling and specifically in predicting the course of the epidemic in Moyo (Schopper, 1992). She noted that Moyo's epidemic had started later than the epidemic in south districts, which are more urbanized and lie along the trans-Africa highway. Citing researchers and prevailing statistics, she suggested that Moyo's epidemic would resemble that of the south within several years. The determining factor, she noted, would be changes in sexual behavior.

However, the findings from this 1991 KAP survey painted a rather interesting picture. The mean age of sexual debut was seventeen for women and nineteen for men (Schopper, 1992), higher than the rest of Uganda except for Karamoja. In fact, judging from differences in age groups, the age of debut had been higher before a historically recent decline. The survey also found that 50 percent of men and only 18.5 percent of women reported ever having had premarital sex. Only 5.8 percent reported casual sex, that is, intercourse during the last twelve months with a nonregular partner (15 percent of men and 2 percent of women). Almost all casual sex seemed to occur before the age of twenty-five (Schopper, 1992).

In fact Schopper (1992) compared 1991 and 1992 surveys in Moyo and found that the average number of partners reported by men had decreased significantly. In addition, the proportion of single respondents engaging in casual sex, especially among women, declined from 11.3 percent to 2.7 percent. Condom ever-use was only 13.5 percent in 1991: 11 percent women, 15 percent men (Schopper, 1992).

If Moyo's epidemic were in fact to have resembled that of the districts of the south, HIV infection rates would have risen to 20–30 percent or higher at some point. This did not happen. Seroprevalence in Moyo peaked in 1993, only a year or two later than the southern districts, and it peaked at only 5 percent. By 2000, the rate had declined to 2.7 percent, the second lowest seroprevalence rate among Uganda's fifteen sentinel surveillance sites. The author herself seemed surprised that "the overall number of casual partners seems to be extremely low," even wondering aloud about the reliability and validity of her survey data (Schopper, 1991, p. 33).

Of course, as with Karamoja, these data are more tantalizing than definitive. In both areas, we only have behavioral surveys in essentially single periods, one in 1997 and the others in 1991 and 1992. We need more than one study. We would like to see two or more studies from different time periods to better understand trends in seroprevalence decline and any changes in behavior. Certainly sexual behavior in Moyo seems rather conservative (Schopper's own term). The researcher makes useful comparisons of sexual behavior statistics with several other countries (e.g., Côte D'Ivoire and Central African Republic), and we consistently find less risky behavior in Moyo. But we would like to know if it became even less risky after 1992. We would like to know if behavioral changes after 1992 seems to account for the significant reduction in HIV seroprevalence that we find in Moyo.

As with Karamoja, we would like very much to know what motivated any behavior changes in Moyo. As another outlying district remote from Uganda's southern urban centers and capital city, Moyo did not benefit significantly from the better-known, well-documented interventions that Uganda is deservedly known for. From the 1998 district health plans cited earlier in this chapter, we know that—at least in the public sector—Moyo put emphasis on community-based, interpersonal IEC. We also know that Moyo trained traditional healers to help identify and appropriately treat STD cases. Again we see evidence suggestive of the importance of a type of IEC that gets far less recognition than mass media IEC, namely, community-based, interpersonal IEC that relies on local leaders. These preliminary findings call for new research in both Karamoja and Moyo by researchers who are not already committed to the condom paradigm.

The Uganda DHS 2000 seems not to have picked up on unusual behavioral patterns in Kotido or Moyo, nor to have attempted to relate the low HIV infection rates found there to prevailing behavioral patterns. Judging by the published sampling design, there was oversampling in southern and western districts (where USAID–supported projects were operating) and therefore undersampling in the north. Furthermore, northern districts had the highest rate of "failure to interview" due to "finding no competent respondent at home" (DHS, 2001, pp. 204–205). Only 16 percent of those interviewed came from the north. Interesting research still awaits in Kotido and Moyo.

WILL HIV INFECTION RATES RISE AGAIN?

Epidemics have a period of explosive growth characterized by an exponential rise of number of infected persons. But eventually, those at risk are largely infected, achieving a saturation point. In the United States, new infections among MSMs reached low levels by 1989 (Rotello, 1997). Was this due to the impact of prevention efforts or was it simply saturation? Rotello believes it was primarily saturation. Of course, we expect there to be different saturation levels based on distinctive patterns of risk factors, such as those that characterize Pattern I populations when considering gay men and IDUs, and those that characterize Pattern II populations when considering sub-Saharan African populations. And using ANC surveillance data, we see that the national seroprevalence rate of Uganda was about 21 percent in the early 1990s (or more like 15%, if rural/urban proportion are taken into consideration), whereas by 2000, a few countries in southern Africa had reached infection levels exceeding 30 percent, as measured in ANCs. This suggests that 21 percent may not be considered what we might call the natural high-water mark, or saturation level, of a (mostly uncircumcised) African population.

If risk behavior does not change, a second wave of infection may arise after an initial saturation phase has been reached, thereby raising HIV prevalence again. Some epidemiologists believe Côte D'Ivoire is now experiencing a second wave of HIV infection as seen in the following:

Back-calculation from mortality data suggests that the incidence of HIV in Abidjan rose in the early and mid-1980s, reaching a peak in 1985–1986. It then declined, but rose again to reach a second peak in 1992. The hypothesis put forward by the authors is that the first epidemic "wave" was predominantly associated with transactional sex, while the second resulted from sexual contacts within stable relationships. (Tarantola & Schwartlander, 1997, p. S17)

The same hypothesis has been made for Thailand, but so far, a second wave seems not to have materialized, perhaps or probably because the reproductive number (Ro) in Thailand is one or less. This means that on average, one infected person does not infect more than one other person in Thailand (Chin, 2001a).

What about prospects in Uganda? In fact, after declining for nine to ten years, depending on how national average is calculated, the national HIV prevalence rate rose slightly. The figure in 2001 was 6.5 percent, up slightly from 6.1 percent in 2000. This difference could be statistically insignificant. But it might also spell the end of the decade-long decline in seroprevalence. HIV prevalence seems to be rising in nearby Kagera region, Tanzania, which has had an epidemic similar to that of adjacent Raki district, Uganda (as will be discussed later). In fact, prevalence seems to have started to rise in Rakai, based on information I received there in December 2002. If national prevalence is in fact rising, what are some of the possible reasons?

There has been less decline in HIV infection rates and less reduction in risky sexual behavior among Ugandans over age twenty-four than among younger cohorts. It may be that most current infections are occurring among older Ugandans, in fact among discordant couples in marital or other stable relationships. This may mean that even if government and donors put more emphasis on AIDS prevention intervention targeting those over twenty-four, the behavior change options are more limited. Abstinence and partner reduction seem to be unrealistic, but so does condom use, because married or cohabiting couples do not like to use condoms anywhere. And at least one study in Uganda shows that this remains true even for couples who know their serodiscordant status and are provided condoms (Gray et al., 2001).

At this writing, I do not know if prevalence in the age fifteen to nineteen cohort has increased, decreased, or remained the same as in 2000. If it has increased in this age group, it could indicate disinhibition. We saw earlier in this chapter that there has been a slight erosion of risk avoidance behaviors between 1995 and 2000, according to the two DHS studies, although the change in proportions reporting abstinence may have decreased significantly. This may be due to more Ugandans turning to and relying on condoms during this period, in the belief that they are being fully protected, that this is safe sex. Condom promotion in the early period of national response was low-key and targeted to higher risk groups (Okware, 2003). But when condom social marketing took off in the mid-1990s, the approach became the usual one of the "maximum number of condoms for the maximum number of people."

It would be a tragedy if well-intentioned programs from Western donors is starting to have the effect of disinhibition, of allowing Ugandans to return to riskier behavior in the belief that medical devices or medicines will protect them. It is very likely that Western donors will respond to the upswing in prevalence by intensifying the very programs that may be leading to disinhibition.

Preliminary findings by a few researchers in fact suggest that condom social marketing in Uganda may have led to disinhibition (Ahmed & Mosley, 2003; Hearst & Chen, 2003b; Kirby, 2003).

ARE THE LESSONS FROM UGANDA UNDERSTOOD?

Uganda provides the example of not only the greatest decline in HIV infection rates, but also an atypical model of an AIDS prevention program. As we have seen, President Museveni was very skeptical of condoms as a solution to Uganda's growing AIDS problems. Uganda's national prevention program reflects this, and we see that emphasis was on promoting PBC. There must have been a great deal of behavior change before HIV began to decline in 1991, and this change must have been something unrelated to condoms since there were few condoms in the country and little reported use before 1991. Much as it may pain supporters of the prevention programs currently favored, neither condom social marketing nor VCT nor STD treatment had begun by 1991. These programs have probably still not really reached northern Uganda districts, such as Moyo and Kotido, where there has been a decline of HIV prevalence on the order of 50 percent (unmatched by any other country).

One would expect that those involved in international AIDS prevention would become very interested in PBC and in the Uganda model of how to promote this. Yet this has not happened, at least prior to 2003. For one thing, there has been little acceptance of the version of events as I have laid them out. The dominant view, at least until recently, is that condoms deserve the credit. For example, a special issue of *Population Reports* (Gardner, Blackburn, & Upadhyay, 1999) cites Uganda as a great success story and implies that this was due to condoms. True, there is mention of delay of debut and partner reduction, but the sidebar tells the reader: "Uganda Ministry of Health STD/AIDS Control Progamme: In Uganda condom use increased and HIV prevalence decreased following a national AIDS prevention and condom promotion effort." The next sentence reads, "Yoweri Museveni, Uganda's president since 1986, has been an activist and strong supporter of AIDS prevention programs," implying that Museveni was behind the alleged success of condoms (Gardner, Blackburn, & Upadhyay, 1999). With such propaganda, it is not surprising that there is lack of consensus over what happened in Uganda, or that many AIDS professionals think Uganda's success was due to condoms.

A recent article in *AIDS* tells us, "A pattern has been observed in several areas in Uganda and has been shown to be associated with increased condom use and a decrease in casual sex" (Fylkesnes et al., 2001, p. 931), and then cites three studies for this conclusion, none of which reports that condom use was the first or main response to AIDS or AIDS interventions. It seems that after such an enormous investment of resources and reputation in condoms over twenty years, many analysts are not willing to report findings without attribution to condoms, even if it is not warranted by the data.

There are studies, such as Ntozi, Ahimbisibwe, Mulindwa, Ayiga, & Odwee (2001) that report condom use as the main behavior change among Ugandans, but, as in this case, the study group consisted primarily of CSWs, bartenders, bargirls, street children, and truck drivers. The reader may only remember increased condom use and forget the methodological details of this study.

A recent UNAIDS Epidemic Update (December 2001) devotes a paragraph to Uganda's success. Yet the only behavior change mentioned is condoms (UNAIDS, 2001, p. 21). Inflated condom user rates are offered with no mention of the denominator for the rates, which in the case of casual partners (said to be 31% and 53% in two urban areas) is probably only among 6–8 percent of the population, judging by Ministry of Health surveys and DHS data.

Recently, the Guttmacher Institute released a thirty-four-page memo that reinforces the view that it was mostly condoms that account for Uganda's success (Singh, Darroch, & Bankole, 2002). The authors argue that only DHS data should be considered because only DHS employs a national sample. There are three DHS studies: 1988, 1995, and 2000. The problems with this paper can be summarized as follows:

- The DHS did not ask AIDS-related questions about AIDS in 1988, so we become restricted to comparisons between 1995 and 2000, when most behavior change had already occurred.
- Men were not interviewed in the DHS until 1995.
- The wording of key DHS questions was changed between 1995 and 2000; for example, for the question about nonregular partners, the 1995 survey used a six-month recall period, whereas the 2000 DHS used a twelve-month recall, making comparisons between responses to the two questions problematic.
- The DHS oversampled in the southern districts of Uganda. The biennial KABP survey of the Uganda Ministry of Health is almost exclusively conducted in the southern districts. When results between DHS and these Ministry of Health are compared (as in 1995 and 2000), the results are very similar, meaning that the Ministry of Health surveys, which began in 1989, should not be discounted as sources of data.

These are familiar errors. We have more behavioral data after 1995 and it is more accessible than pre-1995 data. There has been a significant rise in condom use between 1995 and 2000, while there has been an erosion in levels of abstinence and monogamy, according to the DHS. By restricting comparisons to 1995 and 2000, and using DHS, the case can be made that condom use went up while PBC went down slightly. This implication of course is that this is what happened earlier as well. This interpretation does not explain how and why, in the country that remains the example of greatest HIV decline, national HIV decline began before condoms could have made a significant difference. Yet the Guttmacher view of what happened in Uganda is the one that was strongly promoted and accepted at the 2002 global AIDS conference in Barcelona.

At the XII World AIDS Conference in Geneva (June 30, 1998), I met a Ugandan researcher who was telling me with great excitement about his recent research (I will protect his identity). A study he had been involved in had found clear evidence of decline in casual sex, as well as some rise in age of sexual debut. I was interested in seeing his conference abstract at once. His abstract mentioned only condom use. I asked him to explain. He replied sheepishly, "Well, we were funded by the Americans and of course they are most interested in hearing about condoms." I wrote this down at once on a napkin to preserve this little bit of evidence for some future book, since it is not the kind of thing one can publish in a peer-reviewed journal.

Even the Ugandan public may not understand what has reduced AIDS in their country. A front page article in Uganda's *Monitor* (December 3, 2001) reports UNAIDS statistics showing that life expectancy at birth had recently increased by four years due to Uganda's success in combating AIDS. The accompanying cartoon has a lizard in dark glasses holding up a newspaper that says "condom use begins to pay off!"

Other aspects of Uganda's successful prevention model are not well known. This may be in part Uganda's own modesty in describing its program. As mentioned in Chapter 1, there is a tendency in countries who have achieved measures of success to focus on the negative rather than the positive, the stated reason being that the fight is not yet won and we cannot become complacent. For example, the National Strategic Framework for HIV/AIDS Activities in Uganda (2001) states as a problem area "inadequate involvement of PHAs (PLWHAs) and their networks in HIV/AIDS prevention and control" (Ministry of Health/ Uganda AIDS Commission, 2001, p. 27), even though Uganda is likely the leading country in Africa in its active involvement of PLWHAs. I suppose the thinking is we could always do better, and it must be recognized that those who write national AIDS documents usually lack AIDS program experience in other countries, and so are not in a position to know that whatever the shortcomings, their country may be the best in the region or continent.

It must also be kept in mind that government and donor AIDS documents are at least partially intended to raise money, or justify money already allocated to AIDS.

Stoneburner and Low-Beer (2000) reach conclusions compatible with my own. They analyzed trends in behavior in Uganda between 1989 and 1995, and compared these with trends in Kenya, Malawi, and Zambia. In Uganda, they found an increase in the age of sexual debut; an increase in use of condoms particularly in high-risk partnerships; and a reduction in rates of multiple sexual partnerships. In the comparison countries, condom use was comparable or higher, but they did not have significant partner reduction or rise in age of sexual debut. The authors concluded, "The lack of comparable HIV declines in comparison countries with comparable ages of sexual debut and condom use, but with higher rates of multiple sexual partnerships similar to

Uganda's in 1989, suggests that partner reduction is the factor of greatest importance in the interruption of sexual networks and HIV dynamics in Uganda" (Stoneburner & Low-Beer, 2002b, p. 8).

I contacted Stoneburner to see what he thought about the impact of delay of debut, since I believe this also played a crucial role in reducing Uganda's HIV infections. The response: "I put delay of debut (abstinence) broadly into partner reduction, as it is the same/similar behavioral process and so different from condom use. Perhaps I should clarify that" (Stoneburner, personal communication, March 28, 2002).

Incidentally, these authors had a great deal of trouble publishing these findings and conclusions, even being allowed to present these data at the International AIDS Conference in Durban in 2000.

In short, as I have taken pains to demonstrate, Uganda does seem to offer a model of successful AIDS prevention, and it is far more than condom promotion. Elements of this model have been identified in several reports and publications that go beyond largely unwarranted condom attribution (Alwano-Edyegu & Marum, 1999; Green, 1998; Kaleeba et al., 2000; Okware et al., 2002; Sittitrai, 2001; Stoneburner & Low-Beer, 2002b), and they are summarized in the following list which is divided into the two main periods of Uganda's national response. The elements found in the pre-1991 period should be considered carefully, since they may hold the clue for changing behavior and reducing HIV incidence in the absence of those AIDS prevention interventions that have become the standard package around the world. Moreover, the post-1991 elements are found in most countries and most countries cannot be considered successful in AIDS prevention.

Elements Contributing to Seroprevalence Decline:

Pre-1991:

- a strong, activist national response from the highest political level
- sex education and AIDS education in the primary schools, beginning in 1987
- a policy and a program of empowering or "advancing" women and youth
- a national IEC approach that emphasized community-based, face-to-face, interpersonal communication, along with mass media. IEC targeted youth, using youth-friendly approaches
- promoting partner reduction (fidelity, zero-grazing) and delay of sexual debut as key elements of the IEC or BCC approach
- deliberate use of fear arousal in IEC, but not without showing clearly what people can do to avoid AIDS
- early and significant mobilization of religious leaders and organizations, from 1986 onward

- combating stigma and discrimination associated with HIV/AIDS and respecting and protecting the rights of those infected
- PLWHA involvement in AIDS prevention
- strong NGO and CBO response, leading to flexible and creative interventions and widespread involvement of people at different levels of society (e.g., political leaders at all levels, community leaders, teachers, women and youth leaders, PLWHAs, and traditional healers)
- promoting open discussion of both AIDS and sexual behavior

Post-1991:

- a multisectoral response since 1992
- decentralized planning and implementation since 1995
- condom social marketing, starting in the early 1990s
- voluntary counseling and testing starting in a few districts in the early 1990s
- investment in local level human resources, for example, provision of financial incentives for peer educators and community health educators and workers (instead of expecting them to be volunteers, or be compensated only by profits from the sale of condoms)
- programs of finding and treating curable STIs
- special programs for high-risk groups (CSWs, soldiers, drivers, bar girls, police, etc.)

Adding together all AIDS-related contributions from all sources, total donor support between 1989 and 1998 was found to be approximately $180 million, or $1.80 per adult per year. Donor contributions were estimated to amount to 70 percent of total expenditures on AIDS prevention and care in Uganda (Marum & Madraa, 2000). USAID has been the main donor overall and its AIDS Education and Control Project, formerly the APCP, can be credited with contributing to some of Uganda's more innovative programs. However Uganda itself, both the public and private sectors, must be credited with developing much of the successful prevention model, namely, community mobilization and mass awareness, emphasis on zero grazing and delay of sexual debut, bold IEC in primary schools, involvement of religious organizations as well as PLWHAs, and VCT that combined testing, care, support, and prevention.

No one seems to have estimated the cost of prevention interventions in the period 1987–1991, when sexual behavior changed sufficiently to alter the course of an explosive epidemic. The costs overall and per person would have been much lower prior to the expensive, donor-funded prevention projects, such as condom social marketing, mass treatment of STDs, and VCT. Therefore it seems possible to reduce national HIV prevalence quickly and for probably substantially less than $1.80 per person.

There was also a significant difference in how AIDS prevention funds were spent in Uganda. A substantial portion went to local NGOs and CBO frontline educators for small salaries or in-kind compensation (Marum, 2002). Elsewhere in Africa, prevention funds go to commodities, drugs, project vehicles, fuel and maintenance of vehicles, and of course to expensive foreign experts. Peer educators and other community-based educators are usually expected to somehow get along as volunteers. Uganda's support of community-based educators seems to partly explain its achievements in community mobilization and mass awareness.

Is $1.80 per adult per year a little or a lot? By comparison, the state of Massachusetts spent $6.50 per person per year between 1992 and 1999 for its successful tobacco control program (Biener, Harris, & Hamiliton, 2000). For a poor country in Africa which may spend only $5 per person per year on all health care, $1.80 may seem to be a lot. But for a deadly disease that was infecting 21 percent of the population, and affecting an even higher percentage, the cost seems justified if funds can be found. And it is far less costly than the hundreds of dollars per person per year that is being advocated for the cost of ARV drugs for the HIV infected, including for African countries where 30 percent or more of the sexually active population may be HIV infected. It is important to remember that it is not the amount of money that was spent in Uganda, but how it was spent. Instead of spending $35,000 on one more project vehicle, and another $10,000 on fuel and maintenance, why not support, supervise, and supply scores of community-based health workers for several years? We should not worry unduly about sustainability when we are in an emergency situation, and how sustainable are high-maintenance vehicles by comparison?

The important lesson here is that it seems possible to reduce national HIV prevalence quickly, for probably substantially less than $1.80 per person.

It must be remembered that many of the elements of Uganda's response, namely, decentralized planning and multisectoral responses, do not impact HIV infection rates directly. Behavior must change for this to happen (the contribution of STD treatment or prevention in Uganda is still being assessed, but it seems not to have contributed significantly to prevalence decline). Although fighting stigma or bold political leadership at the highest levels might be cited as major contributing factors in Uganda's success, it must be remembered that these are indirect factors. We must understand which behavior changed, and how and why they changed if a Uganda model of prevention is to be replicated elsewhere. And it is precisely these aspects of behavior change that are now so poorly understood and heatedly debated.

We should not be put off by the vast cultural diversity argument that countries (cultures) are so diverse that no one model could fit all. In cultural elements of importance to AIDS prevention (health systems, health KABP, level of economic development, rural settlement patterns, types of communications channels available, role of religion in society in general and in schools and health care in particular, etc.), health-related cultural differences between African countries are far less than differences between African and non-African countries. This of course does not mean that there should not be efforts to adapt a Ugandan model to particular circumstances.

Stoneburner and Low-Beer (2002) suggest that once we clear away the biases and blinders that often obstruct understanding of what happened in Uganda, we indeed find a model of prevention—and for that matter of care and support—that can be adopted by other countries in Africa and elsewhere. A Uganda model has the potential to "provide a 'social vaccine' for AIDS with perhaps 80 percent efficacy . . . that could avert millions of deaths and prove as effective as any potential biomedical approach" (Stoneburner & Low-Beer, 2002b, p. 12). In fact, they estimated that 3.2 million lives could be saved in a ten-year period in South Africa alone (Stoneburner & Low-Beer, 1998).

I posted an observation about the Museveni approach to AIDS prevention on the Internet. A Ugandan AIDS worker wrote me the following response:

I was in Uganda when Museveni stepped up the campaign against HIV/AIDS. There was nothing else he could have done as one who was concerned about the welfare of his people. He had just come from the "bush war" and had seen a lot of suffering. We were also perishing. The disease was wiping out whole communities (villages) particularly in the southern part of central Uganda. Museveni took it upon himself to get everybody else talking about HIV/AIDS and sex. Government officials, church leaders, and students were all talking about AIDS everywhere, even at funerals. There was a time when catechists would tell us what killed the deceased and they appealed to those remaining to abstain from sex. It is true that the "Museveni Approach" worked for Ugandans. It will certainly work for others too.

I am convinced that the longer one takes before getting into sexual intercourse the more careful they get before getting into it at a later stage as they become adults or mature. If we convince our children and youths to abstain for now, they will certainly make better choices when they finally decide to get into sex. The same applies to adults. Those who have told themselves that the condom is not the solution are not easily taken for a sexual ride. Abstinence is a better approach than throwing condoms around and expecting people to use them all the time. (Ssemwogerere, 2002)

I have mentioned some of the arguments against the interpretation that PBC was the main cause of prevalence decline in Uganda. Some critics are now conceding that this may have been true in the 1980s, but that this has little relevance for what Uganda needs now. This may be called the "stages of epidemic" argument. That is, PBC might have occurred in the 1980s, especially among younger unmarried Ugandans, but now most infections are among older married or in-union discordant couples, that is, couples in which one partner is HIV infected. Therefore, the argument goes, there needs to be vigorous condom promotion to married or in-union couples to prevent infection.

There are at least two problems with this line of thinking. One is that married couples rarely use condoms with any consistency, even if they know one partner is HIV infected. Studies from Rakai suggest that consistent condom use in his group may not rise above 2 percent. The implication of another Rakai study suggests that male circumcision might prevent transmission (Quinn, Gray, & Sewankambo, 2000).

Also, most African countries are far from being at Uganda's stage of epidemic. In most countries, there is still a great deal of casual and premarital sex. Thus the Uganda model of broad, fundamental behavior change is exactly what most countries need.

At this writing, the Uganda model has begun to be embraced by the Bush administration. Although I am a liberal, I have been providing the evidence in this book to conservative and religious leaders because they have been willing to listen. They may have been willing to listen for ideological or political reasons, but still they have been receptive. My feeling was, If fellow liberals are unwilling to listen, then I will send the information to conservatives. The important thing is to get people to start looking at the evidence.

WHAT CAN BE LEARNED FROM A DISTRICT BORDERING UGANDA

Let us return briefly to the view held by some who believe that Uganda's decline in HIV infection rates has been due primarily or entirely to the stage of its epidemic rather than to interventions of any sort. Some point to Kagera region, Tanzania, to support this viewpoint. Kagera lies in the northwest of Tanzania, adjacent to Rakai, Uganda. Kagera is the region where AIDS first exploded in Tanzania in the 1980s. There were military incursions by Ugandan soldiers (under Idi Amin) in 1977, resulting in the rape of Tanzanian women and girls. In response, President Nyerere sent 45,000 Tanzanian soldiers, mostly young conscripts, to Kagera. They later invaded Uganda and overthrew Idi Amin. Whatever else can be said about both Kagera and neighboring Rakai district at this time, there was a lot of sexual mixing between Ugandans and Tanzanians. Some analysts believe that this was the main factor that explains why Rakai and Kagera became the epicenter of AIDS in East Africa (Hooper, 1999).

In addition, Kagera has historically been an area of plantation employment and relatively high salaries, trade and commerce in the Lake Victoria area, commercial sex, and the highest STD rates in Tanzania (Killewo, 1994). Indeed both commercial sex and high rates of STDs, especially syphilis, were described as special problems among the Haya-populated districts of Bukoba and Muleba as early as the 1920s. Explanations for high venereal disease rates offered at the time (and using the language reported at the time) include the traffic of prostitutes back and forth across Lake Victoria; a relatively high age of marriage among Haya men; moral lassitude; alcoholism; and lack of male circumcision. More recent explanations for both the prevalence of prostitution and STDs include the exploitation and oppression of Haya women, especially in marriage; material deprivation in a stratified, hierarchical, cash-dependant society; and the economic decline of the *kibanja* (commercial coffee plantation) system (Kaijage, 1989).

The populations of Kagera and Rakai are similar ethno-linguistically, epidemiologically (e.g., men are uncircumcised), and economically. Like neighboring Rakai, and indeed the rest of Uganda, HIV infection rates fell in Kagera after the early 1990s. In one study, population-based blood tests were conducted to see if and how HIV infection rates derived this way might differ from data derived from ANCs. They found little significant difference, as follows:

Age-adjusted prevalence among antenatal care attenders decreased from 22.4%... in 1990 to 16.1% . . . in 1993 and further to 13.7% . . . in 1996. These results closely resemble those of the majority population of adult women in the clinic's catchment area (the town of Bukoba) where the age-adjusted prevalence of 29.1% . . . in 1987 showed a decrease in the studies in 1993 18.7% . . . and in 1996 14.9%. (Kwesigabo et al., 2000, p. 410)

As in Uganda, there are also incidence data. These studies have shown a downward trend in incidence from 47.5 per thousand per year in 1989 (much higher than Uganda data I have seen) to 9.1 per thousand per year in 1996. And in Bukoba urban district of Kagera, incidence fell from 8.2 per thousand per year in 1989 to 3.9 per thousand per year in 2000 (Kwesigabo, 2001). Note that the 2000 urban rate is very similar to the 3.2 per thousand per year rate found in Kyamulibwa, Uganda, in 1998, as we saw previously.

To some epidemiologists, this evidence is used to argue that HIV rates simply go down after they reach a certain high level; those at risk of infection have already been infected, so rates have nowhere to go but down and we don't need to look to interventions to explain the decreases. Like Uganda, seroprevalence in Kagera fell most markedly among men and women ages fifteen to twenty-four, but even more so among females.

However, this does not explain why HIV prevalence levels have not declined in other countries in the region, including those where infection rates are higher than those of Uganda or Kagera ever were. If we find that interventions in Kagera closely resemble those in Rakai and elsewhere in Uganda, this might be taken as evidence that interventions relate in some causal way with prevalence decline. Let us consider some preliminary evidence of this sort.

More than 200 NGOs and local community-based organizations have been engaged in AIDS prevention in Kagera since 1989. There has been a greater concentration of prevention efforts here than any other region of Tanzania (Kapiga, 2002). There have been diverse forms of AIDS preventive education aimed at various target groups, HIV testing and counseling, spiritual counseling from religious organizations, systemic or structural interventions, such as restricting the duration of night ceremonies (where there are opportunities for casual sex), provision of home-based care, and the like (Kwesigabo et al., 1998). Although there is an apparent need for more behavioral studies, one epidemiological study concluded the following:

Behavioral change, especially postponement of sexual activity by young girls as a result of the demands from the Church for premarital HIV-1 testing, may account for the observed decline in younger women. Increased condom use (although discouraged by the Catholic Church) and decreased number of sexual partners may have accounted for the tendency of the prevalence to decline in other age groups. (Kwesigabo et al., 1998, p. 267)

In another population-based survey by the same lead author (Kwesigabo, 2001), 96 percent of men and women of Kagera said that they were taking precautions to avoid AIDS, namely, "sticking to one partner described as no sex outside marriage, condom use for casual sex and for individuals who are still single, abstinence coupled with voluntary counseling and testing (VCT) when they want to get married" (Annex II, p. 17). The average number of sexual partners did not change between 1993 and 1996 (between 1.1 and 1.3 partners per year), but urban condom use rose during this period from 23.1 percent to

30.2 percent. Condom use was not defined, but if it refers to male ever-use, it is higher than current male ever-use condom rates in Uganda. If it refers to use with the last nonregular partner, then rates are lower than those of Uganda as a whole.

It would be very useful to conduct research to see if the proportions reporting multiple partners, or not sticking to one partner, have changed since 1996. In fact, it would be most useful to have some measures of multiple partners in 1989, when incidence was 47.5 per thousand per year. I have not found these data in the published literature.

Gideon Kwesigabo and his research colleagues believe that preventive interventions probably account for incidence and prevalence decline in Kagera, although they admit they are unable to measure which programs have had what kind of specific effect "because of the multiplicity of interventions in the region that have largely been unsystematic and uncoordinated" (Kwesigabo et al., 1998, p. 267). Moreover, Kwesigabo and his colleagues found that declines in incidence and prevalence were uniform regardless of the baseline levels of infection (high, medium, or low) found in different parts of the region, suggesting that it was not merely stage of the local epidemic, fear of AIDS, or knowing someone with AIDS that led to decline in HIV seroprevalence. This can be seen in the following:

It is therefore concluded that there has been a decline in the prevalence and incidence of HIV-1 infection in areas of varying levels of HIV-1 infection in the Kagera region, especially so among young women. These findings with a declining trend in HIV-infection also in low-prevalence areas, where the epidemic could not have reached saturation, indicate that behavioural changes at individual level have resulted into this decline in the epidemic. (Kwesigabo, 2001, section IV)

Still, the behavioral data are incomplete. As in Karamoja and Moyo, Uganda, much could be learned about the impact of different interventions and about behavior change from further qualitative and quantitative behavioral studies in Kagera.

NOTES

1. These data were not published in the 1995 Uganda DHS but were for the 2000 DHS (DHS/Uganda, 2000). I was able to request the 1995 data from DHS and I asked if they would create a column for the percentage monogamous or abstaining. My request was granted but I was asked, Why would you want to ask that?

2. Thanks are due to Dr. Saifuddin Ahmed for noticing these data.

3. When the health issue is AIDS, the example of the solution is virtually always condoms.

7

Some Other African
Success Stories

SENEGAL

Senegal is another country often recognized as an AIDS success story. With Uganda, it was one of the first countries in Africa to openly acknowledge AIDS as a serious problem and to begin implementing significant AIDS prevention and control programs. There is debate over whether there has been prevalence decline in Senegal in recent years. The U.S. Bureau of the Census compiles global HIV prevalence data, and its latest HIV/AIDS profile for Senegal suggests no clear trend. HIV-1 prevalence at Dakar ANCs has remained at 0.5 percent or lower since 1996. At least it is possible to say that HIV prevalence seems not to be rising and Senegal has one of the lowest rates in sub-Saharan Africa. The census bureau profile begins, "Senegal has been a success story, as the government has managed to keep the epidemic from getting out of control" (BUCEN, 2000, p. 1). Unlike the great majority of sub-Saharan African countries, Senegal's epidemic is classified as concentrated rather than generalized. This means that most HIV is found concentrated in a few defined high-risk groups, such as sex workers and their clients.

There were significant declines in STD rates among women between 1991 and 1996: chlamydia fell from 11.7 percent to 6.1 percent; gonorrhea fell from 2.9 percent to 0.9 percent; syphilis fell from 7.5 percent to 4.4 percent; and trichomoniasis fell from 30.1 percent to 18.1 percent (Sittitrai, 2001). Chancroid was found, especially in CSWs, and it is reported to have declined markedly (Steen, 2001).

As with the president of Uganda, President Abdou Diouf of Senegal acknowledged the presence of AIDS and began implementing a national AIDS prevention and control program in 1987, about the same time Uganda began its program. Unlike Uganda, Senegal only had a few cases of HIV in 1987. It seems very likely that starting an effective AIDS control program at such an early epidemic stage made a big difference. Yet some special factors have also helped to keep infection rates down in Senegal. The first is male circumcision. Another may be the prevalence of HIV-2, another form of HIV found in parts of West Africa. It seems that presence of HIV-2 may somehow provide some degree of protection against HIV-1 infection (Kanki, 2002).

Outreach to CSWs

What was done in Senegal to prevent AIDS? Let us start with interventions aimed at high-risk groups and then turn to the majority population. There were early efforts aimed at high-risk groups that in fact did prove in later years to be core transmitters in the African mosaic of epidemics. Senegal already had what deserves to be called a public health-enlightened program for CSWs who have been registered with the government since 1970 as part of a national public health program. Since 1986, CSWs have received free physician health care, along with AIDS and STD education and care for their children and families (Kanki, 2002). There are some 2,500 registered sex workers in Dakar and several groups of about 200 each in other cities around the country. Moreover there appears to have been strong condom promotion to CSWs. By the late 1990s, 98 percent of CSWs reported using a condom at last sex with a regular client and 94 percent reported using a condom with a new client (Meda et al., 2000).

These efforts directed at CSWs—along with the biological factors mentioned—may have kept HIV infection rates from climbing to the rates found among CSWs in other African cities. Prevalence among CSWs was recently about 12 percent in Dakar, where most sex work is concentrated, in 2000 (Kanki, 2002).

This outreach to CSWs seems similar to programs in the Philippines and Indonesia where HIV infection among CSWs has also remained relatively low by regional and global standards. It may be argued that HIV prevalence has not—or not yet—really started in these two Asian countries, even though the first case of HIV in Asia was found in the Philippines. Some countries where HIV rates have risen, then stabilized or declined, such as the Dominican Republic and Thailand, also reached out to sex workers with peer education, condom provision, and STD treatment programs (Welsh, Puello, Meade, Kome, & Nutley, 2001).

Other interventions aimed at high-risk groups seem to have had impact. For example, a longitudinal study of male clients of Senegalese CSWs ("transportation workers") found that AIDS preventive education through peer education led to both condom use and perhaps partner reduction, as seen in the following:

Significant increases in men's HIV-related knowledge, previous use of condoms (30.4–53.5%), and consistent condom use with regular sex partners were documented over the study period, as were significant declines in perceived barriers to condom use. Though men reported significantly fewer sexual encounters with casual and commercial partners at follow-up compared to baseline, these data were unreliable. (Leonard et al., 2000, p. 21)

Behavior Change in the Majority Population

Turning to the majority population, let us first consider the evidence of behavioral change and then to the question of how and why change may have come about. Researchers compared two cross-sectional surveys using standardized questionnaires conducted in 1990–1992 and again in 1994. Even by 1994, "the proportion of men who declared casual sex partners in the past 12 months decreased from 39% to 21% (P = 0.01). However, the proportion remained stable for women (from 15% to 18%)" (Lagarde, Pison, & Enel, 1997). Condom use (ever-used) was 3.6 percent in 1993, similar to Uganda's level at that time (UNAIDS, 2000b). By 1998, the proportion of surveyed people reporting condom use during last intercourse with a risky partner was 58 percent for employed men, and 55 percent for women ages fourteen to seventy-five (UNAIDS, 2000b). But only a relatively small group of Senegalese have sex with high-risk partners, and this group constitutes the denominator here (see next section).

As often happens with Uganda, articles in prestigious journals like *AIDS* are likely to attribute Senegal's success to aggressive condom promotion, along with political commitment and community participation, ignoring the role of PBC (e.g., Darrow, 2001). Yet a 1997 survey of women in Dakar, where condom use might be expected to be the highest in Senegal, found that 23 percent of women ages sixteen to fifty reported ever using a condom (UNAIDS, 2000b).

Sittitrai (2001), of UNAIDS, is more balanced in explaining Senegal's success. She first cites the relatively late age of sexual debut, followed by partner reduction. Increased condom use and apparently quite effective STD control are also credited. Let us look at the evidence more closely.

Delaying Sexual Intercourse

According to DHS surveys (Macro International, CESDEM, PROFAMILIA, & ONAPLAN, 1997), the median age of female sexual debut has risen somewhat in Senegal, from 18.6 in 1992–1993 to 19.2 in

1997. For the youngest Senegalese women (ages fifteen to twenty-four), the median age of debut rose from 17.5 to 18.8. This means that by 1997, the average age of debut of younger women was nearly nineteen, perhaps evidence that those at whom the delay message is targeted were in fact responding. In fact, the median age of debut of urban Senegalese women ages twenty to twenty-four was 22.3, according to the 1997 DHS.

Recall that the DHS was—and at the time of writing this, still is—calculating median age of debut on the basis of only those who have had a debut, meaning that the actual age, if all delayers of sexual debut were counted as well, would be higher.

For age-specific comparisons, median age of debut for females ages twenty to twenty-four rose from 17.5 in 1993 to eighteen by 1997. For females ages forty-five to forty-nine, debut rose from 15.8 in 1993 to seventeen by 1997. DHS data seem lacking for males before 1997, but by 1997 age of debut ranged between eighteen and twenty, depending on the age group (UNAIDS, 2000b).

From examination of DHS tables in which age of sexual debut is broken down by age group, a trend toward a higher age for younger age groups is evident, suggesting changes in behavior over time. For example, the 1986 DHS shows that women then in the age group forty-five to forty-nine had their first sexual experience at the median age of 15.9, in about 1970.

But as previously discussed, as well as on the DHS Web site, the measures of age of debut used here miss the proportions of respondents who have not had a debut at time of interviewing. For a better measure, only 9 percent of never-married females ages fifteen to twenty-four reported any type of sexual partner in 1997: Seven percent of females in the ages fifteen to nineteen group, and 15 percent in the ages twenty to twenty-four group (DHS/Senegal, 1999). These remarkable data can be viewed on the DHS Web site: http://www.measuredhs.com/hivdata/surveys/survey_ind_data.cfm?survey_id=81&survey_ind_id=1064&ind_id=57. This represents a 25 percent decline from the 1992–1993 Senegal DHS, when 12 percent of never-married females ages fifteen to twenty-four reported any type of sexual partner. This rises to only 17.5 percent among females ages twenty to twenty-four (DHS/Senegal, 1999). More males begin sex at an early age: 35.2 percent in age cohort fifteen to nineteen report a sexual partner (DHS/Senegal, 1999). We also see that these rates are lower in Senegal than in all but a few sub-Saharan African countries. The comparable rates in Botswana are 72 percent (1988) and 62 percent in Côte D'Ivoire (1994).

A 2001 study of never married females in Dakar ages fifteen to twenty-three was conducted by (FHI), with USAID and CDC funding, through the Senegalese Ministry of Health. Only twenty-nine females out of a random sample of 699 reported ever having had intercourse. This means that 95.9 percent were delaying sex; only 4.1 percent were having sex (Hygea/FHI, 2001). This represents a very low proportion of girls and young women having early sex, by almost any country's standard, especially since about 11 percent of the sample is in the age group twenty to twenty-three.

An earlier study by FHI in 1997, under the AIDSCAP project, found very different proportions of sexually active students reporting "at least one sex partner other than a regular partner in the last 12 months." For "pupils" ages thirteen to twenty-four, 21 percent of men and 15 percent of women reported outside partner(s). For "students" ages fifteen to thirty, 40 percent of men and 15 percent of women reported outside partner(s) (UNAIDS/Senegal, 2000, p. 9). This looks very different from the 2001 study which shows that only 4.1 percent of young women had ever had sex. We immediately want to know what proportion of men and women in the 1997 studies were sexually active. Unless we know that, these data can be very misleading. Senegal looks like one of the most multipartneristic countries in the world. Unfortunately I do not know the denominators in these studies. The studies seem to be unpublished and were only summarized in UNAIDS/Senegal (2000, p. 9).

Still, we see again that the better indicator to capture delay of sexual debut, and to serve as a measure of the proportion of vulnerable young women who are at-risk, is the proportion of sexually active females in age cohort fifteen to nineteen or fifteen to twenty-three. It is useful to capture both those who have ever had intercourse and those who have had any intercourse in the past year.

Most (55%) of the twenty-nine young women in the FHI study who reported having any number of partners in the 2001 study reported just one partner (Hygea/FHI, 2001). More than incidentally, 85 percent of the women who reported a sexual debut said that the debut was involuntary, against their will and wishes.

The report of this study, typically, goes on to discuss for many pages its findings about male and female condoms, although with so few females reporting intercourse, there are few data to report. It almost seems like the abstinence findings caught the researchers by surprise, except that the 1997 DHS in Senegal shows that same pattern. One wonders if the instrument for this study was pretested. With so few women having any sexual experience, why would one waste time and money on asking so many condom questions? Surely, the big story in this survey is how few women have ever had sex. Surely, one would want to follow up on this unexpected discovery and find out why there is so little sexual experience and then look for explanations from all sources.

In fact, the 2001 findings could not have taken the researchers by surprise because the same organizations that conducted this study, FHI and Hygea, had done BSS surveys among presumed high-risk groups earlier, in both 1997 and 1998. FHI explains this type of survey in the following:

Behavioral Surveillance Surveys (BSS) provide valuable data about HIV/AIDS-related knowledge, attitudes, and behaviors. The BSS methodology is a monitoring and evaluation tool designed to track trends in HIV/AIDS-related knowledge, attitudes, and behaviors in subpopulations at particular risk of HIV infection, such as female sex workers, injection drug users, migrant men, and youth. Based on classic HIV and sexually transmitted disease (STD) serologic surveillance methods, BSS consist of repeated cross-sectional surveys conducted systematically to monitor changes in HIV/STD risk behaviors. (Hygea/FHI, 1998, p. 1)

Urban students between ages fifteen and nineteen were presumed to be high-risk groups, along with female sex workers. The groups listed in Table 7.1 were interviewed.

Regarding sexual behavior, the two waves of research found the following:

The majority of females in both waves had never had sexual intercourse, and that percentage increased from almost 88 percent in wave one to almost 95 percent in wave two. On the other hand, approximately one-third of male students had had sexual intercourse, and this level remained stable across the two survey waves (34.2 percent in wave one and 35 percent in wave two). Since the level of sexual activity was low among the females surveyed, the remainder of this section will focus on males. (Hygea/FHI, 1998, p. 1)

Most sexually active males reported having only one partner. Males having two or more nonregular partners increased from 14.1 percent to 17.4 percent between 1997 and 1998. Unfortunately, we do not know what this figure is after 1998, but even these somewhat dated figures show that urban Senegalese male students, chosen because they were thought to constitute a high-risk group, report significantly fewer partners than, for example, Zambians, Kenyans, and Swazis.

No doubt condoms play a role in at least Dakar: "The majority of males in both waves reported consistent use of condoms with their non-regular partners. 'Always' use of condoms with non-regular partners increased between waves one and two from 54.3 percent to 63.6 percent" (Hygea/FHI, 1998, p. 1).

Again the situation resembles Uganda: not many men, and even fewer women, have nonregular partners, and those that do—especially if young, urban, and unmarried—tend to use condoms. Also closely

Table 7.1
Groups Interviewed in Senegalese Surveys

Subpopulations	Sample Size		Survey Sites	
	1997	1998	1997	1998
Male students	444	1181	Dakar, Kaolack, Thies, and Ziguinchor provinces	Dakar, Kaolack, Thiés, Ziguinchor, Saint-Louis, Louga, Tambacounda, Fatick, Diourbel, and Kolda provinces
Female students	478	1179		
Female sex workers (FSWs)	449	681		

Source: Hygea/FHI, 1998.

resembling Uganda is the finding that fewer than 3 percent of sexually active male respondents reported sex with a female sex worker. In Uganda, 1.6 percent of males reported paying for sex in the previous twelve months (Macro International, 2001, p. 186), but this is from a national sample rather than one of urban male students.

The other high-risk group in the two waves of BSS was female sex workers. The study found that FSWs had significantly earlier sexual debuts than women on the average, and that "always" use of condoms with regular clients was over 90 percent during both waves, rising to almost 98 percent of FSWs with one-time clients in wave two, up from 93.9 percent in wave one (Hygea/FHI, 1998). This again is very similar to FSW condom user rates in the large cities of Uganda.

Why Behavior Change?

A group of Senegalese and UNAIDS researchers posed a question in the title of their article, "Low and stable HIV infection rates in Senegal: natural course of the epidemic or evidence for success of prevention?" They concluded, "From available data, Senegal can rightfully claim to have contained the spread of HIV by intervening early and comprehensively to increase knowledge and awareness of HIV/AIDS and to promote safe sexual behaviour" (Meda et al., 2000, p. 1276). They noted the following:

From 1989 to 1996, the levels of HIV infection estimated in four sentinel urban regions remained stable at around 1.2% in the population of pregnant women. . . .

A strong political and community commitment led to an early response to the HIV/AIDS epidemic that has been extended since 1986. Blood transfusion safety was established at the start of the HIV epidemic. The level of knowledge of preventive practices relating to HIV/AIDS among the majority population exceeded 90% in the early 1990s. From 1991 to 1996, a 30% to 66% decrease of the STD prevalence rates was observed in pregnant women and sex workers in Dakar. In 1997, 33% of men aged 15–49 years in Dakar reported having had sex with non-regular partners. (Meda et al., 2000, p. 1276)

Ng (2000) agrees that "strong, sustained prevention campaigns have kept the virus under relative control" (p. 2) in Senegal.

What might account for this containment of AIDS, low prevalence rates and apparent behavior change in Senegal? The argument cannot be made that high mortality, and fear resulting from this, were contributing factors, since infection rates remained so low. One factor is that the government acted without delay to address the problem. And when it began to act, 1987, there were very few HIV cases in Senegal. Early interventions aimed at high-risk groups, notably CSWs, no doubt helped prevent HIV transmission to the majority population.

Meanwhile the majority population, especially women, already seemed to exhibit less risk factors than women in most of Africa. Moreover there were Uganda-like interventions aimed at the majority population. As in Uganda, FBOs became involved in HIV/AIDS prevention from early in the epidemic in Senegal. A conservative Muslim organization, Jamra, approached the national AIDS program in 1989 to discuss prevention strategies (UNAIDS, 1999a). As in Uganda, there was initial disagreement about the role of FBOs in condom promotion. The government conducted a survey of Muslim and Christian leaders to better define a role for them in AIDS mitigation. The survey found that religious leaders needed and wanted more information about HIV/AIDS, so that they in turn could educate those in the respective religious communities. The response can be seen in the following:

In response, educational materials were designed to meet the needs of religious leaders. They focused in part on testimonials from people living with AIDS—the human face of the epidemic, often hidden where prevalence remains low. Training sessions about HIV were organized for Imams and teachers of Arabic, and brochures were produced to help them disseminate information. AIDS became a regular topic in Friday sermons in mosques throughout Senegal, and senior religious figures addressed the issue on television and radio. (UNAIDS, 1999a, p. 12)

A Catholic NGO, SIDA, also became involved in prevention as well as counseling and psychosocial support. In 1996, a meeting on AIDS prevention was held for Christian leaders; every bishop in Senegal attended and consensus was reached that AIDS prevention was an important national priority (UNAIDS, 1999a). The following year, Senegal hosted the First International Colloquium on AIDS and Religion, held in Dakar in late 1997. It was attended by some 250 persons from thirty-three countries, including Muslim, Christian, and Buddhist religious leaders and the ministers of health of five African countries (Ladame, 1998). The impact on Senegalese religious leaders of all faiths seems to have been to empower them "to act freely in the promotion of prevention strategies" (Diouf, Paul, Leopold, & Ibra, 2000). Yet there was much to overcome before this was possible, as seen in the following:

During the first stages of the AIDS epidemic the majority of religious (leaders) condemned those infected with the virus, calling the illness a divine curse. This attitude made AIDS shameful and a positive diagnosis difficult. Religion systematically condemned certain modes of prevention as well as certain individual and group behaviour. (Diouf et al., 2000)

A recent *Los Angeles Times* article describes the role of FBOs and religious leaders today as follows:

Conservative Islamic leaders are supporting AIDS prevention activities. Imams have started making AIDS a regular topic in Friday sermons throughout Senegal, where more than 90% of the population is Muslim.

While the religious leaders insist that they encourage abstinence over the use of condoms, they acknowledge the importance of dispelling myths about the disease, such as the common theory that AIDS is a curse or a punishment by God. (Simmons, 2001, p. A1)

It may be argued that sexual behavior in Senegal, especially that of women, is unusually low risk, therefore perhaps it is preexisting norms and values rather than the impact of any interventions that have kept infection rates low. Furthermore, widespread male circumcision among Senegalese men certainly helps prevent heterosexual transmission of HIV. It may even be that the presence of HIV-2 in Senegal and the region has the effect of inhibiting HIV-1 transmission. And there are some virologists who believe the predominant HIV-1 subtype, clade A (actually the variant HIV-1 A-G is the predominant clade), is less infective than clade C which predominates in many of the high-prevalence countries of southern Africa. It may also be that there is less alcohol consumption in Senegal than in most of sub-Saharan Africa, due in part to religious influence (Sankale, personal communication, October 24, 2001). But none of these considerations explain why HIV infection rates have risen in countries neighboring Senegal, countries comparable with regard to the factors just mentioned, including religious profiles. They do not explain why Senegal's rates have remained constant, or have declined.

As in Uganda, it is impossible to isolate the contribution of FBOs from other factors in AIDS prevention, especially since there has been so little attention to FBOs by AIDS researchers anywhere in the world. The authors of one cross-sectional survey in Senegal conclude that religion (defined by answer to a survey question intended to measure if religion is very important to respondents) has led to greater likelihood of fidelity to a single partner on the part of respondents (Lagarde et al., 1999). More research is certainly needed, both related to the role of FBOs and to all of the possible causal factors related to primary behavior change.

Pisani (1999) from UNAIDS summarizes the factors that seem to account for low prevalence in Senegal.

There are three factors that determined exposure to HIV infection and the recorded low levels in the country. (1) Sexual activity begins relatively late and extramarital sex is relatively limited; (2) condom use during extramarital sex, and especially during commercial sex, is high; and (3) sexually transmitted disease control programs are apparently quite effective. These findings suggest that Senegal's early and comprehensive prevention efforts have made a major contribution to keeping HIV infection at low rates. These efforts include: political, religious, and community leadership; provision of information to communities at high risk, especially sex workers and young people; and a pragmatic approach to public health emphasizing prevention and the provision of health services. (p. 25)

I feel this is a fair characterization, although it does not mention male circumcision or other factors not addressed by interventions. In fact, analysts seem to understand the elements of Senegal's success quite well. Another analyst attributes success to the following elements:

The early response to AIDS, vigorous preventive action, care of AIDS patients, and the mobilization of people at all levels have contributed to the success against the spread of HIV in Senegal. Democracy and freedom of the press have also allowed open discussion of the problems and easy access to information. In addition, the systematic screening of donated blood, programs against sexually transmitted diseases, allocation of budgetary resources, and incorporation of AIDS education in school curricula are among the initiatives responsible for keeping HIV infections low in the country. Promoting contraceptives through peer education has proven to be effective in overcoming sexual taboos. Moreover, the active engagement of religious leaders in the battle against AIDS has changed the attitude of the people toward contraception and reduced risky practices. Within the military and private businesses several preventive measures have been taken against HIV infection, such as training concerning AIDS and seminars stressing the importance of disseminating information on AIDS. (Lom, 2001, p. 24)

Note the similarity with Uganda: public discussion in a relatively free, open atmosphere; relative democracy and freedom of the press; and easy access to information.

The wonder is that there is not more discussion about the experience of Senegal. Aside from the occasional nod toward Senegal as an AIDS success story, it seems not to be mentioned often and, most important, its lessons seem not to be have been learned by most who work in international AIDS. In fact, Senegal seems to present a model of the right balance between A, B, C, and even D (for drugs) interventions: condoms and treatment of STDs were targeted at high-risk populations, and this had measurable impact on CSW condom user rates, and on STD rates, including notably chancroid. There are in fact several countries in West Africa where the difference between CSWs and the majority population in HIV prevalence is striking—more so than in southern or East Africa. In such areas, it makes a lot of public health sense to target CSWs with interventions designed to prevent CSWs from infecting their clients.

Meanwhile primary behavior change has been directed at the majority Senegalese population through promoting widespread awareness, peer education, mobilization of religious leaders, and incorporation of AIDS education in schools. Note that Senegal has held a number of international symposia on AIDS, on, for example, the prevention of mother-to-child transmission of HIV, role of religious leaders, role of traditional healers, AIDS research priorities and methodologies, and the like. This suggests that a number of outside AIDS experts have visited Senegal and were exposed to its program of well-balanced interventions.

ZAMBIA

HIV prevalence increased rapidly in Zambia in the 1980s, and then seemed to stabilize in the early 1990s (Bessinger & Akwara, 2003). National prevalence among fifteen to forty-nine year olds was estimated at 20 percent in 1998 and at 16 percent in 2001–2002, although the difference may be due at least in part to the populations sampled. The latter figure is derived from a population-based sero survey that was part of the 2001–2002 DHS. In the absence of cohorts tracking incidence in Zambian populations, epidemiologist Steve Hodgins of USAID/Zambia has developed a model using a variety of known information sources, such as prevalence data, census figures, data from DHS on adult mortality, literature from elsewhere on expected vertical transmission rates, and the like. He believes that national seroincidence began declining before 1995, and has been prevalent since 1999 (Hodgins, 2003). Tables compiled by the U.S. Census Bureau (not shown) indicate that prevalence at ANC sites has fallen, or fallen most, among the youngest age cohort (fifteen to nineteen years).

In the mid-1990s, the number of sentinel surveillance sites was increased to expand geographic coverage of the ANC-based sentinel system to all provinces. A parallel system of population-based HIV surveys among selected sentinel populations was established so that HIV infection, social, and behavioral data could also be collected and compared with ANC data (Fylkesnes et al., 2001). After rounds of data collection in 1996 and 1999, both ANC and population based, researchers concluded the following:

The ANC-based data showed a dominant trend of significant declines in HIV prevalence in the 15–19 years age group, and for urban sites also in age group 20–24 years and overall when rates were adjusted for overrepresentation of women with low education. In the majority population prevalence declined significantly in urban women aged 15–29 years whereas it showed a tendency to decline among rural women aged 15–24 years. Prominent decline in prevalence was associated with higher education, stable or rising prevalence with low education. (Fylkesnes et al., 2001, p. 907)

Thus we see a trend in HIV decline in young cohorts, but not a national trend. As seen in several other African countries, the highest rate of prevalence decline is in youth, the cohort for whom it would be least likely that AIDS-related mortality would have accounted for the decline. There was more prevalence decline among those with more education, a pattern found elsewhere in Africa, including Uganda, South Africa, and Ethiopia.

Behavioral Findings

Looking at behavioral change findings for total populations surveyed, ages fifteen to forty-nine years, we see from the ANC-based surveys that:

Urban men and women reported less sexual activity, fewer multiple sexual partners, and more consistent use of condoms in 1999 compared with 1996. Changes in sexual activity were most pronounced in the younger age groups. The proportion of urban men aged 15–19 years reporting any sexual activity in the last 12 months declined from 47 to 23%, whereas the proportion with two or more sexual partners fell from 52 to 38%. In contrast, no evident change was revealed in most behavioural indicators in the rural population (except that more than 90% reported to have less sexual partners compared with some years ago). (Fylkesnes et al., 2001, p. 912)

Notice the little significance given to the 90 percent of the sample who decreased casual sex. Urban condom use with nonregular partner rose

43 to 46 percent in males and 29 to 33 percent in females (Fylkesnes et al., 2001, p. 912). Corresponding rural rates were 23 to 17 percent for men and 10 to 9 percent for women.

Behavioral trends from the ANC-based surveys are summarized in Table 7.2.

Table 7.2
Changes in Sexual Behavior, 1996-1999, Zambian Population-Based Surveys

Condom used with last nonregular partners

	Males 15-49		Females 15-49	
	1996	1999	1996	1999
Urban	43 %	46 %	29 %	33 %
Rural	23 %	17 %	10 %	9 %

Sexually active in the past 12 months

	Males 15-49		Females 15-49	
	1996	1999	1996	1999
Urban	79 %	73 %	80 %	72 %
Rural	95 %	84 %	93 %	84 %

>2 sexual partners in past 12 months

	Males 15-49		Females 15-49	
	1996	1999	1996	1999
Urban	38 %	31 %	8 %	5 %
Rural	40 %	37 %	6 %	7 %

Sexually active in the past 12 months with >2 sexual partners

	Males 15-19		Females 15-19	
	1996	1999	1996	1999
Urban	47 %	23 %	52 %	38 %

Source: Fylkesnes et al., 2001, p. 913.

If we compare DHS behavioral data for Zambian female youth between 1992 and 1996, reported premarital sex declined from 42 percent to 36 percent. We have no 1992 data for men but 57 percent reported premarital sex. The newly available Zambia DHS 2001–2002 shows that the median age at first sex is about the same for women as it was in 1996 (seventeen for women ages fifteen to twenty-four), but it is higher for men: eighteen compared to 16.2 in 1996 (ORC Macro, 2003, p. 98).

Comparing DHS data in Zambia between 1996 and 1998 (available on the DHS/Measure Web site), the proportion reporting "higher risk sex" in the past twelve months decreased from 23 percent to 17 percent among women, and from 49 percent to 31 percent among men. Condom use in last sex with spouse or cohabiting partner actually decreased during this two-year period, although it rose for condom use in high-risk encounters.

Among the group whose HIV prevalence decline was greatest and statistically significant and whose behavior changed the most, namely, young urban females, "Delayed age at first birth was found among urban women aged 17–22 years ($P < 0.001$), a delay that had resulted in a 40% decline in fertility in the age group 15–24 years (measured as number of children ever given birth to, $P < 0.001$). No similar change was found among rural women" (Fylkesnes et al., 2001, p. 913). It is a pity there were no direct measures of delay of sexual debut in these surveys, but increased abstinence in the young age groups, as well as delayed age at first birth should reflect a trend of later debut.

In another measure of regular condom use, reported condom use at last sex with a nonmarital or noncohabiting partner, there has been some increase, especially among young females between the mid-1990s and later, according to DHS studies. Using this measure, male use rose from 33 percent to 39 percent between 1996 and 2002 (compare 70% in Zimbabwe, 59% in Uganda, 44% in Kenya, 29% in Cameroon) (Bessinger & Akwara, 2003).

The Carolina Population Center, the Zambian Central Statistical Office, and the University of Zambia analyzed data from several sources: the 1990 WHO/GPA, the DHS of 1992 and 1996, and the 1998 Zambia Sexual Behavior Survey (ZSBS). This study described trends in knowledge and sexual behavior in urban Lusaka from 1990 to 1998, and in Zambia as a whole between 1996 and 1998. They found a decline in premarital sexual activity in Lusaka:

In 1990, 50% of never married women reported no sexual experience, compared with 60% in 1998 (p = .003); among men, the figures were 38% and 53%, respectively (p < .001). Fewer women (1990, 8%; 1998, 2%; p < .001) and men (1990, 31%; 1998, 19%; p = .07) had extramarital partners. The bulk of change observed in urban Lusaka took place from 1990 to 1996; the changes in men's behavior observed between 1996 and 1998 were also observed in the national estimates for those years. (Bloom et al., 2000, p. 77)

The authors note that the declines "could not be explained by earlier age at marriage and appear to concur with other studies in Africa that have first observed changes in sexual behavior among adolescents" (Bloom et al., 2000, p. 83). National figures for other indicators between 1992 and 1998 were less encouraging. Fewer men had premarital sex from 1996 to 1998 (1996, 64%; 1998, 46%; p < .001), but there was no change in women's sexual behavior. Condom use with nonregular partners decreased among men (1996, 38%; 1998, 29%; p = .02), although there was an increase in ever-use of condoms (Bloom et al., 2000, p. 77).

A study of Lusaka youths (ages ten to twenty-four) found that girls were having first sexual experience later than boys, at a median age of sixteen rather than fifteen. Moreover, "A higher proportion of males than females reported having had sex in the 10–14 and 15–19 year age groups, but the proportions were similar among 20–24 year-olds" (Magnani et al., 2002, pp. 79–80). Condom use in Africa tends to be highest among the young and single. In the present study:

Only a minority of respondents (38.7% of males and 27.7% of females) reported having used a condom during their last sexual encounter. Yet smaller proportions reported using a condom "always" or "almost always" with their current/most recent regular partner (27.8% of males and 16.7% of females). Thus, although a large majority of respondents recognized condom use as an effective means of preventing HIV transmission and most agreed that condoms were easy to use, consistent condom use appears to be practiced by a only small a minority of Lusakan youth. (Magnani et al., 2002, p. 81)

A Youth Campaign Promoting Abstinence and Condoms

It is useful to look at an AIDS prevention intervention aimed at Zambian youth to better understand the various factors involved in promoting behavior change, as well as possible causal relationships between them. A recent television campaign aimed at Zambian youths taught abstinence and condom use as ways to protect against HIV infection and AIDS. Fidelity or partner reduction was not part of the message. The campaign was called Helping Each Other Act Responsibly Together (HEART), and it is said to have been "designed specifically for youth and by youth. . . . Young people age 13–19 were the intended audience for the campaign" (Underwood, Hachonda, Serlemitsos, & Bharath, 2001).

Some of the media spots dealt with abstinence, such as the following, in the words of the report:

- Choices I Make, with abstinent boys reminding their peers of why they choose to be abstinent
- "When He Says . . . ," with a series of lines from boys to which girls can reply, "no to sex," and maintain their "virgin power/virgin pride" (Underwood et al., 2001, p. 11)

To evaluate the campaign, a quasi-experimental, pretest and posttest design was used. The pretest survey was conducted from July to November 1999 and the posttest was fielded in August 2000. The evaluation report is well worth reading and it certainly deserves publication and broad dissemination. For one thing, it shows that both abstinence and condoms can be promoted in the same youth campaign and show positive results in achieving both types of targeted behavior change. This alone is an important finding because those who favor abstinence promotion sometimes argue that promotion of this along with condoms (A and C, so to speak) sends a mixed message. Or they may argue that condom promotion undermines the abstinence or delay-of-debut message, so it may make more sense to promote one or the other, but not both at the same time.

The evaluation found that 75 percent of males and 68 percent of females who were exposed to the campaign began talking with others about AIDS, abstinence, and using condoms as a result of the campaign. Among the notable behavior change findings were the following:

- Among women who are sexually experienced, 82 percent of campaign viewers contrasted with 69 percent of baseline and 64 percent of impact survey nonviewers reported they feel confident that they have the ability to say no to unwanted sex.
- Using logistic regression and holding the independent variables age, educational attainment, urban/rural residence, and sex constant, data show that viewers are 1.68 times more likely to report primary or secondary abstinence than were nonviewers.
- There was a dose effect: The more health communication spots recalled, the greater the likelihood that the respondent is abstinent.
- Logistic regression analysis found that viewers were 1.91 times more likely to have ever used a condom and 1.63 times more likely to report condom use during last sex when contrasted with nonviewers (holding sex, age, residence, and education constant). Older, better-educated respondents were more likely than others were to use condoms.
- Interestingly, women were more likely to report condom use than were men when background characteristics were held constant. (Underwood, Hachonda, Serlemitsos, & Bharath, 2001, p. 7)

The evaluators found that 28.6 percent of all surveyed reported adopting abstinence, while about half, 14.6 percent, adopted condom use. "Viewers were asked what action, if any, they took as a result of viewing the various spots. The fact that respondents were more likely to say they chose 'to abstain' than to report that they decided to use a condom as a result of viewership, needs to be further explored" (Underwood et al., 2001, p. 22). Note that some of the youths surveyed may have already been abstaining/delaying, and some may already have been using condoms.

Among the study's recommendations were the following:

- Continue to support and encourage abstinence or a "return to abstinence" as a viable alternative
- Convey the idea that abstinence is a social norm among young people
- Portray the use of consistent condom use as a social norm (Underwood et al., 2001, p. 8)

Fear of HIV infection was the main reason abstainers gave for abstaining from sex. Abstainers who had not been exposed to the campaign were more likely to cite not having a partner or the opportunity for sex. The study also suggests that young people in areas of high HIV prevalence will respond to delay/abstinence messages, and a significant number will choose this behavior change (or maintenance) option.

The HEART campaign was high-tech, but the evaluation report notes that it "is one among a range of programs designed to enable young people to protect their reproductive health. Community mobilization efforts, faith-based projects, school curricula, and several media programs have addressed many of the issues central to the HEART Campaign" (Underwood et al., 2001, p. 8).

However, the abstract from a Barcelona paper, presented by Carol Underwood, states the findings differently from this same study, namely, "holding sex, age, residence and education constant, logistic regression analysis revealed that those who had seen the campaign (viewers) were 46% more likely to report abstinence than were those who had not seen the campaign (non-viewers). The data also demonstrated that sexually active viewers were 67% more likely to report condom use during last sex than were non-viewers" (Van Lith, Hachonda, & Underwood, 2002).

Is the difference due to the denominator used in the full study report including everyone, whereas in the abstract it is only the sexually active? And in the abstract, does condom use refer to ever-use of condoms, so this includes those who may have been using condoms before the campaign? These divergent findings need to be clarified. In spite of these problems, this project and its evaluation are important because abstinence and condom promotion messages need not necessarily exclude one another. They can both be successfully promoted in the same campaign, resulting in higher levels of both behaviors. This is not to deny that there is some inherent contradiction in the simultaneous promotion of abstinence and condom use.

Note that the time frame in this evaluation is short. If these results can be achieved in less than a year, it should not be surprising that high proportions of youth in Uganda are abstaining and delaying after years of hearing this message from mass media (e.g., Straight Talk radio spots and programs), from primary school onward (e.g., SHEP and Life Skills), from FBO efforts (e.g., CHUSA, IMAU, Teen Star), and a host of other community-based efforts.

Zambia Peer Sexual Education Intervention

Another abstinence/condom education program, the Zambia Peer Sexual Education Intervention, relied on peer educators rather than mass media. The project was implemented in secondary schools in Zambia by the Society for Family Health/Zambia, a social marketing organization, with support from Population Services International. Male and female secondary students were exposed to a brief educational session (1 hour, 45 minutes) about abstinence and condoms conducted by peer educators. After six months, student beliefs and (self-reported) behavior from both experimental and control groups were compared. Those who were exposed to peer education exhibited positive changes in normative beliefs about abstinence.

In a baseline survey, there were few differences in knowledge, attitudes, and beliefs between the intervention and control site. In comparison of findings from two cross-sectional surveys conducted in Lusaka between 1996 and 1999, researchers found statistically significant reductions in casual partnerships among men and women as seen in the following:

Approximately 7% of women reported having had last sex with a casual partner in 1996, compared with 3% in 1999; approximately 27% of men reported having had last sex with a casual partner in 1996, compared with 19% in 1999. Declines in casual sex were especially large for respondents who reported not having a partner at the time of the survey: 41% of women with no current partner reported having last sex with a casual partner in 1996, compared with 13% in 1999; 73% of men who did not have a current partner in 1996 reported having last sex with a casual partner, compared with 49% in 1999. (Agha, 2002, p. 293)

Condom use (during last sex act) increased to 21 percent (women) and 28 percent (men) in 1999. Decline in casual sex was associated with higher socioeconomic status. There was little change in levels of abstinence, seemingly because at baseline, nearly 80 percent of adolescents were already abstaining in both the intervention and control sites (Ahga & Van Rossem, 2002). It is of interest that abstinence and condoms were emphasized in preventive education, yet partner reduction was the main behavior change outcome.

The evaluation study, conducted by PSI, concluded, "Our analysis of data from two rounds of representative household surveys of Lusaka has shown that there was a significant reduction in casual sex among both women and men between 1996 and 1999. Although condom use in last sex with any partner increased during this period, the increase was not statistically significant" (Agha, 2002, p. 291).

Some Qualitative Rapid Research on Behavior Change

It is always desirable to triangulate or corroborate three types of data: survey, biological or epidemiological, and qualitative. We have considered the first two. I conducted some rapid qualitative research about AIDS and behavior change in Zambia in early 1995. I had been asked to evaluate a collaborative, community-based AIDS prevention program involving traditional healers in Zambia, a component of the Morehouse School of Medicine/Zambia AIDS Prevention Project (Tulane University was a partner in the project and study and in charge of the traditional healer and youth components). I was also asked to design and direct two surveys in Zambia, for traditional healers and for the general population (cf. Green, 1999a, for details and results). I additionally spent three weeks in Zambia in April 1995 conducting interviews with traditional healers, health workers, and other informants, and observing a workshop for healers on AIDS and STDs. The following are some notes from this latter that pertain to behavior change. I had found that interviewing Ugandan health workers about STD trends and behavior change in 1993 provided insights that turned out to be very accurate. I felt that interviewing traditional healers, who tend to see most STD cases in Africa, might provide even more insights.

Notes from Open-Ended Interviews in Zambia, 1995

I asked Mrs. Shinondo, a workshop-trained diviner near Ndola, if she thought STDs were increasing or decreasing in her community. Overall, she felt that in the last year or so there have been fewer STD cases in her community. She said people are changing their behavior in two ways: They are sticking to their partner and not sleeping around, and they are starting to use condoms. Both behavior changes might be occurring equally, but the ones adopting condoms are mostly the younger men. Older people are reluctant to use condoms.

I asked the same question to Mr. Lowipa, a herbalist practicing near Ndola since 1949. Although he himself is getting more STD cases as a result of his training under the project, he said he has definitely noticed a decline of STD cases in his community. He attributes this decline to people becoming afraid to sleep around, not as much to condoms.

Mrs. Mambo, a community nurse in Ndola told me she feels that STDs are declining among people in this area: "Something is happening." She feels that people are settling down to marriage or at least faithful relationships. She said, "There's a lot more marriages taking place than before. This weekend I have two marriages to attend." She characterized condom use as sporadic and a practice which is not sustained after the first few episodes of intercourse within the same relationship. Mostly she said it's adolescents who are using condoms (Tanzanian truck drivers en route to Morogoro said the same thing to me in 1993).

For a view from an informant in a different part of the country (Chongwe), one of the community nurses working closely with healers told me that chancroid and syphilis are definitely declining and not just in the clinics. She said that gonorrhea was still high but the cases tend to come from the same patients who are probably HIV positive. They try all the different antibiotics available (at her clinic at least there seem to be five or more different antibiotics), but the patients tend to come back in a month or two. I asked her if she felt STDs were truly declining and whether this might be connected with any changes in behavior. She said she thought people were abstaining or remaining faithful to their partners—at least not running around as they used to. She felt that condom use was not particularly widespread although they were becoming popular with some adolescent groups.

Both Samson Muvuma, district health officer in Chongwe, and "Dr." Vongo, a traditional healer and president of THPAZ (a national healers association), told me that there are considerably fewer STD cases in the last year or two. Mr. Vongo thinks this (apparent) phenomenon is due to more abstinence and to some use of condoms.

A different view came from Wadi Chiponya, a Lala diviner (*mashave*) from Central Province who was trained in a AIDS workshop in the Copperbelt. He said that he is getting more STD patients nowadays, something like 4–6 a month now compared to 2–3 a month previously. In answer to my question, he said that his training under the program has probably helped establish him as more of an authority in this area and to attract new patients. I asked him whether STDs in the community seem to be going up or down in the last one year. He said up, but the way he phrased his answer made it clear that he was thinking in a timeframe of longer than one year. Also there are many truck drivers and forestry workers and other men without wives in the peri-urban area where he practices.

Just before the beginning of the STD section of the workshop for traditional healers near Kitwe, I took the opportunity to ask the group of 35 healers about trends among the three common STDs. Using the Bemba names for GUD, gonorrhea and syphilis, I commented that these diseases have been increasing all over the world for the past 25 years. I now wanted to ask them about what they have been able to observe in their own experience in the last 1–2 years. I first asked them whether GUD seems to be decreasing, staying the same or increasing in the last 1–2 years. 35 hands went up to say that it has been decreasing. For syphilis, 32 said it is decreasing and 3 said it is increasing. For gonorrhea, 33 said it is decreasing and 2 said it is increasing. Before I asked anything further, a woman healer rose to explain that "all three diseases are in the same family" and the other healers clapped their agreement. The implication seemed to be that obviously these three illnesses would vary together. I asked the healers why these three diseases seem to be decreasing. Two or three healers gave essentially the same reason: Each of these diseases is curable and both healers and hospitals have been busy treating cases. One woman commented that hospital medicine does not always "finish off" the disease and so healers have to do that.

Since no one had mentioned behavior change after several opportunities, I prompted: Do healers think people are beginning to use condoms or avoid casual sex? A female healer said, "All this information on the radio about AIDS has made people more careful."

(Project head) Karen Romano was concerned that the healers might have taken my question to mean, in effect, are healers doing their job that they should be in their communities? Patrick Mubiana didn't think that the healers took the question this way, but he took the precaution of talking a bit further with a couple of healers. One healer clarified that he has seen no *bolabola* in the last six months, compared to quite a few cases a year ago. (Green, 1995)

In our later survey of Zambian healers' knowledge, attitudes, beliefs, and behavior related to STDs and AIDS, we found that when considering a longer time frame, such as the previous five years, healers felt that STD rates had risen overall (Green, 1999a). Reasons provided by healers included people disregarding taboos and traditions in general, and the advice of traditional healers; youth beginning sexual activity at an earlier age; the titillating influence of foreign videos, films and other mass entertainment/media; the rise of new illnesses (chancroid, AIDS); increases in immorality, prostitution, casual sex, promiscuity and drinking alcohol; increase in abortions (a term that might include miscarriage) and therefore of men having sex with women who are "contaminated with death"; growth in population and increase in foreigners carrying illnesses; condom advertisements on television; lack of preventive education by health workers; and teaching sex in the schools.

Many traditional healers expressed skepticism about condoms. Many believed they are of limited usefulness because they can burst or fall off, an obstacle to condom use cited in a great many parts of Africa.

One healer said, "The condom does not cover all the penis hence leaving a certain area exposed to insects." (The insect concept parallels biomedical germ theory, that is, insects in this sense are conceived as animate carriers of contagious disease; cf. Green, 1999a, pp. 148–159). There is truth to this—facts that many AIDS educators who promote condoms are unaware of. For example, chancroid and venereal warts are not fully preventable by condom use.

One female healer from Monze, who treats many STDs, commented that immorality has been on the rise. An interviewer described her comments (these and other translated comments are unedited) as follows:

She blamed the condom adverts to have caused a lot of harm to the Zambian people, more especially to the young people. They now have been made to believe that as long as that person has a condom, then he is free to go anywhere without looking at the dangers of using a condom. She also blamed foreigners for sleeping with Zambian women. . . . They are the ones who are making these diseases to be on the increase.

Other healers said that condoms can prevent sexually transmitted illnesses but even they commented that condoms are not perfect as they can burst during sexual intercourse.

It should be noted that Zambia's religious leaders opposed condoms quite vigorously and openly. The following comments are taken from an article on this opposition:

Church leaders . . . said that the advertisements, some of which feature school students talking about the use of condoms, were in fact contributing to the spread of the disease by endorsing casual sex.

Ignatius Mwebe, a priest and spokesman for the Roman Catholic Church, said, "The advertisements are justifying casual sex using a condom, [suggesting] that you can have sex anyhow so long as you have a condom. . . . The people being used in the advertisements are so young that they should not have anything to do with sex at their age."

He added that it would be helpful if the advertisements simply gave factual information about the dangers of AIDS.

The Christian Council of Zambia (CCZ) said in a statement that the advertisements had "moved from AIDS prevention, which can only be achieved through abstinence, to allowing people to have sex anyhow. This is basically business for those selling condoms."

Joshua Banda, a pastor and vice-national superintendent of the Pentecostal churches in Zambia, told ENI: "The advertisements are promoting the wrong moral values. The emphasis in the advertisements was on marketing condoms rather than halting the disease." However, he explained that he did not support a "blanket ban on condoms. What we are against are lopsided anti-AIDS messages that don't give a positive alternative to casual sex."

Another pastor, Thomas Lumba, who is executive director of the Evangelical Fellowship of Zambia, said: "People should be told to avoid casual sex. After all, condoms are not 100 percent safe." (Kunda, 2001, http://www.christianity today.com/ct/2001/102/56.0.html)

It would be very useful for unbiased research to explore the question of whether these African religious leaders and traditional healers are right, or partly right, about the impact of condom promotion on youth. Does aggressive condom promotion to youth, or males of all ages, lead to more casual sex than would otherwise be the case? In fact, there has been little research on how the A, B, and C elements of prevention might work either synergistically or at cross-purposes with each other. In this Zambia section we have seen that A and C can be promoted together, even though the message, "Abstain, but here are your condoms," might appear to send a contradictory message.

Before research on how ABC messages might interact there first has to be acceptance of abstinence and partner reduction as legitimate research subjects. This means that public and private donors and funding organizations have to overcome their biases.

Recognition of Zambia's Progress

In advance of the 2001 ICASA (International Conference on AIDS and Sexually Transmitted Infections in Africa), an editorial was written in SAT News Bulletin to suggest that Zambia seems to be winning its war against AIDS. After showing how the previous president (Kenneth Kaunda) was relatively outspoken in the right manner about AIDS (probably because his son died of AIDS), the editorial remarks that Kaunda's successor, President Chilube, did little to help the situation. However, it continues with the following:

Zambia does have a story to tell. It is a story of a strong, active, and highly developed community response to AIDS. The mission hospitals in rural Zambia have been on the forefront of innovative approaches to the continuum of prevention and care. The Copperbelt Health Education Project has shown the way on how to reach men in a workplace setting. Urban community mobilisation programmes such as the Human Resources Trust have conclusively demonstrated their impact on STD incidence. And youth peer action was practically invented in Zambia by the Family Health Trust.

If another success is celebrated at the ICASA, let us look closely at its determinants. We may find that what made the difference in Zambia were many people working together away from the clamour of national programmes and politics. Thousands of dedicated volunteers, hundreds of small community organisations. Who knows, if we take another look at Uganda and Senegal we may find that things there are not at all different. (Anonymous, 2001, p. 1)

Zambia's response to AIDS seems to resemble that of Uganda's in some key features: grassroots community involvement, youth focus, peer education, involvement of religious groups and mission hospitals (not discussed here) as well as local leaders and organizations, and relatively open and widespread public discussion about AIDS. Yet these elements can also be found in other countries. It is difficult to quantify the scale or intensity of these interventions. Fieldwork, which should include interviews with informants who have worked for many years in public and private sector AIDS prevention, as well as examination of costs of programs, should help characterize Zambia's response in terms of ABC balance with more precision. Certainly much more research is needed to better understand the relationship between certain types of intervention and specific behavioral changes at the national level. Still, evaluations of the two youth projects summarized here are instructive. They suggest that abstinence (the actual term used) and condoms can both be promoted through familiar interventions (mass media, peer education), and higher levels of these behaviors, as well as partner reduction (therefore A, B, and C), can all result.

As this book was going to press, I spent two weeks in Zambia. The just-released "ANC Sentinel Surveillance of HIV/Syphilis Trends in Zambia" shows trends between 1994 and 2002. It shows (p. 19) that HIV prevalence went down significantly among youth 15 to 19 in the 1990s (i.e., a decrease of 20 percent in urban antenatal clinics) but then rose again after 1998 (and increase of 15 percent in urban ANCs and 8 percent in rural sites). This suggests that the new cohort entering their sexually active years did not practice the same risk avoidance or reduction behaviors of the cohort a few years older than themselves. Why? Some Zambian informants from NGOs and FBOs thought it was because "the message for youth changed" from one that emphasized abstinence in the earlier period (when youth messages were very influenced by FBOs and a national school program run by an indigenous NGO, the Family Health Trust) to one that was more condom focused. Also in the earlier years, there were fear-arousal messages such as skull and crossbones posters, with the message "AIDS Kills," which messages were removed when they fell into disfavor with AIDS experts. The same surveillance report study also found that for the overall population, HIV prevalence at ANC clinics (not necesarily representative of the Zambian population) remained at 20 percent between 1998 and 2002. However, prevalence among those who used condoms during their last intercourse rose from 25 percent in 1998 to 31 percent in 2002

(p. 46). Obviously, this whole important topic needs to be carefully researched before any conclusions can be reached.

We should remember that ANC data only come from those sexually active. According to the Zambia DHS 2001-2 (p. 220), about 64 percent of unmarried Zambians 15 to 19 did not report any sexual partners in the past year, and among those that did, the great majority reported only one partner. Yet in a sample of recent print materials from U.S. AIDS organizations, there is a handout called "Why Haven't Youth Changed Their Behavior?" Bullet #2 reads as follows: "The majority do not believe they are at risk because they have reduced their number of partners. They have selected the 'B' from the 'ABC,' and reached the false conclusion that partner reduction is enough to prevent HIV. However, partner reduction is a subjective concept, and it only takes one infected partner to get HIV" (p. 3). Another handout states what it calls "the reality about condoms: "if used consistently they provide close to 100% protection against HIV."

Let me reiterate that USAID/Zambia is doing more than most USAID programs, especially through the mass media abstinence campaign it funds on TV and radio (that runs along with mass media condom promotion). But the AIDS prevention emphasis of USAID-funded groups has been primarily on condom promotion.

FOOTNOTE ON KENYA

Dr. Mohammed Abdullah, chairman of the Kenya National AIDS Control Council, made a presentation to USAID on February 19, 2003, to show the current status of Kenya's AIDS epidemic and to outline the national response. The presentation showed that by far the major response to AIDS before 1999 was condom supply and promotion. A vast quantity of condoms were brought into Kenya before 1999 (and more since). Yet nothing happened to prevalence except increase during all those years of greater condom availability and relatively high use. Finally, under intense political pressure, ex-President Moi began to take certain steps in 1999.

Remember that Moi was very disliked by most in his country and everywhere by 1999. He certainly did not have the stature of President Museveni in 1986, that is, the liberator of the people, after the bloody years of Idi Amin and Milton Obote. This means that an African head of state does not necessarily have to have credibility and charisma to sound the AIDS alarm.

And what did Moi do? According to Dr. Abdullah, Kenya implemented an ABC program with some real emphasis on A and B; it mobilized the faith-based groups; it went into the schools with AIDS education; it underscored the seriousness of the epidemic, speaking in terms of a national emergency; and government officials were told that they must mention AIDS every time they had a public meeting, or else they'd be in trouble. According to Dr. Abdullah, national prevalence began to be impacted within a year or two. He claims that 2002 ANC data show a decline, although these data are not yet publicly available.

If the findings in this presentation are corroborated, Kenya's recent experience seems to validate the ABC approach or the Uganda model. National HIV prevalence turned around quickly once President Moi took the broad, general steps that President Museveni took in 1986 and that President Diouf of Senegal took in 1987.

To summarize this chapter, we see evidence that parallels Uganda's. That is, there have been varying degrees of primary behavior change and declines in HIV prevalence that may be related to interventions that promote PBC. In the case of Senegal and the two northern areas of Uganda, levels of risk behavior were relatively low at the beginning of AIDS, accounting for relatively lower HIV prevalence rates in these populations. (In the case of Senegal, high levels of male circumcision helped keep infection rates low.) But even in these areas, there was still behavioral change as well as declines in HIV prevalence. In the case of Zambia, the behavioral and epidemiological evidence was mostly restricted to youth.

One of the main take-home messages from this chapter is that the ABC approach and PBC cannot be written off as cultural–historical–geographical anomalies of Uganda. They can happen, and have happened, elsewhere in Africa. And, as we are about to see, in other parts of the world as well.

8

What Can We Learn from Jamaica?

The Caribbean is the region with the second highest HIV prevalence rates after sub-Saharan Africa. The predominant pattern of HIV transmission is heterosexual, although there is also substantial MSM and IDU transmission in some countries. There seems to be stabilization or decline of HIV rates in at least one country, Jamaica, therefore it should be instructive to look at interventions and behavior change there. Something similar may have occurred in the Dominican Republic, but I have less information on interventions there. What I can say is that, like Jamaica, the Dominican Republic has shown evidence of male primary behavior change (Green & Conde, 2000). It also has achieved relatively high condom user rates among those at higher risk. According to DHS data available online, the age of sexual debut is relatively high for females, 18.7 according to the 1996 DHS. It would be useful to see recent data on the percentage of youth ages fifteen to nineteen that are sexually active.

HIV seroprevalence and rates of sexually transmitted infections have stabilized in the Dominican Republic. Sentinel surveillance data from rural and urban ANCs between 1991 and 1998 suggest that HIV prevalence in the general population is about 2 to 2.5 percent. The official figure used by UNAIDS in 2001 was 2.8 percent, yet a sero-survey component of the 2002 Demographic and Health Survey found that national prevalence was 0.96 percent among women and 0.88 percent among men. For young men ages fifteen to nineteen, prevalence was 0.3 percent. For young women ages fifteen to nineteen, HIV prevalence was 0.4 percent (Macro International, 2002).

In short, the Dominican Republic would seem to be a good country to conduct research focused on sexual behavior, behavioral change, and possibly falling HIV prevalence.

JAMAICA

Risk factors are found in Jamaica that would predict relatively high HIV infection rates: an early age of sexual debut (median age of fourteen for boys and girls), multiple sexual partners, a pattern of teenage girls having sexual contact with older men, a robust sex industry linked with tourism, lack of male circumcision, presence of chancroid, age disparity between partners (a pattern of older men having transactional or coerced sex with younger girls), African descent,[1] relatively high levels of alcohol and drug use, and related factors such as poverty, labor emigration, male absenteeism, violence, homophobia, and major stigma associated with AIDS. Yet Jamaica has rather low seroprevalence by regional standards, namely, 1.6 percent or lower among the majority population in 2000, down from 1.98 percent in 1996, according to the U.S. Bureau of the Census data. ANC infection rates are considerably higher than five other groups that might approximate the majority population of Jamaica (Amarasingham, Green, & Royes). In fact, the most recent seroprevalence estimate (2002) by the U.S. Bureau of the Census for the capital or major city is 1.0 percent. (See Table 8.1 for prevalence data pertaining to several Jamaican groups.)

USAID funded the AIDS/STD Prevention and Control Project beginning in August 1988 under the AIDSCAP project. By 1996, the Jamaican government felt that it had enough expertise to design and implement its own program. It said to USAID, in effect, give us a chance to run the show and we will produce the results we all want. And if we fail to do so, you can give us American technical experts again. The USAID mission agreed to this. The national AIDS program, for which USAID was the main but not the only donor, was evaluated in September 2000. I had the good fortune to be one of the evaluators. It is my theory that Jamaica developed more Uganda-like program elements in its prevention program in part because it was able to have more control over its own program.

Our evaluation team found that Jamaica's relatively low and apparently stabilized rates of HIV seem to be attributable to: (1) programs of STD case finding and syndromic management (resulting in declining infection rates of virtually all STIs); and (2) BCC programs that have resulted in reduction in sexual partners, high rates of condom use and—noting the imperfection of the measure—a slight rise in the median age of sexual debut (Amarasingham, Green, & Royes, 2000).

Table 8.1
HIV Prevalence in Jamaica among Groups That Might Approximate the
General Population

	1996	1997	1998	1999	2000 Jan-Mar	2000 Apr-Jun
Farm Workers	0.01	0.02	0.02	0.02	0.02	0.03
Blood Donors	0.42	0.36	0.4	0.43	0.53	0.43
USA Visas	0.09	0.14	0.17	0.24	0.26	0.38
Life Ins Co Ass	0.17	0.18	0.14	0.24	0.32	0.21
Private Labs	0.53	0.63	0.6	0.82	0.79	0.53
ANC Clinics	1.98	1.96	1.7	1.6	1.6	1.6

Source: Amarasingham, Green, and Royes, 2000; Figueroa et al., 1998.

On the intervention side, we find two prominent elements in common with Uganda's response: AIDS education in schools (starting with early grades) and involvement of religious leaders and groups. Another intervention element shared with Uganda is that there was a great deal of community-based, face-to-face AIDS education, in addition to the more usual awareness promotion through mass media. A 2000 KABP survey found the following:

A significant increase in participation in HIV/AIDS intervention, including face-to-face intervention was recorded (from 27% in 1996 to 35% in 2000). Notably here was the citing of "community" intervention (15.7%) for the first time in a KABP survey. This undoubtedly is a reflection of the increased emphasis on face-to-face intervention in the communities. In fact this is second to intervention in schools (48%), as the next most important source of intervention and is the most important source for men 20 years and over. (Hope Enterprises, 2000, p. 7)

AIDS EDUCATION IN SCHOOLS

The Ministry of Education and several NGOs have worked together to reach youth ages ten to nineteen through their schools. By 2000, some sixty-three school guidance counselors, seventy-five peer educators in reproductive health (in St. James parish alone), and twenty Child Health Education Program teachers had been trained in BCC. Teachers and counselors had reached an estimated 10,000 students.

Let me quote the following at length from our 2000 evaluation report (Amarasingham, Green, & Royes, 2000; cf. Figueroa et al., 2000, p. 17):

Jamaican schools have implemented some aspects of sex education (family life education) and life coping skills (which should include negotiation of safe sex, or not having sex) as part of the school curriculum. However, the degree to which the curriculum is actually carried out seems to depend on individual principals and teachers or guidance counselors. Many school staff feel uncomfortable discussing sex or STDs in any manner. It helps if school staff have been trained in HIV/STIs, but this is no insurance that sex education will be taught.

Sometimes BCC peer educators or CIs (contact investigators, who follow up on STD cases and provide HIV/STD education) or others trained under the project are invited into schools to conduct sex education, including HIV/STD education. For example, in Portland parish, 90% of guidance counselors have been trained in HIV/AIDS education, which helps make the local volunteer peer educators welcome in the schools. These PEs [peer educators], in effect, do the work of teachers or counselors for them, since the Ministry of Education has mandated that schools teach life coping skills. However, these are at best one-time sessions.

There is general agreement that sex and HIV/STD education needs to be improved in the schools. Still, the program is making an impact. The majority of Jamaicans age 15–19 in the 2000 national KABP survey cited "school" as their primary source of information about HIV/AIDS and STIs, a finding supported by recent qualitative research.

At least one recent study of school-based programs has shown positive impact, finding that, "Over the two-year period, knowledge of at least two HIV prevention methods increased significantly ($p < .001$) among both boys (71% to 99%) and girls (70% to 94%). Many more adolescent boys reported sexual experience and recent sexual activity than girls. However, declines were reported in boys sexually experienced (59% to 41%, $p < .001$) and sexually active in the past 12 months (40% to 33%, $p = .08$). Ten percent of girls reported being sexually experienced (from 11%) and 7% sexually active (from 6%)." (Wedderburn, Amon, & Figueroa, 1998, p. 191)

It was unfortunate that data were not available for ages younger than fifteen, since it would be important to know the impact of school-based AIDS education on youth from ages ten to fourteen. We see that even though there have been problems with AIDS education in schools, the program seems to have had positive impact.

INVOLVEMENT OF FAITH-BASED GROUPS

From the early stages of Jamaica's epidemic, religious leaders and churches have been involved in two main areas of Jamaica's National HIV/AIDS Control Program: Care and Counseling and BCC. The control program has targeted church organizations and congregations for awareness and prevention programs. There have been considerable numbers of clergy involved in the National AIDS Committee (or sub-committees), or in local (parish) AIDS committees (or subcommittees), sometimes as chairpersons. As in Uganda, Jamaican FBOs have been especially interested in promoting fidelity, which as we have seen can result in reduction in number of nonregular partners, if not in mo-nogamy, as well as abstinence, which can result in delay in the age of first sexual experience if not abstinence after sexual debut. This was done through HIV/AIDS education among congregations of major churches (Anglican, Roman Catholic, Methodist, and Baptist), often using community peer educators, and through similar programs in schools (Amarasingham, Green, & Royes, 2000). Some school officials have allowed condoms to be discussed and shown in schools, others have not. But it seems that none opposed AIDS education emphasiz-ing the abstinence and fidelity messages. The focus of USAID's AIDS program in Jamaica has been on youth.

Community peer educators interviewed by the recent USAID evalu-ation team (Amarasingham, Green, & Royes, 2000) reported that main-stream Jamaican churches, listed previously, have been particularly cooperative in their AIDS education efforts. With some churches, there was resistance at first. But it took only pointing out that members of a particular church were becoming infected with HIV to change these attitudes. The result is that Jamaica has had good, supportive rela-tions between FBOs and national AIDS efforts in both the public or private sector, for many years. The evaluation team was unable to find direct evidence of any clergy or religious organizations opposing the work of the national AIDS program. There were occasional allegations that fundamentalist or Pentecostal churches criticized the promotion of condoms, but no real evidence of this emerged anywhere. On the contrary, individual clergy and FBOs were cited virtually everywhere as helpful not only in the care, support, and counseling of PLWHAs, but also in AIDS prevention efforts. Even the former manager of the government's condom social marketing program was able to promote condoms among church groups on several occasions, and she found no church opposition to any of the program's condom promotion ef-forts. However, as elsewhere, Jamaican FBOs have preferred to pro-mote fidelity and abstinence rather than condom use.

A small survey was conducted in greater Kingston in June 1999 to assess the level of participation of churches in HIV/AIDS prevention in Jamaica (Gebre, 1999). Findings are as follows:

- 9.5 percent of churches had a special HIV/AIDS ministry or special service for HIV/AIDS.

- 19.5 percent of religious leaders (e.g., pastors, deacons, elders) had participated in HIV/AIDS programs. Types of programs were as follows: Support (50%), Education (50%), Counseling (33%).

- 98 percent of religious leaders expressed future plans to participate in HIV/AIDS prevention.

- Types of service to be provided in their plans were as follows: Advocacy (9.5%), Education (33%), Counseling (19.5%), Care (9.5%), Support Groups (14.3%).

Unfortunately, the only paper on the role of FBOs in Jamaican AIDS mitigation at the 2000 global AIDS conference in Durban was one which overlooked all positive contributions and instead criticized some churches for being anti-condom, and for forbidding Christian burial of those suspected of having died of AIDS (Gunter & Hue, 2000). As noted, FBOs in Jamaica have been relatively open about condom education and promotion.

Has promotion of PBC resulted in change? As usual, the causal variables have yet to be sorted out, but the recent national population-based KABP survey of Jamaicans ages fifteen to forty-nine shows that there has been significant reduction in the proportion reporting two or more sexual partners in the past twelve months. The evidence is worth reviewing.

SEXUAL BEHAVIOR CHANGE IN JAMAICA

The proportion of men ages fifteen to forty-nine reporting sex with a nonregular partner declined from 35 percent in 1994 to 26 percent in 1996 (Figueroa et al., 1998). The proportion of both males and females who reported two or more partners for the previous three-month period declined sharply in 2000, compared to 1996. There was a decrease among all age groups with the exception of females ages fifteen to nineteen (4.5% versus 3.8% existing at time of 1996 survey). However the general trend is encouraging, as Table 8.2 shows. In fact, if the question had been phrased about number of partners in the last three months instead of percentage reporting two or more partners currently in 1996, the 1996 groups might have been even higher, making the 1996–2000 differences even greater.

The mean age of sexual debut rose from thirteen to fourteen for males between 1996 and 2000; it remained fourteen for females, according to a recent KABP survey (Hope Enterprises, 2000). Earlier population-based, quantitative evidence (the 1997 reproductive health survey) showed that 50 percent of females ages fifteen to nineteen had had sexual experience, down from 59 percent in 1993. However, the 2000 Hope Enterprises survey found fewer among fifteen to nineteen years reporting

Table 8.2
Change in Casual Sex in Jamaica, 1996-2000

Percent reporting 2 or more	Age groups			
partners in last 3 months	15-19	20-24	30-39	40-49
MALE	(N=196)	(N=337)	(N=88)	(N=48)
2000 survey	24.0	31.8	26.1	12.8
1996 survey	36.8	36.9	32.3	13.6
FEMALE	(N=132)	(N=306)	(N=113)	(N=44)
2000 survey	4.5	5.2	7.1	2.3
1996 survey	3.8	7.0	9.3	6.8

Source: Hope Enterprises, 2000.

delaying initiation of sexual activity (males: 24% versus 34% in 1996; females: 46% versus 57% in 1996). Yet all other age groups reported a trend toward delaying sexual debut (Hope Enterprises, 2000). Therefore we have a somewhat mixed picture with regard to delay of debut and abstinence.

There is evidence from a recent qualitative study that some young people believed that fifteen or sixteen is the earliest that Jamaicans should begin to have intercourse (Chevannes & Gayle, 2000). A focus group of "suburban" boys (those from higher-income neighborhoods) believed that ages eighteen to twenty-five is ideal for first sexual experience. Yet sexual debut is at an earlier age. This means that there is a gap between beliefs, values, and behavior, a gap that FBOs can do even more to focus on in BCC approaches. The same study showed that boys who delayed first intercourse tended to be "raised in a Christian home" suggesting the influence of religion in delay of sexual debut (Chevannes & Gayle, 2000, p. 25).[2]

CONDOM USE AND STD TREATMENT

Condom user rates in Jamaica are high by any country's standards. Over 90 percent of sex workers regularly use condoms with clients, and some 77 percent of men, and between 57 and 79 percent of women (depending on age group) reported using a condom during their last sexual encounter with a nonregular partner. Even condom use among regular partners is high by international standards, increasing among males from 47 percent in 1996 to 52 percent in 2000, using the same measure: whether a condom was used in the last sexual encounter (BSS, 1999; Hope Enterprises, 2000). A recent survey of sexual behavior among 1,100 students at the University of the West Indies, Jamaica, found that 42.9 percent reported condom use during last sex with steady partners and 74.8 percent with nonsteady partners (Norman & Gebre, 2002). The authors characterized these reported rates of protective sexual behaviors as low, although by African standards they would be relatively high.

Moreover Jamaica has an excellent STD control program that includes syndromic management, plus an unusually effective program of contact tracing and HIV counseling and testing. STD treatment centers were established in each of the thirteen parishes and health workers received training in syndromic management of STDs. As an apparent result, prevalence and incidence (when data for the latter are available) of most STDs has declined markedly for several years. It is established that STDs, particularly of the ulcerative type, are facilitating factors in HIV transmission, therefore falling STD rates ought to have contributed to stabilization of HIV infection rates, especially in populations with relatively low HIV infection rates.

In sum, we find in Jamaica stabilized HIV prevalence and falling STD prevalence, as well as partner reduction, rather high condom user rates, and an effective STD case-finding and treatment program. Of course, it is not easy to attribute certain types of interventions or behavior changes to impact on HIV and STD prevalence. Still, Jamaica may be a country where changes in A, B, C, as well as D (drugs, a shorthand way of referring to STD treatment) can all be credited with contributing to HIV stabilizaion.

IS JAMAICA RECOGNIZED IN AIDS CIRCLES OR BY THE PUBLIC?

Jamaica's success in at least stabilizing HIV infection rates, and decreasing STD rates significantly, is a well-kept secret, even among those who ought to know about HIV trends. Part of the reason is that Jamaican officials with whom I spoke fear that donor funds will shift elsewhere if the story got out. Officials are likely to stress doom and gloom in order to keep attention on Jamaica's plight and keep funds flowing. A recent front-page article in the *Washingon Post* by Karen DeYoung ("A Deadly Stigma in the Caribbean") was based on interviews with officials (so perhaps we should not blame the visiting journalist). We are told the following: "AIDS is already the leading cause of death in the Caribbean for those aged 15 to 45, and the number of cases is growing at an 'exponential' rate, 'doubling every two or three years,'" said C. James

Hospedales, director of the Caribbean Epidemiology Center, the leading regional institution monitoring the disease (DeYoung, 2001, p. A01).

The article focuses on Jamaica but sometimes adds broader statistics like this, leaving the impression that Jamaica's epidemic is growing at an exponential rate. The article continues with the following:

In Jamaica, "we listen to music about sex, we dress sexy and we dance sexy. But nobody talks about sex," said Verity Rushton, who heads the quasi-governmental National AIDS Committee. But what nobody talks about, most people apparently do—early, often and with many others. The average age of first sexual experience in the Caribbean is 12 to 14. "Many men and women have multiple sex partners; social and cultural norms condone and even encourage this," according to last year's report by the Caribbean Task Force on HIV/AIDS, the most comprehensive assessment compiled by U.N. and regional organizations. (DeYoung, 2001, p. A01)

A recent article in the *Journal of the American Medical Association* continues the theme of alleged underreporting of HIV in the Caribbean and warns with the following:

Experts on this subject forecast that the withdrawal of economic support from the former Soviet Union coupled with the rise in tourism will increase commercial sex and other high-risk practices. Furthermore, the region has missed the opportunity for the prevention of the epidemic in 1970s [sic] because of ignorance and fear of breached confidentiality and discrimination. (Voelker, 2001, p. 2961)

This seems typical of the kind of reporting one gets about the Caribbean and Jamaica in particular, even from professionals. Only two papers from or concerning Jamaica were presented at the global AIDS conference in Durban. Neither mentioned improving epidemiological trends, and one begins with the seemingly obligatory, "Worldwide, the Caribbean and Latin America rank just below Sub-Saharan Africa and Southeast Asia with regard to cumulative AIDS deaths through 1999" (Kepka, 2000, p. 1). Thus it is not surprising that few people have recognized that Jamaica has had a good AIDS prevention (and STD treatment) program, and that things are looking better there.

NOTES

1. It has been found recently that CCR-5 mutation, which is observed in 10 percent of whites but is much less common among people of African descent, is associated with a reduced risk of HIV infection (Samson et al., 1996).

2. Survey research elsewhere has also shown this relationship, for example, a study of university students in the Philippines, found that (83%) of the students were sexually abstinent, and that abstinence depends on degree of religiosity, in this case mostly Catholicism (Sy et al., 1996).

9

What Can We Learn from Thailand?

Patterns of transmission in Asia are different from those in sub-Saharan Africa and the Caribbean. The difference is that between Pattern II and Pattern IV, and the short way to characterize the patterns is to note that in sub-Saharan Africa and the Caribbean, most HIV infections are found in the majority population, whereas in Asia, most are found in distinct high-risk groups. A recent conference (6th ICAAP [International Conference on AIDS in Asia and the Pacific]: Strategies for HIV Prevention in Low Prevalence Settings, posted on sea-aids@ healthdev.net on October 7, 2001) concluded that "all countries in Asia have low prevalence in their majority populations, although several countries have 'concentrated' epidemics." Most infections in Asia are concentrated in high (or higher) risk groups, namely, MSM, CSWs and perhaps their clients, and IDUs.[1]

My argument is that primary behavior change interventions should be emphasized in majority populations while risk reduction interventions may be more justifiably emphasized with high-risk groups. However, in principal, all behavior change options should be presented to all groups, in spite of where emphasis should lie, for a number of reasons, including cost-effectiveness of interventions and appropriateness to the target audience. Put another way, a full range of preventive interventions ought to be available to virtually all groups, but this does not mean we ought to use the same prevention strategy for CSWs and primary school students who are not yet sexually active.

The *reductio ad absurdum* argument that might arise at this point is: Oh, should we teach abstinence or partner reduction to prostitutes? In fact, while this is an extreme example and CSWs are by no means the only high-risk group, there have been programs designed to help women leave sex work by teaching income-generating skills (e.g., the FHI-supported project in Morogoro, Tanzania, which I was involved in). The Ministry of Health's BCC project in Jamaica even promoted the fewer partners message to CSWs, as quixotic as that might sound. In any case, I will not devote much space to Asia because the primary focus of this book is on Pattern II countries and on the overlooked and uncredited role of PBC.

The headlines about AIDS in Asia typically warn that this region will soon overtake Africa in numbers of AIDS cases, that we have only seen the tip of the iceberg, that IDU cases are exploding, that all types of HIV cases are exploding, and the like. Epidemiologist Jim Chin once wrote this way himself, but changed his thinking as more data became available. He recently wrote the following:

HIV/AIDS programs and policies in Asia have been driven primarily by the belief that in Asian countries with current low HIV prevalence, epidemic HIV transmission into most of these majority populations is inevitable, i.e., it is only a matter of time. However, based on epidemiological observations in this region over the past 15 years an alternative scenario is that HIV has, to a great extent, already spread as much as it can in most Asian-Pacific populations according to the prevailing patterns and prevalence of HIV risk behaviors.

According to this new HIV/AIDS paradigm for Asia, the general patterns and prevalence of heterosexual HIV-risk behaviors in most Asian populations are insufficient to fuel any extensive or sustained spread of HIV outside of those population groups with the highest HIV-risk behaviors. In the few Asian countries where extensive HIV transmission has occurred during the past decade (Cambodia, Myanmar, Thailand, and parts of India), the most recent HIV surveillance data indicate that HIV prevalence peaked in these countries during the mid-to-late 1990s. However, during the coming decade, HIV prevalence in these countries is not expected to decrease rapidly but will likely persist at around 2–3% because HIV transmission from infected FSW and infected male clients of FSW to their regular sex partners will continue to occur at a slow but steady pace. (Chin, 2001a, p. 50)

The concept of reproductive number, Ro, used by epidemiologists, helps explain why heterosexually transmitted HIV infections tend not to grow in majority populations in Asia, where premarital and extra-marital sexual activity for females is relatively low. This can be seen in the following:

The spread of HIV can be assessed at a population level as well. Anderson and May have described the risk of secondary (new) cases of HIV as Ro, where Ro = beta x C x delta, with beta representing the efficiency of transmission, C the number of sexual partners, and delta the duration of infectiousness of the index case. When Ro exceeds 1, new, secondary cases of HIV occur, and the epidemic continues. Successful prevention strategies must reduce Ro to less than 1 and include lowering the rate of partner change, reducing the efficiency of transmission, and shortening the duration of infectiousness. This model offers an excellent conceptual framework to approach HIV prevention and a tool to examine the success of interventions. (Cohen & Eron, 2001)

Epidemiologist Jim Chin has found it useful to make the following basic distinction between two basic patterns of sexual HIV transmission:

1. The epidemic pattern, where Ro of HIV is > 1, has only occurred where there are: (a) high-risk patterns of sex partner exchange and mixing, i.e., having multiple and concurrent sex partners; and (b) a high prevalence of factors that can facilitate the sexual transmission of HIV.
2. The non-epidemic pattern, where Ro of HIV is < 1, generally occurs from HIV-infected persons (regardless of how they were infected) to his/her regular sex partner. Further HIV spread from these regular partners can only occur if these partners have other sex partners. (Chin, 2003, p. 3)

Chin believes that most or all Asian countries exhibit a nonepidemic pattern, referring here to the majority populations of these countries. This does not mean numbers of infected persons cannot grow quite large in countries like India and China, or that infection rates among groups like IDUs cannot become formidable.

Ro seems to be less than 1 in Thailand, due to relatively low-risk behavior in the majority population. Thailand was nevertheless the first country in Asia to document HIV epidemics among IDUs, and among sex workers and their clients (FHI, 1996; UNAIDS/Thailand, 2002). This pattern was later recognized as characteristic of most of Asia, with MSM constituting another reservoir of HIV infections in some countries. During the period 1985–1988, reports emerged of full-blown AIDS cases in Thailand. The saga of one HIV-infected person (Cha-on, known later as the Thai Rock Hudson, a factory guard infected by blood transfusion) was broadcast widely through mass media, putting a personal face on the new disease and confronting any denial that existed (Porapakkham et al., 1996). A better parallel might be with Philly Lutaya, the Ugandan singer who, like Cha-on, allowed his story to be widely told in order to teach people about the reality of AIDS. Between 1989–1990, some shocking prevalence figures emerged and were allowed to be broadcast to the public, such as 1989 findings that 44 percent of Chaing Mai brothel workers were HIV+ (Porapakkham et al., 1996).

Thailand's national response to AIDS also began in 1989. It was initially directed by Mechai Viravaidya and involved the Population and

Community Development Association (PDA) he directed. Mechai and his family planning association had already achieved success in promoting contraception in Thailand. To combat AIDS, the PDA used short television and radio spots to raise awareness and motivate behavior change. The primary target groups were adolescents, CSWs, clients of CSWs, and "wives of 'promiscuous' men" (Pattalung & Bennett, 1990, p. 3). Among the messages were the seriousness and fatality of AIDS, "the risks of promiscuity," and the impossibility of knowing who might be infected. The PDA initially soft-pedaled its message, using the image of a teenage couple holding hands. This seemed to be having little impact, so "both the television and radio spots used fear arousal messages to attract attention, to convey the core information that AIDS is fatal but can be prevented by using condoms" (Pattalung & Bennett, 1990, p. 4).

Mechai also made speeches during his national tours, calling for partner reduction as well as condom use. "His joke to military audiences was this: 'Take the number of sex partners you have right now and divide by two. That should be your goal'" (A. Bennett, personal communication, January 10, 2003).

The PDA gained the cooperation of the Ministry of Interior and disseminated standardized information about AIDS and prevention through networks of district governors, subdistrict chiefs, and village headmen throughout rural Thailand. Similar dissemination occurred through the police force, and community development and social welfare administrations, which fall under the Ministry of the Interior (Pattalung & Bennett, 1990).

AIDS education was incorporated into school curricula in 1990. This education evolved to include life skills empowerment (Phoolcharoen, 1998). Thai religious leaders, along with other community leaders, "became involved in contributing to policy dialogue, resource mobilization and the local implementation of activities" (Sittitrai, 2001, p. 14). By 1991, Thailand's new prime minister became directly involved in AIDS control. He worked with technocrats and activists, chaired the national AIDS committee, established a national AIDS budget, and helped develop a five-year plan (Porapakkham et al., 1996).

The USAID–funded AIDSTECH project was active in Thailand from 1988 to 1991. It sponsored a number of small but influential pilot projects and research studies which the Ministry of Health and other donors built upon. It funded the first expansion of the 100 percent condom program from one province to nine before it was nationalized. AIDSTECH funded Mechai's "AIDS in the Workplace" project; a peer education program for Bangkok IDUs; educational flip charts for Shan populations; mobile entertainment discotheque programs for rural youth; sex networking research; and the like. None of these alone would have had national impact. But combined with other projects they formed a lattice of action that moved Thailand's AIDS control agenda along at a quicker pace (A. Bennett, personal communication, January 21, 2003).

Thailand developed a national sentinel surveillance system which covered both the majority population and high-risk groups. Surveillance data indicate that HIV prevalence peaked at ANC sites, as well as among FSWs and their clients, in the mid-1990s and has been slowly decreasing since then (UNAIDS/Thailand, 2002). New HIV infections in Thailand declined from 143,000 in 1991 to 20,000 in 2000. HIV infection levels among pregnant women have dropped from 2 percent in the mid-1990s to 1.5 percent in 2001 (Sharma, 2001). Prevalence among military conscripts fell from a range of 3.5–4.0 percent in 1993 to a range of 1.6–1.3 percent in 1998–1999, according to the HIV/AIDS surveillance database compiled by the U.S. Census Bureau.

Population-based surveys provided evidence of broad behavioral change in the general (male) population soon after Thailand's initial response to AIDS (there was far less need for behavioral change among most females). Phoolcharoen, Ungchusak, Sittitrai, and Brown (1998) summarize this behavioral change as follows:

Over the next few years, numerous behavioral studies found evidence of major risk reduction in the Thai population resulting from the extensive societywide efforts to promote safer behavior [37]. Comparison of two national behavioral surveys in 1990 and 1993 [12, 41] showed that the fraction of men reporting any premarital or extramarital sex in the last year fell from 28% to 15%, the percentage visiting sex workers dropped from 22% to 10%, and the consistent condom use (reporting always using condoms in commercial sex) rose from 36% to 71%. (Phoolcharoen et al., 1998)

Thus there is early evidence of delay of debut (or premarital abstinence), partner reduction by males (most but not all of which involved commercial sex), and increased condom use. We see in Figure 9.1 that decline in commercial sex between 1990 and 1993 occurred in all age groups.

Most (82.5%) HIV transmission is heterosexual in Thailand, followed by 4.8 percent IDU and 4.6 percent perinatal (UNAIDS/Thailand, 2002). Because most HIV transmissions were occurring through commercial sex, considerable resources were focused on promoting 100 percent condom use in all commercial and casual sexual contacts in order to choke off the epidemic before it spread to the majority population (Rojanapithayakorn & Hanenberg, 1996). Reported condom use in Thai brothels rose from roughly 10 percent in 1989 to over 90 percent by 1992, a remarkably short period of time (UNAIDS, 1998c). There were also efforts to reduce multiple partner sexual behavior, including specifically the number of males visiting FSWs, as seen in the following:

Figure 9.1
Age Structure of Reduction in Use of Commercial Sex by Thai Males between 1990 and 1993

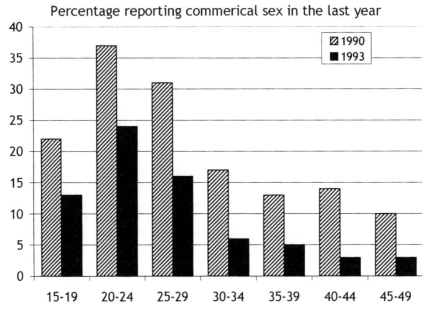

Percentage reporting commerical sex in the last year

Source: Thailand Ministry of Public Health; Chitwarikorn (2002).

The percentage of adult men visiting FSWs has fallen from almost 25% of the population to roughly 10%, and condom use when visiting sex workers has become the norm. The success of Thailand's "100% condom programme" has not had much effect on the slow but steady transmission of HIV from infected male clients of FSWs or from infected male IDUs to their regular sex partners. There has also been limited success in reducing HIV prevalence among the IDU population. (UNAIDS/Thailand, 2002, p. 2)

Using a repeated cross-sectional survey design with a structured (BSS) questionnaire, Mills and colleagues also found that reported patronage of commercial sex by the three male groups declined by an overall average of 48 percent between 1993 and 1996 (Mills et al., 1997). There was also a reduction in the number of clients per sex worker (Stoneburner & Low-Beer, 2002a; UNAIDS, 1999b).

Table 9.1 shows data from USAID–supported BSS research on condom use trends over time for men and women in Bangkok. It is important to note that the samples in BSS surveys are not necessarily representative of the entire population of Bangkok or Thailand. BSS sampling tends to select for higher-risk population segments. Regard-

Table 9.1
Reported Condom Use 1993-1996 among Groups in Thailand

Populations	T1 1993	T2 1994	T3 mid-1995	T4 late-1995	T5 mid-1996
% of men who reported using condoms with last CSW:					
service worker	89.2	92.7	89.1	92.9	93.7
office worker	88.4	96.0	-	-	-
student	92.0	83.3	95.7	95.2	94.4
% of indirect CSWs who reported using condoms:					
service worker	89.2	92.7	89.1	92.9	93.7
office worker	88.4	96.0	-	-	-
student	92.0	83.3	95.7	95.2	94.4
% of single women (non-CSW) who used condoms for last sex:					
all groups combined	18.6	23.1	20.5	19.5	18.9

Source: FHI data from Family Health International Web site.

ing condom trends among such groups, a FHI evaluation report notes the following:

Condom use levels in commercial sex confirm that use has become a norm and that accessibility does not seem to be a barrier for either male customers or the female CSWs. What stands out however are the poor levels of condom use among nonpaying partners of CSWs and among men with non-CSW single female partners. To the extent that these male partners are infected or engaged in risky sex with multiple partners posing a continuing and significant risk for their female partners, both commercial and noncommercial (sic). Some improvements are noted, although modest, for condom use by indirect CSWs with nonpaying partners. Ominously though, no improvements are noted for condom use among partners of single, sexually active Thai women who are not CSWs. (FHI, 2002)

The FHI final report just quoted also provides some outcome data indicating higher levels of abstinence among higher-risk groups. Since little seems to be known about abstinence interventions in Thailand, the following are excerpts from peer education materials for male and female youth in the citywide AIDSCAP Bangkok program:

Guidance for Male Youth [Remember that, in Thailand, customarily the first sex is with a sex worker, although this is changing.]

"Abstinence is easy if you're determined"

1. Try to avoid those things which would make you go to sex workers in the first place such as:

   - Drinking: Which can make you want to go to a brothel; reducing or quitting your drinking can help. Lowering the amount you drink is also good for your pocketbook and health.

   - Peer Pressure from Friends: Try to find ways to turn down invitations to brothels without offending your friends, or find ways to excuse yourself from the party scene before it moves on to the brothel.

Guidance for Female Youth

"Three steps you can use to help calm him down"

If you are not ready to have sex with your boyfriend because you don't think it's worth the risk of pregnancy and disease, or because you would like to keep your virginity until you are sure that your boyfriend is committed to you, then you should avoid situations or an environment that promote intimacy by trying some of the following tricks:

1. Close the door on the mood: You shouldn't let yourselves remain alone together out of the sight of others or in places where sexual desires would have a chance to fulfill themselves, because the sex drive between men and women is a hard thing to trust. If you don't want to take risks then you shouldn't give in to men's or your own desires. If you have to be together, choose places where there are lots of people or invite some friends along too.

2. Talk openly together.

3. Revise the relationship. (Bennett, personal communication, January 21, 2003)

This material is presented not to diminish the role of widespread condom use in commercial sex but to illuminate a part of Thailand's prevention program that seems to have gone largely unnoticed outside of Thailand.

In view of the evidence reviewed, HIV prevalence decline in Thailand seems at least partly attributable to the following behavioral factors: (1) high condom use among FSWs and their clients; (2) significant reduction in levels of premarital and extramarital sex in the majority population, mostly (perhaps two-thirds) on the part of males involved in some form of commercial sex; and (3) relatively low-risk behaviors on the part of women, even before the appearance of AIDS.

A fourth factor, or intervention, may also have had significant impact on HIV prevalence, namely, control and prevention of STIs. Thailand's AIDS prevention program was to some extent "built upon the foundations of Thailand's 45-year-old venereal disease prevention program" (FHI, 1996, p. 1). Even before the AIDS epidemic, "VD Units, based in every province, served two main functions. First, they provided STD services to the majority population, both male and female, and to CSWs, who were treated and urged to stop receiving customers until they were cured. Second, they provided contact tracing of the STDs back to the sexual partner" (FHI, 1996, p. 2).

The following are the words of Tony Bennett of FHI, who lived and worked for many years in Thailand:

A key, but often overlooked, intervention was the national network of provincial and district government STD clinics. No other country in Asia had . . . such an extensive network. These clinics were established since the 1960's, expanded nationwide in the 1970's and, by the 1980's, they provided rapid, state-of-the-art diagnosis and treatment of STDs to the lower income urban and rural population. These clinics also provided free condoms and educational materials to the most vulnerable populations; conducted outreach and contact tracing; and mapped all commercial sex establishments in every province and district of the country. The hundreds of staff of these clinics were, in fact, the ones who implemented the 100% condom program as well. (Bennett, personal communication, January 21, 2003)

Thailand had another advantage prior to the outbreak of AIDS, namely, an effective and highly developed family planning program. Thailand's mature family planning program helped in the implementation of a national condom program (which was nevertheless targeted), because people were already quite familiar with condoms, and contraceptive distribution systems were already in place.[2]

In sum, we see in Thailand considerable ABC behavior changes as well as a comprehensive AIDS control program that included A and B interventions to some extent, as well as C and D for drugs (for STD control) interventions. Its interventions targeting partner reduction and delay/abstinence seem to be not well-known outside of Thailand.

It is hard to not find parallels between Thailand and Uganda despite their different epidemic patterns. In both countries, an early and vigorous response to the threat of AIDS was developed and implemented, largely by nationals from those countries (although with limited foreign financial assistance). By the time foreign technical experts arrived in significant numbers, prevention programs were already in place; significant behavior change had occurred; and HIV prevalence had recently peaked. Perceived risk of HIV infection and knowledge of what to do to avoid infection (self-efficacy) was widespread, including in rural areas. In both countries, this was achieved within a time-frame of four to five years.

The predominant strategy of Thailand may have been 100 percent condom use (at least for social marketing, or sound-bite purposes), whereas zero-grazing may have been Uganda's. Yet there was ABC promotion in both countries, as well as ABC behavioral changes in the majority populations (except as noted, abstinence levels among Thai women were already quite high).

It is worth mentioning that Buddhism is the primary religion of Thailand and Buddhist monks have participated in AIDS mitigation programs. In an overview assessment of what contributed to the HIV reduction successes of Thailand (as well as Uganda and Senegal), Sittitrai (2001) notes that Thai religious leaders, along with other community leaders, "became involved in contributing to policy dialogue, resource mobilization and the local implementation of activities" (p. 14).

How much effort by how many of which groups is needed to reverse the upward surge of an AIDS epidemic? In closing the section on Thailand, it is interesting to note that the same Thai AIDS expert just quoted on explaining success did not think Thailand was doing enough even at the time that HIV prevalence was being reversed, as seen in the following:

Present national efforts and achievements in response to the already enormous size of the AIDS epidemic in Thailand are grossly inadequate. The Thai government is still trying to handle the situation without having to resort to radical measures or mobilize resources to an extent which would be economically painful. Nongovernmental organization (NGO) achievements are also negligible given the size of the problem. The government needs to waste no more time in responding to the growing crisis and instead bring all available resources to bear in an effort to radically change sexual behavior, protect the human rights of infected individuals, and prepare for the future medical, social, and economic needs of families already affected by the epidemic. (Ungphakorn & Sittitrai, 1994, p. S155)

NOTES

1. Of course, Asian countries want their share of AIDS money. It also makes public health sense to err on the side of caution. Some at this conference cautioned that the local epidemic simply may not have taken off yet; those at risk may not yet be found; HIV may simply not have entered the majority population yet; or surveillance may have been inadequate to detect reservoirs of HIV.

2. Still, the rate of condom use for contraception among married couples has never exceeded 2 percent (Knodel & Pramualratana, 1996, p. 97).

10

Common Factors in Success

As we conclude examination of particular countries that have had varying degrees of success in AIDS prevention, looking for common elements that may explain success, it is surprising that such an exercise has not been done before, and often. If there were 500 water and sanitation projects that failed and a handful that were successful, wouldn't we look carefully at those that worked to see what we could learn? The only exercises quite like my own that I am aware of have been some papers, or paper sections, by UNAIDS that attempt to generalize about the common elements in the first three countries generally recognized as AIDS success stories, namely, Uganda, Thailand, and Senegal. Sittitrai (2001) actually points to the same elements that have been identified in this book: primary behavior change, government commitment, and a multisectoral and multilevel response. Sittitrai asks, "What are some essential features of effective programmes which are shared by the three countries? In each one, national AIDS programmes share a package of common features that UNAIDS regards as 'best practice.'" He continues by naming them as follows:

- Strong political commitment at the highest level to dealing with the epidemic (this ensures policies and funding to address the epidemic)
- Multisectoral approaches to prevention and care and, at government level, involvement by multiple ministries
- Multilevel responses (at national, provincial, district, and community levels)
- Effective monitoring of the epidemic and risk behaviours, and dissemination of the findings both to improve policies and programmes and to sustain awareness

- A combination of efforts aimed at the majority population and focused on groups at high risk, at the same time
- Implementation on a large scale
- Integrated prevention and care. (Sittitrai, 2001, p. 5)

As useful as this list is, they really just identify recommendations for a general approach. They do not identify specific programs or provide clues to what specifically causes behavioral change, the proximal causes of incidence or prevalence decline. Still, in the analyses by individual country, programs that may relate to behavioral change are identified or implied. For example, the first four of seven elements of Senegal's response are as follows:

- As in Uganda and Thailand, politicians in Senegal were quick to move against the epidemic once the first cases appeared in the second half of the 1980s.
- Since 93 percent of Senegalese are Muslims, the government made efforts to involve religious leaders, HIV/AIDS became a regular topic in Friday sermons in mosques, and senior religious figures talked about it on television and radio.
- Many other levels of Senegalese society joined in. By 1995, 200 NGOs were active in the response, as were women's groups with about half a million members.
- HIV prevention was included when sex education was introduced in schools. Parallel efforts reached out to young people who are not in school. (Sittitrai, 2001, p. 9)

For both Uganda and Senegal, a rise in age of sexual debut is identified, perhaps reflecting the importance this UNAIDS author attributes to this behavioral response. The author notes the following: "Sengalese women in their early 20s did not have sex until they were almost 19 or older. For their mothers' generation—the women who were between 40 and 49 in 1997—the median age was closer to 16" (Sittitrai, 2001, p. 11).

In listing the probable reasons for Uganda's early and decisive downturn in seroprevalence, the UNAIDS author mentions the presidential commitment to dealing with the AIDS problem first, followed by its multisectoral approach, then its wide involvement of people at different levels of society, specifically its political, community, and religious leaders.

There is widespread agreement that high-level political commitment is an essential ingredient in a successful anti-AIDS program, perhaps a *sine qua non* I agree. Unfortunately, such commitment has been rare in the part of the world that most needs such programs: Africa. This is summed up in the following:

Table 10.2
AIDS Prevention Behavior

Country	Women, all ages					
	No change in sexual behavior	Kept virginity	Stopped sex	Began using condoms	Restricted sex to:	
					...one partner	...fewer partners
Benin 1996	48.7	7	2.5	1.8	24.7	1.6
Burkina Faso 1998-99	47	6.9	1.1	3.4	34.1	1.3
Cameroon 1998	42.3	4.9	2.7	6.7	36.4	7.4
CAR 1994-95	22.8	-	5	4.1	55.4	9.3
Chad 1997	33.5	8.4	4.5	1	19.2	1.4
Comoros 1996	29.4	24.5	2.1	5.1	29.4	3.6
Eritrea 1995	58.3	10.5	2.7	0.9	8.6	0.4
Ghana 1998	21.3	8.4	4.3	6.4	56.7	3.4
Guinea 1999	14.4	8.1	2.4	3.3	62.7	8.6
Kenya 1998	22.6	12.7	6.3	2.6	46.7	5.3
Madagascar 1997	43.8	3	1	0.9	15.8	2.1
Mali 1996	50.2	4.9	1.5	2.1	39.1	1
Mozambique 1997	23	3.5	2.4	3	39.3	5.2
Niger 1998	54.4	10.5	3.4	1.1	26.5	0.5
Tanzania 1996	18.1	12.8	6.6	2	48.9	14.5
Togo 1998	47.5	6	3.3	3.6	32.9	3.1
Uganda 1995	-	-	9.3	1.9	47.7	3.3
Zambia 1996	19.9	10.2	9.9	2.4	56.5	2.5
Zimbabwe 1994	78.9	-	3.3	4.2	9.9	1.8

Source: DHS/Measure Web site, http://www.measuredhs.com.

condoms are not readily available, condoms may be associated with lack of trust between partners, and all the other reasons we have reviewed? It is astonishing that these and other data pointing to PBC have been ignored so long.

In fact, PBC seems to be the natural response to concern over, or fear of, HIV infection. It is the behavior change that most people choose for themselves, whether or not it is promoted. I do not want to overstate influence of religious groups, school authorities, or anyone else in achieving significant behavior change and lower HIV prevalence rates. I say this because survey findings show that people opt for PBC over condom use on the order of at least four or five to one everywhere. But where it is actively promoted with even a fraction of the resources that normally go to risk reduction, such as in Uganda and Senegal, there tends to be even more PBC. My point about FBOs is that they are particularly suited to PBC promotion for several reasons, but they are not the only organizations so suited.

It conforms to the findings and principles of diffusion of innovation theory to build upon what people already do rather than try to promote alien ideas or technology. Specifically, one of the attributes of innovations that determines acceptability and adoption of innovation is its compatibility with existing values, norms, and behavior. Another is its lack of complexity (Rogers & Shoemaker, 1971). Condom technology is fairly complex. It involves learning behaviors sufficiently well to provide protection, and then adopting those behaviors for an indefinite period of time. It involves monetary and other costs, such as reduction in sexual pleasure. Condoms (and drugs for STD treatment) need to be constantly resupplied in vast quantities, raising complex logistical and sustainability challenges. Condoms also require a system for their safe and hygienic disposal, a factor often overlooked. Condom use is usually not compatible with existing norms, in fact they seem to contradict fundamental norms regarding behavior among youth. And these norms are often closely linked with religious beliefs and values.

In short, it is only common sense that PBC could or would be adopted more readily than condoms or medications. Yet common sense is precisely what is so often missing in promotion of any sort of innovations across cultural barriers. Fidelity and delay of debut ("premarital chastity" in the words of some religious groups) are behaviors which are familiar, sustainable, compatible with prevailing social and religious norms (formal, communitywide norms, if not informal adolescent norms), and incur no monetary costs or technological challenges. Indeed, sexual abstinence for fertility regulation is a tradition found throughout Africa (Blanc & Poukouta, 1997).

Based on evidence from Uganda, Senegal, Thailand, and Jamaica in particular, interventions based on PBC may also be the natural response of Third World governments as well as many of their citizens. These efforts are too often thwarted or at least diluted by well-meaning foreign experts (people like myself) who are sure we have the only proven interventions. PBC may be the natural government response in resource-poor countries for several reasons that ought to be explored further, namely, because it makes sense; it is what people do anyway; it is more compatible with culture; and religious leaders and education authorities tend to support PBC and remain opposed to condoms. Furthermore, where we have Pattern II or generalized epidemics, we are often talking about countries with authoritarian leaders and tradition-based societies. The leaders tend to agree with religious authorities (of whatever religion) that condom promotion to youth sends the wrong message, one that seems to assume or even condone premarital sex. It makes more sense to political leaders in religious and tradition-bound societies to avoid political risks, to promote premarital abstinence among youth and fidelity among the married.

In addition to the DHS data summarized in Gardner, Blackburn, and Upadhyay (1999), two authorities of the Harvard AIDS Institute made the following observation about global findings of sexual behavior change:

In several countries, studies have documented that the average age at first sexual intercourse for women is slowly rising, the number of men and women reporting non-regular and/or multiple sexual partners is declining, the age differential between occasional sexual partners is narrowing (although still involving the pairing of younger women and older men) and the frequency of transactional sex is declining in several populations of young adult males. In contrast, few favorable trends have been noted concerning regular condom use. (Tarantola & Schwartlander, 1997, p. S15)

Yet papers like this are exceptions, and seem to have had little or no impact on official thinking. Still, a U.N. report issued five years later let the cat out of the bag once again, summarizing what we have learned from DHS data and putting this in the report's executive summary as follows:

- In all countries surveyed, a large majority of men, ranging from 60 to 90 percent, reported that they had changed their behaviour to avoid AIDS. In contrast, in only half the countries have a majority of female respondents made a behavioural change.

- Among those respondents, whether male or female, who did change their behavior, the most frequently cited change had entailed confining sexual activity to one partner.

- Only a small percentage of respondents began using condoms to prevent HIV transmission. Fewer than 8 percent of women in all countries surveyed report that they have changed their behaviour by using condoms. Among married women, the percentages are particularly low. Figures are usually higher for men, ranging between 15 and 25 percent in most countries. (United Nations, 2002, Section IX)

Even though these empirical findings have now been spelled out several times, the donors keep funding condom and drug programs. Data that contradict the prevailing paradigm or challenge Western, urban values tend to simply be ignored. We turn now to an egregious example of just that.

CAN SURVEYS MEASURE CHANGES IN SEXUAL BEHAVIOR?

For over a decade, surveys such as the DHS asked a pair of questions: Since you heard of AIDS, have you changed your sexual behavior to prevent getting AIDS? followed by, If so, in what ways? As already noted, the most common answer by far was that men and women were moving toward having only one partner. Younger respondents reported they are waiting until they are older to begin sex. Responses mentioning condoms came in last or nearly last. These were not the answers the AIDS professionals wanted to hear. The questions that elicited these answers were discontinued by the DHS in 2000. I was told in an e-mail from the Measure Project (that conducts the DHS) that these questions were dropped because it was felt they don't elicit valid information. In another e-mail from the same project, "I learned that as I understand things, a 1999 meeting of AIDS experts convened and determined that these questions . . . the old wording was not relevant, since previous studies indicated that self assessments of behavior change did not correspond to actual changes in behavior" (Croft, 2001).

I am not certain of the reference here, but there was a joint Impact, UNAIDS, and FHI workshop in May 1998 (Pisani, Brown, Saidel, Rehle, & Carael, 1998) which in fact concluded that when we corroborate self-reported data with other reported survey data, qualitative findings, and biological data, we actually have something quite useful (Pisani et al., 1998, p. 19). Moreover,

One reason more behavioural data has not been collected in the past is that many people are deeply skeptical about the validity of self-reported data on sexual behavior. "Everyone lies about their sex lives," the reasoning goes, "so why bother asking?" The same was said of asking about contraceptive use just 20 years ago, but fertility and reproductive health surveys are now routinely conducted on every continent. (p. 19)

Recently there seems to be a growing consensus that surveys on self-reported sexual behavior can be useful. Even if there is systematic distortion, such as exaggeration upward or downward of one's number of sexual partners, this probably endures over time, and so trends in one direction or another, rather than exact numbers, are worth paying attention to. While it is not possible to validate data on sexual behavior through direct observation, "It is, however, possible to triangulate them with data from other sources to see whether the picture presented is consistent and credible," as concluded by the FHI/UNAIDS workshop. Such corroborative evidence includes qualitative research, such as in-depth, key-informant interviews and focus group discussions. Change in new HIV infection rates is the most desirable corroborator.

This sort of triangulation has become an accepted research norm. For example, in the UNAIDS Multisite study, researchers used internal validity checks, such as comparing biological data on STDs with self-reported behavior; comparing reports of spouses; and comparing numbers of sex partners reported by both men and women (Buvé et al., 2001). In any case, why is it that we should believe self-reported sexual behavior when it involves condoms (and there are many condom-related questions in the DHS AIDS questionnaire), but not when it involves the number of sexual partners or abstaining from intercourse for a defined period of time?

Perhaps potential problems have to do with self-assessments involving *change*, even if they provide a time frame for change, as distinct from simpler descriptions of behavior with shorter time frames (did you have a nonmarital, noncohabiting partner in the past twelve months?). One problem is that if asked about change in sexual behavior due to AIDS in the past five years, wouldn't someone who had made major changes six or seven years ago also answer affirmatively? Or if such a person answered "no" and yet had made significant changes a bit earlier than the time frame provided, would that be misleading information?

Perhaps the way to overcome this problem could be to ask respondents these questions without a specific time limit, by substituting "in recent years" instead of "in the past five years." Or even "since you became aware of AIDS." In fact, the current KABP questionnaire of the Uganda Ministry of Health (Uganda Ministry of Health, 2001, p. 17), allows for respondents to reply that they started making these changes "more than five years ago," even though the wording of the question asks about the past five years.

Barton (1997), in his review of behavioral studies in Uganda, commented that "difficulty arises in disentangling persons 'maintaining' safe, faithful behaviour versus those persons 'changing' their behaviour to include faithfulness after previously engaging in casual (non-regular) sex" (Barton, 1997, p. 29). This distinction between maintained and changed behavior is one of the reasons questions about change are asked, especially if comparisons from earlier baselines are not available. One rationale to abandon the change questions is that it seems better to establish a baseline and then ask direct questions about behavior within a recent time frame, and compare the results to establish change (but see later discussion). The trouble is, the DHS and some other surveys have often changed the questions, or question wording, of the time period parameters for a question, so that comparisons are impossible or fraught with peril. This may be especially true with questions about multiple partners, but it is even true with condom questions. This is one of the arguments for keeping the behavior change questions, whatever their shortcomings.

There seems to be a curious double standard at work here. Major donor organizations decide to drop behavior change survey questions because of concern over the concept of change. Yet BCC remains one of the areas of significant funding and spending for AIDS prevention. We dedicate ourselves to changing behavior, and of course we know what is best for Africans and others. We decided at the outset, and by definition, that behavior had to *change*, based on the assumption that all Africans were engaging in risky practices, which we defined as having "unprotected" sex. As it happens, we had just the technology and the technical know-how to correct this widespread problem. After all, we had decades of experience in contraception. We did not allow for the possibility that many Africans and others were already monogamous or having a relatively late sexual debut. In fact, our focus was not on these behaviors but on condom use, which we already knew was low.

Now to shift to a more positive viewpoint. The behavior change questions would seem to have value for several reasons. The main one is that they tell us if there has been any sort of behavior change attributable to AIDS—useful information itself—and then we hear unprompted what type of change it has been. There is value in asking an open-ended question about sexual behavior, one that does not prompt answers related to condoms, last nonregular partners, partner reduction, or anything else. Even if the time period for change is inexact, and even if we cannot necessarily take the proportions identifying particular change options as reflecting the exact prevalence of condom use or abstinence in a population, we at least learn something about the relative choice or even prevalence of behavioral options.

In a survey such as the current DHS that asks explicitly about condoms, mentioning this word twenty-nine times in various questions, the behavior change questions would provide an opportunity for respondents to tell interviewers about some other types of behavior not asked for or rarely asked for. And however inexact the particular measures might be, they tell us in at least a general way about trends over time. These behavior change questions have been asked in the Uganda Ministry of Health population-based surveys since at least 1991, and so there are data on this covering a decade. In districts known to have particularly low condom availability and low user rates, such as Kotido (ever-use is 3%), responses to the behavior change questions show that the condom option is only mentioned by 0.8 percent. Meanwhile in Mpigi district (condom ever-use is 33.9%), the condom option is mentioned by 13.9 percent. Thus we see a relationship between mention of the condom option and reported condom use, even though the proportions seem always to be lower in the retrospective question.

The truth is that we don't know if the retrospective behavior change questions provide underestimates of certain behaviors, or if the more direct questions (Have you ever used a condom?; Did you use a condom with your last nonregular partner?) provide overestimates. A study in the United States compared two methods of assessing behavior change: the retrospective change method, which asks respondents about change explicitly by asking whether they have made any changes in their sexual behavior in a past time period; and the longitudinal or panel method, which asks respondents at two different times about their sexual behavior and then compares the two sets of answers. The study found that among heterosexual men and women, as well as among gay men, the two methods of measuring change in condom use produced very similar answers (kappa of 0.38). And "among both heterosexuals and gay men, the two methods of measuring change in number of partners had a small but significant level of disagreement. Among heterosexuals, kappa was –0.14; among gay men, kappa was –0.16. Where the two types of change measures disagree, the data do not permit the authors to say which measure is more valid" (Stone, Catania, & Binson, 1999, p. 102).

If these findings hold for Africa and elsewhere as well, results from behavior change questions over the years suggest that not only is condom use low in Africa, but it may be lower than reported from other, more direct types of questions. For example, most recent surveys in Uganda suggest that condom ever-use is about 20 percent. Yet data from five southern districts (where condoms are more available and promoted than elsewhere) show that between 4 percent and 15 percent report condom adoption as a recent behavior change over the past five years (Ministry of Health, 2000–2001). This could be accurate if most condom adoption occurred earlier than five years prior to interviewing. The lower figures might also provide a measure of more consistent use than questions about use on last occasion with a certain type of partner.

One might speculate (since in fact I have heard this said) that the behavior change questions were dropped because there was so much reporting of partner reduction and abstinence, and researchers simply found this hard to believe. They concluded that there must be something wrong with the questions, since everyone knows that behavior doesn't change in this way. A more cynical, less charitable view might be that the questions were dropped because so few people anywhere reported choosing the condom option, and this conflicted not only with the AIDS prevention mindset ("everyone knows that only condoms can prevent AIDS") and the fact that donor organizations have spent countless millions on the condom solution. It also conflicts with the rosy reports that social marketers and others have been providing about ever-growing condom sales. Likewise a cynic might speculate that most USAID- and UNAIDS-funded surveys dropped questions on ever-use of condoms because use was found to be so low, and scarcely growing. By asking instead about use with last nonregular partner, condom use could look a lot better, as long as the denominator of these figures is seldom mentioned.

Finally, some critics of the change questions argue that those surveyed tend to tell interviewers what they think is expected. True enough, and the polite response factor should be factored in to all survey data. Answers about condoms, abstinence, and faithfulness are probably all exaggerated to some extent. This is why we look for trends over time and do not take any answers as absolute. But the fact remains: No matter who conducts the survey, the proportions of those reporting A and B rather than C changes are several times higher. Although there may be methodological problems with the behavior change questions, it seems to me culturally arrogant for donors to simply decide these are of no value and to ignore the evidence. I suggest that the evidence from these questions has some value, at least no less value than questions that supply words like condom.

It has been argued specifically that since Uganda emphasized A and B behaviors so much in its early prevention program, this led to higher levels of A and B answers to survey questions. However, this does not explain why other countries in Africa and beyond also produce high levels of A and B answers. The most recent study results I have seen come from Mozambique, a country whose overall AIDS prevention program has emphasized condoms and STD treatment with little attention to A and B, at least prior to 2002. In spite of this, a survey in Sofala and Zambezia provinces found that "reducing the number of sexual partners was reported by respondents from both Sofala (62.2%) and Zambezia (71.6%) as the most important behavioral change they have adopted to stem transmission and spread of HIV/AIDS" (Bukali & Mesa, 2002, p. 71). This compares with reported condom use of 21.1 percent in Zambezia and 6.5 percent in Sofala.

In sum, as we consider data from Uganda, Senegal, and elsewhere in the previous chapters, we need to take all self-reported data on sexual behavior with a few grains of salt, and that includes condom reporting as well as PBC. When it is possible to link or triangulate survey data with qualitative findings, biological data, and AIDS prevention interventions, I do so. When I do not do so, it is because I lack the information, but this does not necessarily mean it does not exist.

THE ROLE OF FBOS IN HIV/AIDS PREVENTION

During the early years of the HIV/AIDS pandemic, many people who worked in HIV/AIDS prevention thought of religious leaders and organizations as naturally antagonistic to what they were trying to accomplish. In many minds, the stereotype of a religious leader was that of a conservative moralist who disapproved of any form of sexual behavior outside of marriage, to say nothing of nonstandard sexual practices. They were also thought or known to disapprove of what was seen as the only solution to HIV infection, namely, condoms. An example of the tendency to stereotype the attitudes of religious leaders toward HIV/AIDS is seen in the following comment by Kaleeba, Namulondo, Kalinki, and Williams (2000) who note that some religious leaders "have also added to the misery of people living with HIV by condemning them as 'wrong-doers' or 'sinners,' thus contributing to the stigma to which they were already subjected from other sections of society" (p. 58). Organized religion was also seen as an impediment to sex education in schools. A recent UNAIDS report puts it the following way:

Perhaps the greatest obstacle to AIDS prevention activities in many countries has been opposition, or even just the fear of opposition, from religious authorities. The tendency for religious leaders to prescribe abstinence and mutual monogamy in the face of overwhelming evidence that these behaviours are not always the norm has been seen in almost every corner of the world. The fear of offending powerful religious constituencies has created gridlock in some national governments, and for good reason. Conservative lobbies have shown that they can obstruct everything from family life education to condom promotion if they choose. (Pisani, 1999, p. 12)

Presenters at an earlier International AIDS conference point to another issue:

Religious taboos on sexual education have been harassing AIDS prevention throughout Latin America. The confrontation between the condom and abstinence or fidelity has snapped closed any possibility for negotiating joint strategies. It has polarized political stances that clash public opinion and counterattack official efforts for AIDS prevention. (Farill, Romero, Ornelas, & Urbina, 1992)

Keep in mind that there has been longstanding antagonism between the Catholic church and those who work in family planning over artificial contraception, and that many of us who work in global AIDS have backgrounds in family planning (myself included). There are also religious fundamentalists, at least in America, who have proven highly emotional about anything that seems linked in any way to abortion. These fundamentalists often seem to be against all forms of contraception, perhaps—it is suspected by some—because it liberates women from control by husbands. More directly related to AIDS, religious fundamentalists in America and elsewhere sometimes condemned those infected with HIV as sinners, as people who deserve punishment from God for their immoral behavior.

These dated and stereotypic generalizations miss the point that many FBOs have been working patiently, compassionately, and effectively for a number of years in AIDS mitigation, specifically in the following: (1) care, support, and counseling of PLWHAs, including care of AIDS orphans and income-generation projects for PLWHAs and their dependants; and (2) HIV/AIDS prevention. There have been workshops and seminars for leaders of a variety of Christian, Muslim, Hindu, Buddhist, and other FBOs, and these efforts often have resulted in programs aimed at both followers of the religion and others in local communities. These efforts generally demonstrate the ability of FBOs to bring AIDS support and education to communities not being reached by government campaigns, often using creative educational approaches (e.g., Ariyaratne, 1998; Campolino & Adams, 1992; Farill, Romero, Ornelas, & Urbina, 1992; Kagimu et al., 1998; Roesin, 1998). Part of the challenge now is for health workers to overcome their own biases against working with FBOs. "Activists in HIV/AIDS prevention need to purge themselves of their own prejudices and negative attitude towards religious institutions and engage them as partners in breaking the silence" (Iwere, Ojidoh, & Okide, 2000, p. 1).

Recent evaluations have shown that FBOs can have considerable impact in both areas of HIV/AIDS mitigation: prevention and care. This should not be surprising. The following introductory note from "Religious-Based Initiatives" (MAP International, 1997) describes accurately the potential role of religious organizations, even though it confines its remarks to Christian churches in Latin America:

RBIs (religious-based initiatives) are pivotal to the success of prevention and care efforts in Latin America as well as globally. Churches are found in nearly all communities in the region and wield a significant level of cultural, political, social, educational and economic influence. The Church can be viewed as the largest, most stable and most extensively dispersed non-governmental organization in any country. Churches are respected within communities and most have existing resources, structures and systems upon which to build. They possess the human, physical, technical and financial resources needed to support and implement small and large-scale initiatives. They can undertake these actions in a very cost-effective manner, due to their ability to leverage volunteer and other resources with minimal effort. Unfortunately, the resources, capabilities and potential of the Church are considerably neglected or untapped, and it has not been considered part of the solution and/or a driving force in the fight against HIV/AIDS. (MAP International, 1997, p. 1)

Indeed, FBOs are often the only genuine nongovernmental organizations in many rural parts of poor countries, or at least the strongest and most influential. FBOs are able to mobilize people and resources and are able to reach rural or isolated areas because of their vast organizational networks. They have strong, expansive infrastructures and have a good understanding of local social and cultural patterns. Many FBOs have long worked in health care as well as related areas such as education. There are more than 1,000 faith-based hospitals in sub-Saharan Africa alone, and the number of religious schools may be uncountable. In all parts of the world, FBOs have the power to mobilize large numbers of volunteers to contribute to worthy causes. In addition, those who work or volunteer their efforts through an FBO tend to be motivated by faith, idealism, and compassion, rather than merely by salary or career prospects. These former can be powerful and sustaining motivators when working with the sick and dying, under extremely difficult conditions.

FBOs can be very influential in timely policy debates concerning the legal, ethical, and moral issues surrounding AIDS and human rights (Lazzarini, 1998). They can be influential in the debate over introduction of sex education, reproductive health, AIDS, and STDs in schools—and at what level this can occur. In fact, religious leaders and FBOs can be more than merely influential since they provide a substantial proportion of primary and secondary education in many less-developed countries.

It should be mentioned that indigenous or traditional healers also qualify as faith-based groups in many parts of the world, since both the healers and their clients believe that spiritual forces underlie all or most indigenous therapy and healing. But the contribution of traditional healers to AIDS mitigation will not be considered here because there is already a literature on this (cf. Green, 1996; King, 2000 for summaries), and because of the present need to draw attention to the role of internationally recognized religious groups.

Illustrative Experience to Date of USAID FBO Direct Grantees Already Working in HIV/AIDS

From searching the literature, it appears that USAID is the main donor agency that has supported FBOs in international AIDS. Therefore most examples in this book of FBOs working with donor funds are USAID funded. There is another reason for focus on USAID experience. There is currently a major debate over the Bush administration's announced intention to support faith-based initiatives, with the focus of debate being almost exclusively domestic rather than international. Underlying the debate is fear of the unknown: What if support of FBOs opens a Pandora's box that results in unforeseen negative consequences? In fact, USAID has been supporting FBOs in both humanitarian and development efforts for decades, with basically positive results and few if any of the problems of the sort Americans are worried about (see Is There a Downside to FBO Participation, in a later section). The following are some examples of USAID–funded projects implemented by FBOs which address HIV/AIDS.

Catholic Relief Services (CRS) has implemented a variety of HIV/AIDS programs since 1989 with an emphasis on care and support of PLWHAs. In Zimbabwe, the group has assisted the diocese of Mutare in establishing AIDS committees in every parish. Groups of community volunteers visit and care for the sick, perform AIDS preventive education dramas, and engage in income-generating activities. In an area where 25 percent of the adult population is HIV positive, this program has greatly improved the quality of life for PLWHAs, assured dying parents their children will be cared for, and brought support and comfort to families and communities afflicted by AIDS.

In Egypt, CRS has established the country's first anonymous HIV testing and counseling service. The group, together with Caritas Egypt, opened an HIV/AIDS Counseling Center in Cairo in 1995; its drop-in service targets youth, women, IDUs, street children, and sex workers. The center is collaborating with the Ministry of Social Affairs to train hundreds of youth and women peer educators in HIV, AIDS, and STD awareness.

CRS has also established a care facility in New Delhi, India, for recovering drug users who are HIV positive—a model that is being replicated by the government of India at three additional sites in New Delhi.

Another faith-based USAID grantee, *World Vision*, is currently implementing innovative HIV/AIDS prevention strategies in Asia among high-risk groups, such as sex workers, truck drivers, migrant workers, fishermen, and IDUs. The group promotes a variety of prevention modalities, such as condom promotion and distribution, STD syndromic management, and behavior change. Some of its programs are regional and are focused on cross-border populations, and some are active in non-USAID presence countries, such as Burma. World Vision also works with AIDS orphans and PLWHAs in a variety of care and support programs.

The *Salvation Army*, another USAID grantee, provides relief supplies, education and prevention programs, HIV counseling and testing services, and spiritual support for infected and affected communities throughout Africa.

FBO Activities

Among the programs that have been initiated, supported, and organized by various FBOs, with or without USAID funds, are the following:

- Support groups for the purpose of counseling PLWHAs and their families
- Support groups for educating local communities about HIV/AIDS
- Peer educator programs aimed at HIV and STD prevention
- Programs of income generation and vocational training for PLWHAs and their dependants
- Programs of care and support for children orphaned by AIDS
- VCT, depending on linkages with hospitals that can do testing, although CRS provides its own anonymous VCT services in Egypt and perhaps elsewhere)
- Rehabilitation of girls and women who are vulnerable to or are trapped in the trafficking sex trade
- Hospice care
- Drama or music groups for the purpose of AIDS awareness and education
- Fighting against stigma associated with HIV infection at local community levels

Regarding the last, fear and stigma are major obstacles to AIDS prevention or care initiatives, and faith-based groups can be important in reducing the stigma too often associated with HIV/AIDS. Just as open and frank discussion about AIDS by the highest government authorities helped to reduce stigma in Uganda and Senegal, faith-based leaders have the authority and influence to have a similar impact. The Christian Church Association of Lesotho, for example, implemented a project whose objectives were "to prepare communities for accepting and supporting all people with HIV and AIDS, [and to promote] destigmatization of STD/HIV/AIDS patient care" (Barton, Thamae, & Ntoanyane, 1997, p. 8). CRS, which works with partners on more than eighty HIV/AIDS projects in over thirty countries, has facilitated awareness workshops with clergy in several countries in order to demystify and destigmatize HIV/AIDS (C. Stecker, personal communication, February 15, 2003). The Adventist Development and Relief Agency held workshops for clergy, in part to "sensitize church leaders and reduce fear/denial/stigma associated with HIV/AIDS" (ADRA, 2002). Reverend Gideon Byamugisha, for many years the HIV/AIDS coordinator for the Church of Uganda (Anglican), has organized and led many workshops, conferences, and seminars on breaking the silence about AIDS and acceptance of HIV+ people as part of the community of faith. He continues to do so across Africa and elsewhere in his current role as the church liaison of World Vision International's Hope Initiative. As a final example, the Kip & K'Noodle Project of the Global Initiative on AIDS in Africa, a religious-oriented NGO, uses drama in Cameroon to "change the way people think and react to HIV/ AIDS, replacing stigma with love and compassion" (B. Marshall, personal communication, February 15, 2003).

Since most funds targeted toward AIDS are still directed at prevention, it is worth looking at some examples of FBO programs aimed at prevention in countries where impressive changes in sexual behavior have been measured. Moreover, the role of FBOs in prevention is less well-known and documented than their role in care and support.

The country where FBOs have had the most impact is probably Uganda, and this has already been discussed. The contribution of FBOs to AIDS prevention in Jamaica has also been described. The Dominican Republic is another of a handful of countries that seems to have stabilized or even reduced HIV seropositivity at the national level, to have reduced infection rates of standard STIs, and to have achieved positive behavior change, not only in relatively high condom user rates, but in reductions of numbers of partners outside of marriage or consensual union. In the mid-1980s, the Dominican Republic's national STD and AIDS control program (PROCETS) made efforts to preempt church opposition to the program's condom promotion efforts by explaining to Catholic church leaders the lifesaving mission of its AIDS prevention campaign (Green & Conde, 1988). More recently, a variety of churches have participated in training workshops and have become involved in some way in AIDS prevention, including the Episcopal church, Assemblies of God, various Pentecostals and evangelical churches, the Church of the Nazerene, Methodists, Reformed Christians, the Church of the Prophet, and the Movimiento Misionero Mundial.

FBOs as Behavior Change Agents

We see from some of these previously mentioned examples (notably Uganda and Jamaica) that FBOs can influence behavioral change through a variety of methods, ranging from the relatively passive (inviting or allowing AIDS educators to address congregations) to the more active (using the prestige and moral authority of the religion to strongly advocate behavior such as fidelity or abstinence). The moral authority that FBOs bring to promotion of behavior change can influence at least certain types of people more than through what might be called technological approach of condom promotion.

Recent long-term, qualitative research in KwaZulu-Natal (South Africa) attempted to establish whether membership in any religious group affected sexual behavior, using as a measure the degree of extra- and premarital sex (EPMS) found in the population. The researcher found that Pentecostals had the lowest level of EPMS, much lower than mainline Christian churches (the same churches that seem to have influenced EPMS so profoundly in Uganda and Jamaica). Although the KwaZulu research is based on a very small sample and may not be very representative of FBOs, the author's analysis of the mechanisms that seemed to reinforce abstinence and monogamy in the Pentacostal community may shed light on how and why FBOs influence behavior, as seen in the following:

Indoctrination against all types of EPMS is persistent, and is fortified with eschatological incentives and disincentives. Religious experience is subjectively intense; levels of participation in lively, expressive worship are high. Church members are highly socialised, meeting almost daily for prayer, Bible study, music practice or social events; interaction between men and women is over- seen and monitored by senior members. Finally, there is the real risk of exclu- sion (from participation, or even membership) where a breach of the sexual code is suspected or proved. Mainline Christianity may feature these elements, but in much smaller doses. (Garner, 1999, p. 5)

Such interpretation of the mechanisms and antecedents of behavioral change may be considered speculative, mechanistic, even reductionis- tic. It could be argued that it matters less how and why participation in religious groups, along with exposure to religious teachings and leaders, results in positive behavior change; only that it probably does. On the other hand, studies of this sort may help overcome scientific skepticism surrounding abstinence/delay and the role of religious groups.

Some other studies in Africa have suggested that religious affilia- tion is associated with lower HIV seroprevalence or less risky behav- ior. For example, in Kagera, Tanzania, there was more seroprevalence decline during 1987–1993 among Christians than among non-Christians (Kwesigabo et al., 1998). Yet religious affiliation is not always found to be associated with less risky behavior. A study of young men and women (ages 10–24) in Lusaka that looked at the correlates of risky sexual behavior found the following:

Being affiliated with the Protestant or Catholic religions (as compared to "no" or "other" religion) was not associated with ever having had sex or number of lifetime partners, but was protective for number of partners in the 3 months prior to the survey. Regular church attendance, however, a measure of religi- osity, failed to achieve statistical significance on any of the three sexual behav- iors considered. (Magnani et al., 2002, p. 80)

Yet, as seen in the following, this same study pointed to the value of community-based efforts aimed at influencing young people through inculcation of positive values and behavioral norms through peer groups, something religious fellowships are capable of:

The study findings concerning the powerful effects that peer behaviors (actual or perceived) have on youth are also worthy of note. In Lusaka (as elsewhere), adolescents appear to form groups or networks that engage in group behaviors that, in some cases at least, are mutually reinforcing. Overcoming negative influences of peers can indeed be a formidable task. However, associating with peers who engage in "positive" (i.e., socially approved) behaviors has been shown in research in the United States to be protective across a wide range of health and social outcomes. A growing number of observers are of the belief that community-based efforts to change social norms and values surrounding adolescent reproductive health behaviors and issues are likely to be most cost-effective in addressing the adverse effects of negative peer influences in the long run. (Magnani et al., 2002, p. 82)

Impact of FBOs on HIV Infection Rates

Reviewing the experience of the first developing or resource-poor countries where national HIV seroprevalence has stabilized or declined, we see that all have involved religious leaders and FBOs in HIV/AIDS in significant ways. One might hypothesize that in order to change behavior enough to impact HIV seroprevalence at the national level, it may be necessary to have significant involvement from the religious community. In countries where religion is important, faith-based involvement may prove to be at least as necessary as condom social marketing, treatment of STDs, voluntary counseling and testing, and other interventions considered state-of-the-art that characterize the approach of countries serious about AIDS prevention. This is especially true for countries which can be considered highly religious and where FBOs comprise a major part of the nongovernment sector. It certainly makes little sense to mobilize only secular resources in such countries. It might be nearly impossible to prove definitively the hypothesis just suggested, but much could be learned through careful analysis of how behavior came to change in the handful of countries that have stabilized or actually lowered national HIV infection rates. It is necessary to conduct more qualitative studies as well as survey research that includes response categories that can capture answers that refer to all aspects of religion.

In light of the apparent contribution of FBOs to positive behavior change, and possibly to reduced STD and HIV infection rates in countries like Uganda and Jamaica, steps should be taken to overcome any such conflict or antagonism between a faith-based approach and a secular, public health approach. As noted previously, religious organizations ought to be given support in doing what they do best in AIDS prevention: promoting what they call fidelity and abstinence. That is precisely where most of these organizations want to place emphasis. Forcing FBOs to work in condom promotion risks alienating them from AIDS prevention efforts, and thereby losing the great potential they bring to such efforts.

FBOs in Care and Support Roles

The other area of great contribution is care and support of PLWHAs and their families. This has not been emphasized in this book because the role of FBOs in this area is better understood and less controversial. It is less controversial because FBOs have always been involved in care of the sick and needy, and as noted, a great deal of health care and social services in poor countries are already in the hands of FBOs.[1] Once enough members of a particular religious group become HIV infected, that group usually finds a way to help members of the group in more direct ways. In countries with high HIV infection rates, AIDS has been found to affect local communities in various ways, such as stretching health services beyond their capabilities, loss of employment, exacerbation of poverty, increase in the number of widows and orphans needing psychosocial and economic support, increasing the spread of opportunistic infections, increasing the need of mourning rituals and the costs associated with burials, and the list could go on (cf. Girma & Schietinger, 1998). FBOs can and do become involved in some or all of these problem areas, especially if there is little alternative support available. They usually do this with no outside funding.

Although local FBOs in poor countries typically lack in money, they have the capability to mobilize volunteers to address these problems, as noted above. An example, provided by the Victoria Project and implemented by the local Lutheran church with support from a French NGO, can be seen in the following:

Volunteers in Tanzanian villages near Lake Victoria take part in a community effort to care for vulnerable children. Each village elects a 16-member committee to identify needy children, discuss and establish priorities, maintain a register of orphans, and implement the activities. The volunteers provide needy children and families with food, clothing, bedding, and medical care, and pay for school fees, uniforms, books, and lunches. While the program could not function without its paid staff, it also could not function without the many volunteers who perform the daily tasks essential to ensuring that the children and families who are most needy receive services and supplies. (Mukoyogo & Williams, 1991; quoted in Schietinger & Sanei, 1998, p. 5)

In an example of how FBOs assist PLWHAs directly, a model faith-based project emerged in Brazil's largest city, Sao Paulo, in the late 1980s when a Catholic nun, with the support of her local bishop, recruited a group of volunteers to make home visits to PLWHAs. Dubbed Project Hope, the effort spurred the opening of three centers devoted to care and support of the HIV infected. In addition to home visits, the project provides health programs, including nursing care, occupational therapy, and psychological support groups; carries out a variety of fund-raising efforts, including Campaign for Orphans; provides training for volunteers and families of PLWHAs; and implements HIV/AIDS public education campaigns aimed at youth.

Project Hope reaches close to 200 new PLWHAs each year and relies on a large network of volunteers and "godparents" who care for AIDS orphans. The National Program for STDs/AIDS has worked closely with the project and supported the opening of its two additional centers in the cities of Vila Esperanca and Guaianases.

When large, resource-rich, international FBOs assist, they can have major, national impact, as the following final care and support example from Malawi illustrates:

The Catholic Diocese of Mzuzu joined other stakeholders in the fight against HIV/AIDS by initiating the AIDS Education and Home Based Care project. Mzuzu Diocese covers the entire northern region of Malawi, almost one-third of the national territory, with an estimated population of 1.2 million, virtually all of whom are subsistence farmers. In cooperation with seven home based care providers at the parish level, 44 AIDS committees and 149 home visitor volunteers, the project promotes increasing awareness as to the causes of AIDS and the means of its transmission. Specialized training has been provided to all volunteers/committees in order to better prepare them to effectively convey this information to community members through multiple education sessions. The project directly reaches a target population of 2,000 persons positively diagnosed with HIV/AIDS, and indirectly 30,000 people through general education efforts within the community. . . . In the home based care component of the project, the group of volunteers periodically visit the sick, the dying and the orphans left without care when their parents become too ill, and then die. Services provided range from material support such as food, medicine, tuition and clothing, to spiritual support, all in coordination with the network of other institutions dealing with the terrible effects of the AIDS pandemic in Malawi. (CRS Web site, 2001, http://www.catholicrelief.org)

Again, we should ask ourselves who else in poor countries is capable of providing such services? Only traditional healers come to mind, and they are a self-defined type of faith-based group themselves. It has become clear that governments of poor countries with high seroprevalence are unable to respond adequately. Constitutional arguments against public funds going through FBOs in the United States sound academic in a country like Malawi.

Is There a Downside to FBO Participation?

Is there a downside to FBO participation in HIV/AIDS mitigation or to donor support of such efforts? Some drawbacks have been voiced. In fact, since President Bush announced his faith-based initiative as a cornerstone of the new administration's approach to delivery of social and humanitarian services in late 2000, debate about the pros and cons of FBIs prevailed in various news media, at least before September 11, 2001. These issues are worth considering because they might arise in discussion about FBO participation in HIV/AIDS activities.

Concern: Some who work in public health criticize a moral approach to HIV prevention on the grounds that such an approach is judgmental, that it relates to the values of particular groups, and therefore has no place in public health. Regarding the moralizing issue, it may be that sexual behavior, certainly some of the high-risk varieties that involve coercion, rape, and seduction of minors, takes us into the realm of morals or at least ethics, whatever our objections. Issues involving questions of right and wrong (should I or should I not?) may well require an ethical answer. Noted sociologist Amitai Etzioni argued in a *Christian Science Monitor* op-ed that AIDS prevention has become unduly medicalized, when in fact it is largely a behavioral issue (Etzioni, 2003). He argues that the solution to AIDS is fundamental behavioral change leading to monogamy, and that AIDS prevention funds "should be largely granted to educators, community leaders, and faith-based institutions, rather than to medical centers" (Etzioni, 2003). He notes that this is what worked in Uganda. I would add that the strong involvement of religious leaders in Uganda and Senegal, who indeed take a moralizing approach to AIDS prevention, suggest that both a moral and a medical (or value-free) approach to prevention may be what people need. The current language of the National Strategic Framework for HIV/AIDS Activities in Uganda, 2001–2006 still uses words like sexual immorality, defilement, adultery, and indecent assault (Uganda AIDS Commission, 2001). I am not arguing that this Ugandan document or program *should* use such value-laden terms, I am only pointing out that they do, and that this suggests that values may have a place in motivating behavior change. After all, Uganda can show much more evidence of sexual behavioral change than the United States.

Ellen Goodman has also wondered whether in the American transition from a more religious to a more secular society, we have somehow given ourselves a "moral lobotomy." She asks whether, in our reluctance to being (considered) judgmental, "are we disabled from making any judgment at all?" (quoted in Etzioni, 1996, p. 135).

There is also a widespread concern among AIDS activists—perhaps especially in the West—and among some health professionals that promotion of abstinence and fidelity can lead to marginalization, stigmatization, and possibly victimization of those who do not change behavior in these ways. It is true that stigmatization and victimization have been an unfortunate consequence of some of the pronouncements made by some religious leaders, and this happened more often earlier in the pandemic. But because of the mistakes of some religious leaders, this should not be a reason to exclude FBOs forever from AIDS prevention. It has been my own experience that the FBOs who wish to work in AIDS prevention, or are already doing so, are not the fundamentalist variety feared by many AIDS activist groups. They tend to be relatively liberal and open-minded. Perhaps self-selection filters out the more intolerant groups, whether Christian, Muslim, or any other religion.

Concern: Some critics of FBO involvement in AIDS point to examples of religious faith healers who raise false hope by claiming to be able to cure or improve cases of AIDS through prayer, the laying on of hands, and the like. The answer to this is that anyone can claim miraculous AIDS cures: physicians, traditional healers, nutritionists, religious faith healers, and others. This does not mean that all in these groups should be excluded from working with donor funds in AIDS mitigation. Some PLWHA groups might even argue that hope of recovery can help keep people alive who would otherwise die; indeed, it has been documented that depression and helplessness stresses the immune system. This consideration does not mean, of course, that donor funds should go to anyone making unsubstantiated claims of any sort.

Concern: Another possible problem arises in the separation of church and state issue. If USAID or another donor works with one religious group, must it work with all such groups so as not to appear to favor a particular religion? Or if the donor supports one FBO at higher levels of funding than another, could this be taken as evidence of religious bias or favoritism? The answer to this concern in the present international context is that USAID has been funding FBOs like CRS, the Salvation Army, and World Vision, without significant problems of this sort. USAID grants have been awarded on the basis of technical soundness of proposals and the experience of the FBO in carrying out similar projects, as with any other NGO, subtype private, voluntary organization, or PVO. In USAID's view, FBOs are one type of PVO that USAID funds because they bring experience, their own funds, and a record of achievement to international health and other sectors of development.

Concern: USAID and other donors have their own agendas, and these are different from the agendas (purpose, goals) of religious-based groups. By wielding economic power, donors might distort the purpose of at least smaller FBOs with fewer financial resources. The answer: If this has not happened yet in USAID's support of FBOs, it probably won't, at least to a great extent. Usually the technical assistance that PVOs acquire by becoming USAID grantees helps them become more effective in doing what they already want to do and may be doing.

Other FBO-related policy issues and debate points have recently arisen and been much discussed in the U.S. print and electronic media. The debate has focused on possible roles of FBOs in delivering social and health services in the United States, rather than in less-developed countries. Yet the issues are worth considering because they could arise in the context of international health. Illustrative points include the following:

- Public support of FBOs could lead to government favoring some FBOs (such as conservative, Christian ones), and discriminating against others (e.g., Muslim, animist or liberal, activist ones). Or the government might discriminate against FBOs that support policies that are out of favor with the current administration, namely, contraception or choice in abortion. This raises serious constitutional issues of separation of church and state. It might also raise the possibility of lawsuits against branches of government.

- Public support of FBOs could lead to government interference with, or creeping control of, religious institutions. FBOs that rely on government funds would become less independent; more creatures of the changing policies of the government of the day. FBOs would also have to comply with U.S. (or other government) labor laws in hiring, and adhere to other personnel policies that may be quite different from current practices.

- FBOs would probably hire extra staff to carry out new or additional social services. Yet with the irregularities and uncertainties of government funding, FBOs would have to do as much laying off of staff as new hiring. Some FBOs have used this as a reason to not become involved in the first place.

- Public support of FBOs could lead to a corresponding shift away from current government support of nonreligious PVOs, such as CARE International and Save the Children (just to use examples from international health programs).

Promoting the Maximum Range of Prevention Options

In AIDS prevention, there remains an unnecessary conflict in many countries between a medical or realistic approach to AIDS prevention (and to behavior change specifically), and a religious or moral approach. This antagonism is sometimes evident in the popular press and in some of the AIDS literature. This seems to pit medically enlightened progressives who recognize human behavior as it actually is against religious conservatives who simply moralize about how behavior ought to be. The former tend to emphasize condom use and, more recently, the treatment of STIs. The latter emphasize abstinence and fidelity, or sticking to one partner. Since treatment of STDs does not really qualify as behavior change, we end up with condoms being promoted by one group, and a group of behavior options not involving condoms by the other group.

Yet it is well known in public health and behavioral science that people differ, often greatly. One preventive approach to something as complex as human sexual behavior will never appeal to all people, let alone influence their behavior. Some people will continue to have multiple partners, therefore the only preventive options may be condom promotion and the treatment of STDs they might contract.[2] The same may be true to some extent for those already HIV infected. Other men and women seem to respond to the abstinence or delay and fidelity messages. It certainly makes public health sense to reach all categories of people and provide the maximum range of prevention options just as we try to provide the maximum range of methods in contraception.

Donor Funding

In spite of the contributions of FBOs in prevention, as well as in care and support of PLWHAs and their families, extremely few international HIV/AIDS funds have gone to support FBO programs in HIV/AIDS prevention to date. This may in part be due to the absorbtive capacity of FBOs, and the relative paucity of FBOs that have experience working with major donor organizations. But reasons less often acknowledged may be closer to the truth. For example, donors have been reluctant to fund FBOs who wish to emphasize a behavior change approach that many in public health have little faith in (abstinence and fidelity). And there have been refusals to award AIDS grants to FBOs that don't want to promote condoms.

During the XIV International AIDS Conference in Barcelona (July 2002), there was very little recognition of the constructive roles FBOs have played in AIDS mitigation, especially in prevention. In fact, there seemed to be a coordinated effort to sideline and marginalize FBOs at the conference. There was a fair amount of discussion about an article in the *New Republic* (Allen, 2002) that presented a balanced view of the abstinence, delay, and partner reduction ideas and findings that I and a handful of colleagues brought to the attention of the international AIDS community. High-ranking officials from major donor organizations were heard to opine that any such ideas were part of a plot from the religious right. Furthermore, they were heard to say, public health would never yield to right-wing or religious pressure (even if millions of lives could thereby be saved).

Well, neither would I yield to political pressure. But neither I nor my colleagues who have been raising questions of great public health concern come from the religious right. We only ask that our colleagues look at the evidence, use their common sense, and leave Western cultural baggage behind.

Immediately after the XIV International AIDS Conference in Barcelona, there were several postings on international AIDS list-serves criticizing or outright condemning religion and FBOs. The contribution of FBOs to AIDS mitigation was said to be little more than stigmatizing the sick and dying. One man posted a note on INTAIDS urging that we all oppose religion because *"religion kills."* A posting from South Africa said in effect that the only good religious leader is one who gives out condoms.

I submitted the following response to the first posting:

Subj: Re: [intaids] AIDS2002: Religion Kills?

Date: 7/18/02 9:36:37 AM Eastern Daylight Time

Regarding Altman's comments, activism directed against corporations in the interest of public health is fine but let's not get carried away. The admonition that AIDS activists oppose religion may sound like an enlightened and progressive approach to some in Europe and the USA. But the truth is that religion is a power to be reckoned with in Africa and indeed in most resource-poor parts of the world.

In the fight against AIDS it makes no sense to marginalize or alienate the groups that run many of the hospitals, clinics and schools. Obviously it is more effective to work with the powers that be. Experience in countries like Uganda, Senegal, Jamaica, and Thailand suggests that making religious leaders part of the solution means that they are less likely be part of the problem.

A religious group's willingness to promote condoms should not be the litmus test for participation in AIDS prevention. Many are willing to do so, but their preference is to emphasize delay of sexual debut and partner reduction ("fidelity") in their prevention strategies. Examination of which behaviors changed to which degree in the few countries where HIV prevalence has stabilized and declined suggests that all three behavior changes (delay of debut, partner reduction, and condom use) are needed.

Perhaps for the first time on any AIDS list-serve, my note was not posted. In fact, I saw very few if any postconference postings by anyone presenting an alternative view to "religion kills."

My suggestions were apparently considered too radical to get beyond the censor. Deep suspicions about FBOs continue to dominate the AIDS-related Internet discussion groups. For example, a posting by the president of Catholics for a Free Choice dismisses FBIs as a mechanism "which would force-feed the poor with religious propaganda" (Kissling, 2003). I wonder if such people have ever been to a country like Mozambique, where FBOs may be the only health care providers. It doesn't ultimately matter what Westerners imagine about FBOs; they will continue to play an important role in health care among the poor.[3] There may be some proselytizing along with health care from some of these groups, although I have seen little evidence of this myself during thirty years of work in developing countries.

This FBO bashing was not lost on the FBOs. Following the Barcelona conference, the Ecumenical Advocacy Alliance, ecumenical representatives, and other supportive individuals wrote the following to the Secretariat of the World AIDS Conference:

[We] express our serious concern at the near-absence of faith-based groups from the agenda of the 14th International HIV/AIDS Conference in Barcelona. Many submissions were made, under the headings of workshops, satellite meetings, posters, NGO exhibition booths and skill-building events. Almost all submissions were rejected. (http://www.e-alliance.ch/hivaids/actionletters.htm)

Around the same time, twelve members of the U.S. Congress wrote a letter to the secretary of the Department of Health and Human Services (July 17, 2002) complaining about the marginalization of FBOs (among other complaints), questioning whether U.S. taxpayer funds ought to go to sending delegates to such conferences. They wrote the following:

We were also shocked to learn that the Vatican—which cares for one in four people receiving treatment for HIV infection globally—was uninvited to the conference. None of the major speeches or lectures dealt with faith's role in the crisis. And the Associated Press reports that some of the conference's seminars and workshops often became "religion-bashing" sessions.

This letter circulated among interested parties and no doubt fueled paranoia among the AIDS establishment that conservatives have a secret plot to cut off funds to global AIDS programs. This political polarization, already a serious obstacle to common sense and public health prior to Barcelona, only became more pronounced during and after Barcelona. If conservatives in the United States do curtail funds to some programs, I believe this could have been avoided if (1) donors make efforts to include in AIDS prevention all groups that are locally important, including FBOs; (2) we listen to what Africans and others have been telling survey and qualitative researchers for many years, namely, that people often chose A and B behavior change options; and (3) people are given a full range of behavior change options for AIDS prevention, as distinct from a single one, in prevention programs.

In an exchange of e-mail on the role of FBOs in AIDS prevention, a colleague wrote to me a note that suggested working with FBOs in AIDS prevention "promotes religious fundamentalism (both Christian and Islamic) and the anti-sex values that this perspective thrives on." This in turn leads to "homophobia and bigotry" and strengthens the Taliban and "the clash between Christians and Muslims in Nigeria today" (Available at: http://puffin.creighton.edu/aarg/prevention. html).

I think what we see here, apart from paranoid thinking and *reductio ad absurdam* reasoning, is (unintended) cultural hegemony, that is, Americans projecting their urban, postsexual revolution values on Africans and others. Africans are more concerned with staying alive in the AIDS era than with fighting homophobia, a concept with which most are unfamiliar. Indeed, the American AIDS expert just quoted who abhors working with FBOs posted the following outline of his philosophy of the joys of multipartner sex:

Unlike gibbons and some other mammals, humans are not naturally monogamous.

Some major religions make polypartnering (having sex with several partners) a sin in order to promote monogamy. However, there is nothing intrinsically wrong with polypartnering. Indeed, polypartnering allows participants to enjoy a greater variety of sexual behaviors with a greater number of persons, to enhance their lovemaking skills, and it can be very enjoyable for both participants.

Imagine if religions were to dictate that it was morally wrong for people to eat out at different restaurants, requiring its adherents to stick to one restaurant for their entire lives; or to stick to one movie—seeing the same film over and over again, never being allowed to see a new movie or to broaden one's experience.

The ideology of the sexual revolution which occurred in North America and Western Europe during 1965–75 was very important in breaking down the Victorian morality of the past, allowing people to become more sexually free.

I believe this was a positive change in human growth, and we should not use the HIV/AIDS crisis as an excuse to revert back to a monastic view of sex. We need to be more sex positive, and encourage people to feel they can become open to sexual experiences with different people. There is nothing wrong with sex with different partners. The problem is not the sex, but the failure to prevent unwanted pregnancies and sexually transmissible diseases.

Responsible polypartnering requires condoms and birth control as a given at all times. We need to teach those who engage in the joys of polypartnering how to effectively protect themselves from potential dangers.

My comment on polypartnerism to this colleague, posted on the Anthropology and AIDS Research Group list-serve in February 2003 (http://puffin.creighton.edu/aarg/prevention.html), was that it may be all right for Americans to cherish this lifestyle and philosophy but it is not the message needed today in Botswana, where some 40 percent of the sexually active population is HIV infected.

THE ROLE OF AFRICAN HEALERS IN ABC

This section is relevant to AIDS prevention in resource-poor countries where indigenous health practitioners, usually referred to in Africa as traditional healers, take care of a substantial proportion of health care. I will focus here on African healers because Africa has both the highest rates of HIV (as well as sheer numbers of HIV-infected people) and the greatest reliance on indigenous healers by the population, if we compare broad regions of the world.

This section also pertains to the broader issue of cultural compatibility, indigenous responses and life as it really is, even if Westerners or for that matter Africans might prefer it to be different. In matters involving community-based health, it is important to work with and through traditional healers if for no other reason than they are the primary health care providers in Africa.

Most in the religious community in and outside Africa would not be comfortable with this parallel, but viewed objectively, traditional healers constitute a kind of faith-based group, since most of them believe they are empowered to heal through ancestral or other spirits. (God the Creator of the Universe is thought to be too remote from daily human affairs to be directly involved in an activity as mundane as healing.) Viewed anthropologically, traditional healers may be regarded as a kind of indigenous FBO group, based on indigenous religion. Many or possibly most healers nowadays also claim affiliation to world religions, especially Christianity or Islam, and they see little or no contradiction in following both indigenous and formal religions.

In Africa, as in many other parts of the developing world, a basic distinction is often made locally between the herbalist and the diviner-medium. In ideal-typical terms, the former tends to work primarily with natural *materia medica*, while the latter additionally cultivates a relationship with ancestor and other spirits believed to assist in diagnosis and healing. Diviner-mediums may be called *shamans* in parts of Asia and the Americas. There are other types of African indigenous healers, such as religious faith healers, bonesetters, oracles, traditional birth attendants, children's specialists, and the like, as well as newer practitioners who don't really qualify as really traditional in Africa (but they may well be in Asia), such as homeopaths, nutrition therapists, injectionists, massage therapists, or acupuncturists.

We must start this section by asking why AIDS prevention programs ought to collaborate with traditional healers in AIDS prevention. The answers may be summarized as follows:

- At least 80 percent of people in Africa rely primarily or exclusively on traditional healers.
- Traditional healers are respected, their services are available virtually everywhere, and their service is culturally acceptable. A country like Mozambique has a physician to population ratio of 1:50,000, compared to a ratio of 1:200 for traditional healers.
- Traditional healers are eager to learn about Western medicine and to collaborate and cooperate with public health programs.
- Healers are willing to warn about the dangers of multiple partners, and explain this in culturally meaningful terms. They are also potential partners in promotion of later age of sexual debut. They have already proven willing to promote and distribute condoms.
- Working with healers gives AIDS programs access to vast numbers of healers' patients, people who might not ordinarily be reachable through clinic services or even mass media campaigns.
- Traditional healers treat most of the cases of STIs in Africa. (Green, 1994)

In a country like Mozambique, where I have worked with healers in AIDS prevention, a medical doctor theoretically serves about 50,000 people. In practice, coverage is even less. Most doctors live in larger cities, while most rural Africans are lucky if they live within 5–10 kilometers of a clinic staffed by a minimally trained nurse, where medicines may or may not be available. These realities have led some who work in public health to think that healers ought to have some role to play in curbing the spread of AIDS in Africa. Indeed, from a public health viewpoint, this would seem to make a great deal of sense. Traditional healers are not only found everywhere. They are culturally acceptable and they explain illness and misfortune in terms that are familiar, that are part of local belief systems.

What is less well known outside Africa is that they treat most of the cases of STDs in Africa. In fact studies in several countries show that both healers and their patients have a great deal of confidence in plant-derived medicines used to treat locally recognized illnesses that closely resemble gonorrhea, syphilis, genital ulcer disease, and other common STDs. AIDS prevention programs in Africa have lately been putting more effort into the treatment and prevention of standard STDs as a way of preventing the spread of AIDS, since it is now widely accepted that STDs facilitate the transmission of HIV. It must be acknowledged that the medical sciences have neither proven nor disproved that plant-derived medicines might contain enough antibiotic compounds or immune-system enhancing properties to actually cure an STD. This is an area of research deserving urgent attention (Green, 1994, 1999a).

The Nature of Collaboration

A number of collaborative programs involving traditional healers have been attempted in several African countries, including Mozambique, Nigeria, Tanzania, South Africa, Swaziland, Uganda, Zambia, and Zimbabwe. The major objective of these programs has been to develop healers as promoters of condoms. Other objectives are to prevent HIV infection through sterilization of healers' instruments that come into contact with bodily fluids (there is actually little evidence that HIV is spread this way, but hepatitis and tetanus can be); to encourage referrals of healers' STD patients to hospitals (which of course is not in their financial self-interest); and to modify healers' practices that may put themselves at risk of HIV infection. It has also become recognized that traditional healers can play an important role in care and counseling of patients who are already HIV positive. Healers practicing in Dar es Salaam were found to be giving sound advice to AIDS patients about diet and exercise, avoiding alcohol and tobacco, and avoiding despair and depression. Patients were advised to refrain from sexual intercourse because it would spread the disease and waste their survival energy. Healers helped AIDS patients maintain hope and spiritual faith. Hospitals in that city, and elsewhere in Africa, are rarely equipped to provide the same kind of personal attention and understanding to chronic patients (Green, 1994).

USAID, the WHO, the Swiss Development Cooperation, and the European Union are among the international donors who have funded AIDS prevention programs involving traditional healers. Some programs operate in the public sector, typically involving a ministry of health, and may be national in scope (e.g., Uganda). Others may be smaller scale and involve only NGOs. Usually there is a workshop or seminar lasting three to five days or more during which traditional healers and nurses or health educators exchange views and information. Judging by my own experience in these programs in several African countries, the learning should not be only one way (Green, 1999b) . Biomedical health workers need to learn about traditional health beliefs and practices that can have effects on AIDS and STDs. There may be discussion about other players in AIDS or STD treatment, such as un-trained injectionists who give antibiotic shots, perhaps watered down to make the drugs go further. Traditional healers can be enlisted to dis-courage people from seeking this type of treatment (Green, 1994, 1999a).

Are Modern and Traditional Beliefs Compatible?

Some skeptics of these collaborative programs argue that there is too much basic incompatibility between modern medicine and tradi-tional African beliefs regarding illness in general, and perhaps STDs and AIDS, in particular. Moreover, they say traditional healers will never change their practices. Secure in their own minds that they have done the right thing by dismissing African medicine, health officials promote Western allopathic medicine as if there were no medical sys-tem already in place, as if Africa were a blank slate. This is wrong for at least two reasons. The first is obvious: There is a strong, vibrant indigenous system of African health already in place. The second is less obvious, and relates to compatibility between biomedical and Af-rican health belief systems.

It is—or should be—part of the basic approach of collaborative pro-grams that they not be confrontational. Instead, it's best to discover the common ground between the two systems of health and then try to build upon this in an atmosphere of mutual respect and understand-ing. Contrary to widespread opinion, there is quite a bit of common ground to build upon. If one studies indigenous African conceptions of diseases biomedically classifiable as STDs, we see that these are of-ten thought to be illnesses that are not caused by witches, sorcerers, or evil spirits, but instead are caused by having sexual intercourse with a person who is "contaminated" or "dirty" with some sort of dangerous essence (Green, 1999a, 1999b). Often blood, semen, or vaginal fluids are thought to become contaminated, polluted, or—in our terms—in-fected when it comes to this class of disease. Indeed, one often finds parallels to Western germ theory. Sometime STDs and other conta-gious diseases are thought to be transmitted by tiny—often unseen—insects or worms, called *kadoyo* among the Bemba (Zambia); *iciwane* among the Zulu (South Africa); *liciwane* among the Swazi (Swaziland); *atchi-koko* among the Macua of northern Mozambique; *khoma* among the Shona of central Mozambique; or *kokoro* among the Yoruba of Ni-geria (Foster, Osunwole, & Wahab, 1996; Green, 1999a).

Thus we see that there are parallels between biomedical and Afri-can indigenous STD belief systems: Like biomedical theory, African STD theory tends to be naturalistic, based on the idea of sexual inter-course or other intimate contact between people, or contact with blood, causing illness involving genital symptoms. Transmission of sickness might be via a tiny or unseen agent. Whatever the etiologic theory, it tends to be based to a large extent on observed cause-and-effect relationships: A person with the illness has intimate contact with someone without the illness, and some time later acquires the same illness.

The evidence for these indigenous etiologic beliefs of STD are summarized in Green (1999a). I go into this detail to discredit the widely held notion that African theories of AIDS and STDs are based on witchcraft or evil spirits, which justifies dismissal both of indigenous health beliefs and practitioners as being irrelevant in HIV or STD prevention. This intersectoral misunderstanding was exacerbated when a number of indigenous healers did seem to believe, early in the African epidemic, that AIDS might be caused by witchcraft. It must be remembered that AIDS was a new disease, and healers were not alone in speculating about its origin. By the end of the 1980s, it seems that most healers understood that AIDS was a new but deadly type of STD. Meanwhile, there was little understanding on the part of Westerners that STDs were understood by Africans to be naturalistic (nonsupernaturally caused) illnesses.

Certainly the experience in collaborative AIDS prevention programs has shown that traditional healers are almost always open-minded when they are taught biomedical notions about AIDS, especially because it is a new disease. They tend to have no difficulty understanding AIDS as an illness transmitted through sexual intercourse by a dangerous substance found in blood, semen, or vaginal fluids.

Avoiding AIDS by sticking to one partner makes sense to traditional healers because they already interpret locally recognized sexually transmitted illness as resulting, at a broader level, from a violation of the codes that govern proper sexual behavior. They typically feel encouraged and vindicated to learn that their own governments as well as the international community also believe that people should be warned against having sex with "just anyone," with too many people, with strangers, with prostitutes, with someone other than one's wife or husband. One is far more likely to come into contact with "contaminated, polluted," or otherwise dangerous semen or vaginal fluids when one strays from home, so to speak (note again the culturally competent brilliance of Uganda's zero-grazing message).

In fact, my many years of experience of research and collaborative programs with African healers leads me to conclude that African healers are much the same type of AIDS/STD prevention resource as religious leaders: Both are more comfortable and in professional character, so to speak, when they promote PBC (through warning about the dangers of straying sexually from marriage) than when they promote condoms (in accord with outside funding priorities).

Will African Healers Promote Condoms?

But we should still look more closely at condoms. Are African healers willing to promote what is seen as an alien technology from the west? In fact, traditional healers are almost always sufficiently interested in learning about modern medicine and in collaborating with doctors or nurses that they will do this on whatever terms are presented to them. This is in part because they tend to gain prestige in their local communities and respectability in the broader society by having any sort of links with modern medicine. This helps explain why, before AIDS emerged, African healers virtually everywhere were willing to promote oral rehydration salts to combat dehydration from diarrheal diseases. Once the role of condoms is explained—especially if this can be done in ways that make sense in terms of traditional STD beliefs—healers are usually willing to advise at least their STD patients to use them to avoid becoming "contaminated" with the same illness once again, and to avoid catching AIDS.

Yet while healers are willing to promote condoms—and sell them for a small profit in social marketing schemes—they often share many of the same negative perceptions about condoms found in broader African society. For example, healers have been found to believe that AIDS and STDs are actually spread by condoms (could they have made the observation that it is the very sexually active condom users that are more likely to become infected, just as some studies suggest?); that the lubricants in condoms have deleterious effects (Green, Thornton, & Sliep, 2003); that condoms are offensive to African traditions, even taboo; that condoms can cause "bad blood" to back up into the sexual organs.

Even if these beliefs can be overcome, there is always a problem supplying healers (or anyone else) with condoms on a regular basis. Contraceptive social marketing programs have supplied traditional healers in countries like Mozambique and Zambia, although I am not aware of evaluations that demonstrate consistent availability. Healers can make a few cents profit on the sale of condoms in these programs, and of course this is an added incentive to the healer. However, I believe it is a mistake to limit collaboration to the promotion of condoms, both because of the limited impact that condoms have had so far in Africa, and because it fails to tap the distinctive potential of traditional healers to promote PBC.

Program Impact of a Typical Program

How have collaborative programs involving healers fared to date? It must be admitted that there have been few external evaluations of these programs, especially ones involving a control group. A USAID–funded private sector program in South Africa that I helped design and implement underwent an internal evaluation at the end of its first year. The evaluation used survey methods and a semistructured, flexible questionnaire. According to findings, a high percentages of the sampled healers interviewed were able to do the following:

- Define and describe HIV accurately
- Describe three or more correct AIDS symptoms (and not give incorrect symptoms)
- Accurately describe three or more means of HIV transmission and prevention. (Green, Zokwe, & Dupree, 1995)

There was also evidence of positive impact on healers' practices. Almost all healers reported providing correct HIV/AIDS preventive advice as well as demonstrations of condom use. Condom promotion and provision by healers had occurred but had been seriously constrained by lack of condom availability (condom resupply was supposed to have been the government's responsibility). To be sure, these preliminary evaluation data came from traditional healers only. A more thorough evaluation in the future should include interviews with, and direct observations of, the clients of traditional healers exposed to AIDS workshops. This could give a better idea of what advice healers actually provide, whether they really promote or supply condoms. But this program and its evaluation, even though I was deeply involved in both, is what I would call a minimalist approach to collaboration with traditional healers. It does not take advantage of the great opportunity to do far more to influence fundamental change in sexual behavior. And remember that we have not yet seen evidence that rising condom use has had significant impact at national levels, or perhaps even at population levels in Africa.

Programs in the Future

It must be admitted that we still don't know the best way to work with traditional healers in the fight against AIDS. We are still learning. There is often medical opposition to the whole effort, with some doctors arguing that we encourage and lend undeserved and dangerous respectability to traditional healers by having anything to do with them.

Collaborative programs may be implemented in either the public or private sectors. The former have tended to be fragile programs that can easily be derailed and terminated if problems arise, or if a newly appointed minister of health has a curative rather than public health orientation. Yet THETA, Uganda's national collaborative program discussed in Chapter 6, has continued for a long time. It is one of the most durable programs of its kind in Africa. THETA proves that with the right elements, collaborative AIDS programs can survive for years, if not indefinitely. It has helped that Uganda's president apparently recognizes the value of traditional healers and medicine, and that a sympathetic Ministry of Health physician headed the project until recently.[4] There has also been at least one strong supporter of traditional healers and their public health potential in Uganda's national AIDS commission.

Perhaps the most powerful argument for involving traditional healers is that whatever our attitude may be toward them, they enjoy the confidence of most people and most people continue to consult them. It ought to assist AIDS prevention and other public health goals if some type of collaboration that involves these important health care providers and opinion influencers can be developed. There simply aren't enough trained health personnel to do the job, and those we have are too often remote from the population—culturally and socially as well as geographically. There should however be more careful monitoring and evaluation of programs involving healers, so that the fundamental question of whether these programs work and are cost-effective can be answered. And so that the best model of community-based prevention of AIDS and STDs can be defined and presented for adoption on a broader scale.

To my knowledge, the healer programs that have been implemented to date in Africa and other resource-poor countries have not begun to promote PBC. Yet there ought to be great potential here to influence sexual behavior. According to prevailing indigenous etiologic notions of STDs and AIDS, there are numerous reasons not to engage in sex with multiple partners or even sex outside of marriage. The reasons traditional healers give for this are not identical to biomedical explanations. Their explanations may seem exotic, or even like "meaningless pseudo-psychological mumbo-jumbo, which is positively harmful" (Motlana, in Freeman & Motsei, 1992, p. 1186). However, as I have suggested previously and argued at great length elsewhere (Green, 1999a, 1999b, 1994), indigenous STD theories in fact usually involve naturalistic ideas about contact with essences and bodily fluids through sexual intercourse, and the way to prevent this boils down to the Museveni approach to AIDS prevention: Do not graze away from home. Do not have sex with strangers, with prostitutes, with someone else's spouse, or indeed with no one but one's own spouse.

My next comments are based on less systematic research than that which informs the rest of this section. But it seems that traditional healers see their role as primarily curative. Or at least it is curative far more than it is preventive. People come to healers with a problem and healers try to solve the problem, just as biomedical treatment proceeds. When it comes to illnesses locally regarded as related to sexual intercourse, African healers do not ordinarily preach about avoiding sexual risks; they simply treat the illness. They may also prevent further illness by suggesting to the patient that his or her partner also come for treatment, but that often appears to be the extent of their preventive advice or activities. In short, it could be said that their role in STD management is much like that of a physician, at least in its curative and preventive mix.

I discussed this preventive and curative mix with some healers in Zambia in 1995. They told me that if they would have training in AIDS prevention, they would be more than happy to fulfill their responsibility to their communities and preach the word about AIDS prevention (I am using their language). What they meant is that any degree of biomedical training would legitimize healers in new roles as community health educators. It would be understood and well accepted that healers were carrying an important message from the government or from the international community about how to avoid a deadly disease.

This got me thinking more about the potential of healers as proactive community health educators rather than reactive clinicians who may also teach the ABCs of AIDS and even promote condoms when patients happen to be visiting them. Knowing what we now know about the importance of promoting PBC and the limitations of condom promotion in Africa, I believe that future AIDS prevention programs involving traditional healers should not be limited to condom promotion, or to condom promotion plus attempts to refer clients of healers to hospitals, along with a component of ensuring that any razors used by healers are used only once per patient or are sterilized in bleach. These may be useful interventions, but I believe we have not yet begun to tap what may prove to be the greatest AIDS prevention potential of healers: Enlisting them in promotion of PBC, particularly in partner reduction or avoidance of multiple partners.

Commenting on findings from several months of in-depth interviews with traditional healers in KwaZulu-Natal, South Africa, a colleague of mine notes the following:

Of the traditional healers interviewed, 92% expressed the desire to reinstate traditional sexual practices to deal with the problem of HIV and promiscuity, but only one came forth with ideas about how these could be adapted to the present situation. Lack of adherence to cultural prescribed practices is seen as the most important contributing factor to HIV and STD transmission (68%). THs do not seem convinced of the role condoms can play in the general prevention strategy. (Sliep, 2003)

A South African anthropologist with years of experience with traditional healers recently summarized his findings about healer attitudes toward condoms in the following:

Indeed, it seems that many if not most African traditional healers prefer not to recommend condoms, partly because they believe that their own medicines are more effective in preventing HIV transmission or STIs, but also because they believe that condoms present significant dangers. Many people in South Africa believe that lubrication on condoms, or so-called "condom oil" was absorbed by both men and women during sex with condoms and that this led to impurity of the blood that could only be treated with traditional medicines (Wojcicki & Malala, 2001). I have heard, too, that some people fear "worms" in packaged condoms that can be seen if a small amount of water is placed in the condom and it is held up to the sunlight. Others say that condoms can "get inside" women, or that it can "blow up in the uterus" and cause damage or death. Some fear that the semen that ought to flow out is forced back into the man's blood by the condom and thus causes a new form of illness. All of these beliefs limit use of condoms, and thus may have consequences for public health, but they also point towards some important cultural truths. These cases and beliefs suggest strongly that substances—menstrual blood, "pollution" from death and funerals, or substances from the condoms themselves—can be absorbed into the bodies of both sexual partners. Some informants suggest that sex with a condom is not really sex at all. (Thornton, 2003, p. 1)

Given these perceptions and attitudes, which are quite common throughout Africa, why fight the uphill battle of trying to turn healers (or religious leaders) into condom distributors when what they could be best at is promoting PBC? It is often said that everyone has a role to play in AIDS prevention. If this is so, then let people do what they do best. We should not be saying we need everyone to fight this scourge, but religious leaders and traditional healers need not apply. This is especially true since PBC is what seems most likely to bring down national HIV infection rates and so few are currently involved in its promotion.

POVERTY DOES NOT MEAN THAT EFFECTIVE AIDS PREVENTION IS IMPOSSIBLE

One often reads and hears nowadays that poverty underlies AIDS or at least that poverty drives the epidemic. The same is often said of marginalizion. In a recent article, Richard Parker (2002) comments, "In all societies, regardless of their degree of development or prosperity, the HIV/AIDS epidemic continues to rage, but it now affects almost exclusively the most marginalized sectors of society." That presumably means that those primarily infected with HIV may not always be poor, but they are likely to be marginlized, that is, members of groups on the margins of society, such as IDUs, MSM, CSWs, or racial minorities. This may be true for the United States and Brazil (where Parker has done a great deal of AIDS work), but this is not a very accurate statement for Africa.

Let us consider the first proposition. One explanation for why poverty causes or underlies AIDS is that poor women turn to sex work, putting themselves and their partners at risk, risk that would not exist if such women had not had to resort to sex work. Another argument is heard less often, namely, that poverty leads to poor nutrition, which may make people shed more viruses and be more infective if they are already HIV positive (Stillwagon, 2002); or that poor nutrition and weakened immune systems (more related to concurrent infections than to poor nutrition) makes people more susceptible to HIV infection in the first place (Root-Bernstein, 1993). Those who accept that poverty underlies AIDS proposition uncritically can be led to proposing AIDS prevention solutions such as Forgive Africa's Debt and Overthrow the World Bank.

We see at once that there must be more to the story, at least in Africa, because the wealthiest African countries (South Africa, Botswana, Swaziland, and Zimbabwe, until very recently) in fact have the highest HIV infection rates on the continent (25–40%), not the lowest as we might expect. Meanwhile, some of the poorest countries (Somalia, Guinea, Liberia, Mali, Eritrea) have among the lowest rates (under 3% in 1999). Certainly the two African countries that stand out as successful in reversing the direction of HIV infection rates, Uganda and Senegal, cannot be called wealthy. Uganda's gross national product per capita income is about $240, while Senegal's is under $240 (Sittitrai, 2001).

In fact, there is growing evidence that affluence rather than poverty can drive local HIV epidemics. Several studies in Africa (e.g., Over & Piot, 1993; Smith et al., 1999; Vandemoortele & Delamonica, 2000) have shown that there is an association between increased education and income, increased HIV risk behaviors, and increased HIV infection; and, not so incidentally, with increased use of condoms (discussed in Chapter 4). In pondering the notion of an education vaccine against AIDS, Vandemoortele and Delamonica (2001) note:

An inverse association between the disease burden and the level of education exists for most infectious diseases. The incidence of malaria and cholera, for instance, are known to be negatively associated with the level of education. But because of its main propagation channel, HIV/AIDS first affects those with more opportunities, including more educated, mobile and better-off people. (p. 1)

"Better-off" of course means those with higher incomes. The authors note that it is often observed that men who wear a tie do not get cholera. Yet these are often the men in Africa who are most likely to become HIV infected. One even hears of the "three Cs" risk factors for

AIDS: cash, car, and cellphone (Altenroxel, 2003). But why? It appears that higher incomes allow men to pay for commercial or transactional sex or, as is more often the case in Africa, simply to have many sexual partners. A taxi driver in Guinea Bissau might have preempted this whole poverty/AIDS debate in 1987 when he explained to a visiting *New Yorker* journalist that in Africa, "The more money you have, the more women you can get." He made clear he was not talking about commercial sex in the usual, Western sense (Shoumatoff, 1988, p. 155).

Vandemoortele and Delamonica (2001) note that a direct relationship between education and HIV infection rates (i.e., higher levels of education are associated with higher HIV infection rates) tends to be found in countries with high HIV prevalence, whereas there tends to be an inverse relationship in low-prevalence countries. Hence the difference we see between sub-Saharan Africa and, say, Brazil. Others have suggested that the direct relationship between education and HIV infection might only characterize countries in the early stages of an HIV epidemic, that as an epidemic becomes mature, we no longer see it. Yet studies of populations with mature epidemics often show continuation of the inverse relationship. For example, in one study, American and Ugandan researchers examined the association between education (usually linked to income) and HIV prevalence in rural Rakai district, Uganda, based on a cross-sectional analysis of a randomly selected, population-based cohort. The Rakai HIV epidemic must be one of the most mature in the world. They found the following:

Higher levels of education were associated with a higher HIV seroprevalence in bivariate analyses (OR 2.7 for primary and 4.1 for secondary education, relative to no education). The strength of the association was diminished but remained statistically significant after multivariate adjustment for sociodemographic and behavioural variables (adjusted OR of HIV infection 1.6 (95% CI: 1.2–2.1) for primary education and 1.5 (95% CI: 1.0–2.2) for secondary education. (Smith et al., 1999, p. 452)

The authors conclude that higher educational attainment is associated with higher incomes which in turn "facilitate behaviours that place individuals at greater risk," such as more travel and having multiple sex partners (Smith et al., 1999, p. 457).

Another random sample, population-based study of socioeconomic status (defined by possessions, acreage, housing quality, and education) and HIV infection was also conducted in Rakai. The researchers found that "higher economic status and certain occupations were consistently associated with more partners (lifetime or within last year) and higher levels of concurrent partnerships for both sexes" (Ssengonzi et al., 1996).

A study of socioeconomic status and HIV prevalence among pregnant women in Dar es Salaam likewise found that "women of higher socioeconomic status in Dar es Salaam were at greater risk of HIV infection" (Msamanga et al., 1996). Other studies show that lower education and other socioeconomic status indicators are associated with greater risk behaviors, such as not using condoms, but this may not translate into higher HIV infection rates, at least in Africa. Elsewhere, such as in Brazil (Veloso et al., 1998), there tends to be a relationship between lower socioeconomic status and higher HIV infection rates.

Carael, Cleland, Deheneffe, Ferry, and Ingham (1995) reveiwed sample surveys conducted from 1989 to 1993 of male and female respondents ages fifteen to forty-nine years reporting sex with a nonregular partner in the preceding year. Significant positive associations between educational level and risk behavior were found among women as well as men in about half the studies.

This topic was discussed at a regional conference held in Nairobi to discuss young women and HIV/AIDS in eastern and southern Africa. The following is from a conference summary posted on af-aids@health dev.net (December 19, 2002):

The role of education was discussed at length by F. Malola from Malawi. In a presentation that proved to be controversial to some, he outlined how education has contributed to the spread of HIV—not only through providing a venue for men and women to meet but also that with education one is able to secure employment thus money "to woo girls into sexual relations." Much debate was spurred, in and out of session halls, if it was just location (e.g., schools, university) that was the risk factor or the impact of being educated itself.

Some who argue very publicly that poverty drives AIDS epidemics might concede that in Africa, wealth may be even more of a risk factor than poverty for men, but not for women. We have just seen some data that show that socioeconomic status may be associated with higher HIV infection among women as well. But what about the increased risk of women driven to prostitution or transactional sex by poverty? Even this may be more complicated than it appears. Chin, Bennett, and Mills (1998) showed that level of CSW customer turnover (the average of number of clients per week) is a major factor explaining HIV infection levels, at least in Asia. One of the reasons that HIV infection levels may remain low among sex workers in the Philippines is that they have an average of two to three clients per week, compared to more than this per day in some countries.

When I was evaluating the impact of AIDS prevention programs in the Philippines in 2001, infection rates among CSWs were still below 1 percent, in spite of significant economic decline in the previous two years. It appeared from interviews that my colleagues and I conducted and from available data, that while more Filipina women had turned to commercial sex, the number of male clients was the same, or even lower, due to the weak economy and perhaps to the effects of AIDS preventive education. This meant that the number of clients per woman was even lower than it had been before. This would prevent infection rates among CSWs from rising. Incidence, if someone took the trouble to measure this, might even decline, assuming other contributing factors remained roughly the same. On the other hand, poverty may well be one of the causes of the sugar daddy phenomenon in Africa, Jamaica, and elsewhere. This refers to older men offering gifts of cash or kind to young unmarried women in exchange for sexual favors. This has become sufficiently widespread that it often provokes little or no negative social sanction (Gupta & Mahy, 2001). In fact, a good deal of female sexual behavior in Africa can best be understood as strategies for economic survival and adaptation to patterns of male dominance in low-income countries (Cohen & Trussell, 1996; Green, 1994; Guyer, 1994). As Barnett and Blaikie (1992) have summarized it, African women gain access to economic resources through a range of sexual relationships with men, including monogamous and polygamous marriage, long-term relationships lacking *de jure* recognition, stable nonresident relationships involving visits on a regular basis, casual liaisons, and the type of commercial prostitution familiar in industrialized countries. "The economic transaction may not be the main or express aspect of the relationship for the participants, but given women's underlying unequal access to economic resources, sexual favours and reproductive potential are powerful resources—sometimes the only resources—on their side of the transaction" (Barnett & Blaikie, 1992, pp. 77–78).

Thus, we see a widespread pattern of transactional sex in Africa that is not the same as commercial sex in Asia or elsewhere. This is said to be a pattern driving the epidemic in Cameroon, which has one of the highest levels of infection in the West African region (Calvès, 1999).

None of this is to argue that there is no relationship between poverty and HIV infection levels, or becoming HIV infected. But it is not the simple, unidirectional, casual relationship that is usually presented. We have already seen that greater income can, through various mediating factors, underlie higher HIV infection rates. Poverty can lead or even force women into sex work, but poverty can also greatly limit the number of customers, and the proportion of men who are clients of sex workers. There seems to be a relationship between drug abuse and poverty, so it might be said that poverty, along with other social factors, can contribute to the high numbers of IDUs who are then at high risk of acquiring an HIV infection (Chin, 2002). Thus, the evidence suggests that any relationship between poverty and AIDS is complex and multidirectional.

Another part of the issue is that poverty is a difficult factor to influence. Part of the value of the National Research Council table of epidemiologic factors relevant in Pattern II AIDS transmission (Cohen & Trussel, 1996, previously mentioned) is that it reminds us that some desirable changes may not be achievable in the short or medium term, to use the language of the table. For example, poverty, unemployment, and gender inequality are the aspects of AIDS that occupy the attention of many American anthropologists concerned with international AIDS (cf. Schoepf, 2001). Yet it could be argued that little will result from denouncing poverty, at least not as much as putting into place effective, workable prevention programs. In fact, poverty and inequality are an easy set of factors to invoke, since one can argue on the side of the angels yet little can be done to change these factors during anyone's lifetime. For example, it has long been recognized that poverty and gender inequality underlie high fertility and associated problems, and that poverty and unemployment provide the conditions for child diarrheal disease. Yet during the decades this has been known, poverty and unemployment have become worse, not better, in Africa.

It is fine to denounce the evils of poverty and better still to work actively to change the broader social and institutional systems that need changing. But let this not keep us from finding better ways in the short and medium term to prevent HIV transmission, even if delay of sexual debut does not have quite the same visceral appeal as, End poverty, racism, gender inequality and homophobia NOW! Certainly when I was a sophomore, I never would have attended a rally centered on the theme of delayed sexual debut.

The Reverend Eugene Rivers, an African-American social justice and AIDS activist from Boston, met with religious leaders and others in June 2002 in Abuja, Nigeria, to discuss that country's response to AIDS. There was discussion and debate about the true root causes of AIDS, that is, poverty, the status of women, crushing external debts, lack of education, and the like. According to a U.S. Embassy cable describing the event, "Rivers agreed that all these issues must be addressed, but he said there was no time to wait for root causes to be solved. This focus was a distraction or an excuse for no action. The immediate prospect of death for so many millions required immediate, direct action."

This reflects my position. I don't support the simplistic belief that AIDS is caused or driven by poverty, but this in no way means I am against overcoming poverty nor that poverty does not exacerbate HIV epidemics in some ways. We should all seek to overcome injustice but let this not be confused with a sound AIDS prevention strategy.

Poverty does affect the power of people to make health-related choices, in part by limiting these. Poverty is often associated with less education, inferior social position, powerlessness, lack of access to health and other services, and perhaps discrimination on the basis of ethnic group, race, religion, or gender. Both theories and programs of behavior change assume that such change is volitional, that if a person wants to change, this is possible. Obviously in the case of a poor woman who must exchange sex for subsistence, or women in societies where rape or coerced sex goes unpunished by law, behavioral decisions in the direction of condom use or partner reduction are not fully in the hands of these women (UNFPA, 2003, p. 42).

GENDER EQUALITY IS DIFFERENT

The role of gender inequality must be treated somewhat as a separate issue. We saw evidence in our discussion of Uganda that part of that country's success in addressing its AIDS crisis was to empower women and girls so that they became better able to resist unwanted sexual advances and negotiate condom use. Moreover Ugandan women's groups were among the first targeted by IEC programs and many of these became actively involved in AIDS prevention. Uganda's experience suggests that ABC prevention programs, primary behavior change, and women's advancement (to use Museveini's term) are somehow all compatible. A hypothesis arises for empirical testing from Uganda's experience, namely, that raising women's status through various measures helps make PBC possible and thus contributes to HIV prevalence decline.

It may be possible to achieve a degree of PBC without much change in female empowerment, as may have happened in Zambia and Senegal. But it seems easier to achieve PBC and marked national HIV decline if women are empowered to refuse unwanted sex and they have more economic and political power. We cannot pretend that women are adequately protected, and their human rights respected, simply if men use condoms most of the time or even all the time. Women must have the power to refuse unwanted sex and there must be serious legal consequences for rape and sexual coercion.

I have been rather mystified at the lack of interest by Western women's organizations in women's empowerment (to use the Western term) in Uganda. Part of the reason is that this story has not really gotten out. From personal and Internet discussions I have had, the reason seems to mostly be the ethnocentric blinders worn by so many: Anything to which the label "abstinence" can be attached must be a secret plot to end all family planning and restrict women to the kitchen forever.

Gender advocacy groups (such as Gender-aids on the Web) seem to pin most of their hopes and efforts on improving condom negotiating skills or on another technological solution—antimicrobials. Gender-aids puts out a regular news feature called "Microbicides this Week." The development of safe and effective microbicide would be a great help in AIDS prevention, and I have been part of those calling for this since the mid-1980s. But female empowerment must be broader and deeper than control over contraceptives if AIDS is to be effectively prevented. Besides, we do not yet have the needed technology and we need to be preventing HIV transmission now.

There is also interest and discussion among Gender-aids and similar groups about reviving the diaphragm for AIDS prevention, since there is some evidence it protects the cervix, a presumed vulnerable spot for HIV infection (gender-aids@healthdev.net, December 12, 2002). Of course there is interest in the female condom. We see that solutions to AIDS involving women is always about somehow giving them power over technology, over contraceptives. A recent example is this comment from the list-serve "sea-aids," from Bobby Ramakant in India (October 31, 2002): "The only plausible solution is if the prevention options are women-controlled. Only then women can be really empowered to protect themselves not only against HIV/AIDS but also against a broad range of STIs."

All this would be fine if the main solution to AIDS were to be found in technology. There is little discussion of behavior by these groups. I find myself wondering how much pharmaceutical companies might be influencing the agendas of internet discussion groups. Certainly the topics considered permissible for Internet discussion seem limited to those that contribute to corporate profits. I know my comments on the role of behavior have been censored lately on several occasions.

NOTES

1. Where there is controversy is stigma associated with PLWHAs and the degree to which a particular FBO fights or perpetuates this.

2. Arguably, other options might be promotion of male circumcision (Halperin & Bailey, 1999) or finding ways to keep viral loads of PLWHAs below a threshold level of infectivity (Quinn, Wawer et al., 2000).

3. The image that comes across in Internet postings seems to be kind of fire-and-brimstone, Elmer Gantry caricature, pointing an accusing finger at a gay man and talking about eternal damnation. I have not encountered such a figure in Africa over the past quarter century.

4. One of the problems that has plagued these programs has been infighting among healers for leadership positions both in their own associations and in programs involving outside funding. With a sympathetic Ministry of Health physician in charge of the THETA program, it seems that jockeying for power and position by healers was minimalized.

11

Conclusion: New Paradigms for
AIDS Prevention Programs

As I finish writing this book, President Bush has announced that the United States will spend $15 billion on global AIDS, of which $10 billion is newly pledged money. An article in the *New York Times* (Stolberg, 2003) implies that this announcement might not have been possible for this administration unless there had been a way to spend AIDS funds that would be acceptable to conservatives. What is acceptable is the Uganda-style ABC approach, as the article notes. I was quoted in this article on what happened in Uganda (and on how it would be much better to talk about partner reduction and not use the A-term, abstinence, since it is a political lightning rod).

Many people were disappointed that the Global Fund would not be getting more than about $1 billion of the $15 billion.[1] That leaves $14 billion for U.S. bilateral programs. It is not clear right now exactly which U.S. agencies will oversee that spending of the new billions, but at this writing it seems the State Department will be the lead agency. Since USAID is under the State Department, although quite autonomous, it seems that USAID will be the most important agency, even if there is some administrative control from a higher level in State.

As for the GFATM, it has elected a long-term executive director and it has just allocated grants to thirty-one developing countries worth $378 million over two years. It indicated that it soon would approve more two-year grants worth another $238 million. I expect that at least the early grants will go to the same programs that have not been very effective where we find most of the world's AIDS cases and HIV infection rates, Africa and the Caribbean. They will still be Western-designed Pattern I solutions for Pattern II countries, even if much of the design putatively comes from the countries themselves. Nevertheless, there are some new personnel at the GFATM dedicated to ensuring that primary behavior change programs become part of country strategies and programs in the future.

An article in the *Washington Post* ("The AIDS Fund Gets Going," April 29, 2002, p. A20) has the following to say about the GFATM:

Because some of the grants will go to treatment as well as prevention programs, they may mark a conceptual breakthrough. The world finally seems to recognize that treatment is not just a moral obligation but an essential complement to prevention efforts. You can't get people with HIV to change their behavior or even come forward for testing if you have no treatment to offer them.

Whatever the actual, casual relationship proves to be between ARV treatment and prevention (and we don't yet know), we know the last statement is false. People have changed their behavior; it is just that the way it changed did not conform to expectations and so it has been overlooked. And we have seen evidence that treatment availability might work against prevention, might lead to backsliding on behavior change. I am certainly not arguing against provision of treatment, but let us look at things the way they really are with regard to prevention.

If the evidence assembled in this book were given careful consideration, the organizations currently involved nearly exclusively in risk reduction approaches to AIDS prevention could begin designing and implementing more balanced, comprehensive, and effective programs of AIDS and STD prevention. Risk reduction programs should continue, and they should especially target high-risk groups, such as CSWs and their clients, soldiers, and truck drivers, as well as IDUs and MSM. (This is not to say that MSM and perhaps IDUs cannot and even have not reduced partners, as an AIDS prevention strategy.) Meanwhile PBC programs should be supported to a much greater extent, and targeted to general or majority populations. More program impact indicators should be developed to ensure that this really happens, making implementing groups accountable for PBC interventions. Donors such as USAID may now have one indicator to capture partner reduction and one for age of sexual debut. But others are probably needed. For example, the indicator, "proportion reporting one or more nonregular partners in the past twelve months," does not capture serial monogamy. A person could change partners every year and end up with thirty-four partners over the course of the ages between fifteen and forty-nine, yet still qualify as monogamous every year a survey is conducted. But even this worst-case scenario does not negate the PBC argument. Multiple, concurrent partners is known by epidemiologists to be far more dangerous than serial monogamy, than by having a new partner every twelve months.

But how do we design and implement interventions that promote PBC? We don't know exactly. More research is needed to answer this question. My colleagues and I are currently researching this question through the USAID–funded ABC study. But I can suggest now that it is not as hard as many might imagine. From our review of evidence in this book, it seems that whenever some effort and resources go into promotion of PBC, there tend to be at least some results, if not more than those anticipated. That means that however amateurish and in-expert such efforts are—and they are probably often just that—there tend to be some results. Perhaps this is at least in part because, as I noted earlier, PBC seems to be the natural response to concern over, or fear of, HIV infection. When we promote PBC, we are reinforcing and building upon what people may often already doing, as distinct from trying to introduce new, alien behaviors and technologies—always a difficult feat, even when it doesn't involve costs including sacrificing a degree of sexual enjoyment.

When I say "we don't know" how to promote A and B interventions, I refer to the decision makers in the major donor and international health organizations. As can be seen in this book, when given the opportunity, governments and NGOs in countries like Uganda, Senegal, and Jamaica have come up with effective, culturally appropriate ways to address AIDS prevention in their general (i.e., majority) populations. A little humility among the international experts, along with laissez-faire in program design, would probably go a long way toward showing the world how best to design and implement PBC interventions.

We saw examples from Uganda, Senegal, Zambia, and perhaps Jamaica that A interventions (abstinence, delay) can be successfully promoted through schools, perhaps especially when interventions start in primary school. A interventions can even be promoted through the same mass electronic media as condom campaigns, as we saw with the HEART youth program in Zambia, where both abstinence and condom use resulted, but with more of the former reported by respondents than the latter. Programs such as Life Skills and the Sara Initiative (which goes by several names, depending on global region) also promote A and B if not C behavior changes. We have seen in several countries that A and B interventions can be successfully promoted through faith-based groups and through community-based peer education and awareness efforts involving local leaders. Most of this evidence is merely suggestive at this stage; further research is needed to confirm these hypotheses.

It may even be easier to promote PBC than condoms. An evaluation of the Zambian peer education we discussed found the following:

Positive changes in attitudes and beliefs about abstinence were largely sustained until six months after the intervention. Several of the positive changes regarding attitudes and beliefs about condoms and HIV risk perception that were observed soon after the intervention could not be sustained over time.

Conclusions: Stronger and more regular efforts may be required to sustain positive changes in beliefs about condom use than about abstinence. (Agha & Van Rossem, 2002)

International experts need to face some uncomfortable realities about the limited success—or even failure—of their so-called proven interventions before they are ready to be more laissez-faire, or allow host country governments more of a genuine role in selecting and designing interventions. Few experts give credit where it is due. Nor does the general public in wealthier countries. The general public forms its opinion from mass media reports about AIDS in the developing world. And the media message is doom and gloom about both the pandemic and about the capacity of Third World people to handle their problem. The following analysis was made of the "AIDS and the African" series in the *Boston Globe*, October 1999:[2]

The text and the photographs that accompany the stories present uniform images of Africans that are widespread in American mass media. In this series, Africans are portrayed as either passive in the face of the epidemic or as irrational for engaging in high-risk sexual behavior. . . . The passivity of the women and children in these photographs suggests to the American reader that Africans cannot take action themselves to combat the disease. . . . When Africans are cast as actors, they are often granted negative agency as prostitutes. Though the articles in this series briefly mention female sex workers' economic struggles, it is the struggle to make them understand the importance of condom use that is highlighted by the reporters. (Shillinger, 1999, p. A1)

This media analyst observes that these perceptions in turn influence expert thinking: "These examples from mainstream American media highlight the ways that knowledge about AIDS and the Third World is produced and how it can influence policy-making" (Vavrus, 2000).

The image of the helpless, irrational African continuing to have unprotected sex is so unfair because the truth is that the few successes that can be claimed in African AIDS prevention have been due to the insight and ingenuity of Africans themselves, often in spite of the advice of foreign experts and their proven interventions. It is unfortunate that corruption in African governments, which is too often very real, is likely a factor in why donors don't rely more on local technical, social, and cultural expertise in developing countries—even though financial management and AIDS prevention ought to be two separate issues.

One way to free ourselves from the grip of the old paradigm is to rethink the basic assumptions that form the basis of our prevention approaches. These guiding assumptions include:

- Don't try to actually change sexual behavior. Better not to even mention it.
- Don't make people afraid of AIDS; it's counterproductive. The effects of fear arousal are short-lived at best.
- Don't involve FBOs; they are the enemy.
- Remember, sexual behavior does not change. Young people in particular are driven by hormones.
- Remember, (African) men are by nature polygamous. Women have no power to resist the advances of men in patriarchal societies.
- Africans are poor. All sex has a transactional dimension. Transactional sex is how Africans survive. Just use a condom every time.
- Abstinence is great. There is only one problem: It doesn't work.
- People can't abstain forever, so why even consider this as an intervention?
- Why should we care if a girl postpones sexual debut by a year or two? It just delays by this amount of time when she will be HIV infected.

This is not a caricature. I have heard every one of these beliefs expressed by AIDS experts representing major donors and program implementers, and expressed often. They are trotted out to prove why partner reduction and abstinence cannot possibly work. There is a sociocultural or economic basis for many of these assumptions, making them appear valid. Some of them are valid to some extent. Yet each of these beliefs have in fact been challenged by something as simple as ABC. We might say challenged by the simple formula of risk internalization plus self-efficacy equals behavioral change. In other words, in spite of cultural patterns that might be valid, behavior can nevertheless change if the right conditions are present. We know this because it has happened.

NEW OPPORTUNITIES IN AIDS PREVENTION

What about entrenched interests in business as usual? There are consulting firms, universities, for-profit companies, large nonprofits, and sprawling government agencies and organizations that currently benefit from the billion-dollar AIDS enterprise, the prevention part of which is built around risk reduction and technology. There will doubtless be fear and uncertainty at first, judging by resistance to date to look at any evidence that challenges risk reduction approaches. Yet if the issues are thought through, minus the usual fear and loathing, the inclusion of A and B interventions ought to lead to new and expanded opportunities. The new areas of implementation would be additive to, not subtractive from, current business, because A, B, and C would all be given emphasis, not simply C and treatment of STIs. There is now considerably more money available for global AIDS so funding additional interventions is quite feasible. We could be marketing ideas as well as things. The things we are currently marketing for prevention, condoms, cost only pennies apiece; therefore the real costs of marketing and distribution go to personnel. These costs would not change even if all prevention funds were to switch miraculously to A and B interventions, which of course is not what I am suggesting. If only those who resist paradigm modification so vigorously would be willing to think through the source of their fear.

Marketing PBC ought to in fact be much more complex and challenging (and therefore interesting) than promoting a small piece of latex. Delay of sexual debut alone would involve policy and legislative reform (to discourage rape, coerced sex, and seduction of minors); promotion of programs like Life Skills (Sara Initiative, etc.) to empower youth (male and female) to make health-promotive choices in sexual behavior; and programs to address gender inequality and generally raise the status of women. Had there not already been striking achievements of just this sort documented in Uganda, I would be hesitant to even suggest that interventions could be built around delay of sexual debut.

In fact there would be more receptiveness to PBC programs than BCC or social marketing programs have come to expect, especially among certain population segments, such as women, church congregations, schools, and among often-influential opinion leaders and gatekeepers, such as traditional healers and teachers. The short section on Kenya in Chapter 7 provides some evidence of this. Such groups and opinion leaders have often been actively or passively resistant to AIDS prevention programs precisely because of the overemphasis on condom promotion. Donors and program designers in the West often forget that they are implementing programs in Africa and elsewhere among largely rural people who tend to be tradition bound and often very religious. Yet outside program designers expect AIDS prevention programs in these societies to advertise condoms in newspapers and on radio and TV, even if these same designers would be unable to do the same in their own countries.

I sometimes put it this way: It doesn't matter if most of my Western colleagues and I happen to be urban, liberal, and secular; most Africans are rural, conservative, and religious. When we are designing and implementing programs in Africa, we must always remember where we are.

A senior AIDS educator in Mozambique recently told me that in order to simply be accepted by most people in rural areas, AIDS prevention needs to be presented as something other than condom promotion only. Having worked for over two years in that country, I know she is right. A paper presented at the Barcelona conference entitled, "Increasing Condom Use Through Community Mobilization and Social Marketing in Madagascar," likewise concluded the following (unexpectedly, judging by the paper's title) from experience in project implementation:

Current messages for prevention focus on abstinence and fidelity as well as condom use and STI care-seeking behavior, in direct response to expressed community concerns and needs. While these behaviors are not readily measurable, offering a choice for preventive behavior enables communities and individuals to accept the package of messages more readily. (Rossi, Raharisoa, Ny, & Ralison, 2002, from abstract)

One of the most controversial elements of AIDS prevention in resource-poor countries has always been condom promotion to youth. I have already discussed the relative merits of abstinence only versus a balanced ABC approach, and have come down on the side of the latter. However, many or most youth programs have been condoms only programs in all but name, and this can be proven by looking at how funds for such programs are actually spent. African school authorities have often—or usually—resisted AIDS education or sex education in schools precisely because of the emphasis on condoms. Often schools will have no AIDS education because of impasses over condoms.

If there were some balance between PBC and condoms, AIDS programs would be more acceptable to school authorities and to parents, whose beliefs and values cannot be ignored. Even if the only way AIDS education can enter the curriculum is by agreeing to teach PBC only, it is better to have some AIDS education than none. Experience, such as that of Uganda's FBO programs, has taught that once there is an AIDS program that gets people thinking and talking about AIDS, the stage is at least set for further education and awareness. Those for whom PBC are not realistic options will be in a better position to find out about risk reduction approaches.

At the very least, those who believe primarily or solely in condom interventions ought to see their own "Trojan horse" opportunities to get programs into schools under whatever conditions or restrictions may be imposed. There is a fairly good chance that once A and B options are discussed, C options could be conveyed in one or another manner, perhaps indirectly. AIDS educators in Jamaica told me during our evaluation in 2000 that even though they kept their promise to not mention condoms on school grounds (in certain schools), some students would always run over to the departing educators and ask about condoms as they were leaving school property. One point of this argument is that there is no chance that condoms can be promoted in school if there is no program at all, whereas there is quite a good chance if there is any kind of program.

I expressed a conclusion like this, along with supporting evidence, in my 1993 trip report from a quick evaluation of the USAID–supported APCP in Uganda. Among these were some faith-based initiatives in AIDS prevention, perhaps the first ever supported by USAID anywhere. These USAID–supported FBI programs were in their first year at the time, but important lessons were already emerging. These were discussed at a workshop for the APCP project and can be seen in the following from my trip report:

Lessons Learned

Whatever reluctance religious or other so-called conservative groups might express about their involvement in condom promotion, the reality has proven to be that such organizations, as their programs develop and progress, actually desensitize themselves regarding condoms and open discussion of sexual behavior. In other words, as long as an organization is involved in AIDS education, the subject of condoms will emerge and discussion of condoms in some form is inevitable, as is referral to condom outlets even if priests and imams do not distribute condoms themselves. Therefore it makes sense to let organizations get started in AIDS prevention in whatever way they feel comfortable. An example presented at the workshop might illustrate this.

An AIDS educator priest was told by a group of parents that they had never seen a condom package nor indeed were they willing to see one. The priest said fine, and continued his AIDS education presentation without mention of condoms. However later in the program the priest asked the group of parents if they would recognize a packet of condoms if they saw one lying on a desk next to their child's homework. The parents realized they would not and therefore suddenly felt they needed to actually see a packet of condoms if only to monitor their child's behavior. The same priest had been admonished by his bishop not to mention "those you-know-whats" during his first AIDS education workshop. The priest agreed but by the third day for the workshop, the participants were demanding to know something about condoms, at least their role in HIV prevention. Naturally condoms had to be discussed at that point and apparently there was no problem with the bishop over the priest responding to a demand for information from church members themselves.

It was agreed at the workshop that the promise of active promotion of condoms should not be a litmus test for religious or other organizations which seek support from APCP for their AIDS prevention activities. (Green, 1993a, p. 7)

In any case, we have seen enough evidence by now to know that abstinence, delay, and mutual fidelity if sexually active are the messages that young people need, in and out of schools, especially if they can be reached before becoming sexually active. AIDS educators should not simply get their foot in the door by promising to emphasize or restrict themselves to A and B messages; they should really emphasize them.

In the future, condoms should be promoted more the way Ugandans promoted them in the early period, as something one resorts to if PBC is not possible or fails, or if people are already HIV infected. Ugandan educators even put it that way: If you fail, be sure you fail with a condom. My other recommendation is that people should be told the truth about the effectiveness of condoms; condom promotion should not state or imply that condoms are 100 percent effective. If condom programs were confronted with this question, many would say that they are already doing this to some extent. This may be true insofar as official documents in the files of the home office are concerned. But this is often not true where it really counts, namely, actual promotional efforts. Socially marketed condoms have names like Protector, Sure, Shield, and Trust, and there is seldom or never anything in their marketing that warns the target audience about known failure rates from breakage, leakage, slippage, human error, and the like. Programs should give people all the options so that they can make responsible choices—but let them have all the facts.

As Harold Jaffee, chief of epidemiology at the National Centers for Disease Control, has commented, "You just can't tell people it's all right to do whatever you want as long as you wear a condom. It (AIDS) is just too dangerous a disease to say that" (Gruson, 1987, p. 1).

Are programs that give equal emphasis to A, B, and C affordable? We already know that total donor support from all sources between 1989 and 1998 in Uganda was approximately $180 million, or $1.80 per adult per year (Marum & Madraa, 2000). It is safe to assume that most of this money went to programs other than what I have just outlined, since almost all of it was foreign donated and spending reflects donor priorities. But at least we can say with confidence that a program with some reasonable balance between A, B, and C interventions need not cost more than $1.80 per adult per year, and that it is possible to promote A and B interventions and get results.

I must stress that Uganda does not represent anything like a pure model of PBC or anything else. Even today there are many foreign technical experts working in Uganda who have little or no understanding of what has happened in Uganda to dramatically reduce HIV prevalence rates. These are the foreign advisors and experts who direct American- or European-style prevention programs from their offices and rarely visit the field. And when they do, it is often only to see if condoms or health facilities are being used sufficiently. They have control over the programs their organizations fund and these programs are identical to the ones that seem to have had little or no impact on national HIV infection rates elsewhere. It is therefore possible to hypothesize that even if a balanced ABC program (one with a strong

PBC component) is only a part of a national AIDS prevention program, it is still possible to reduce national HIV prevalence by some 66 percent—even where millions (or nowadays billions) of donor dollars go to business-as-usual programs. One can only wonder what might have happened in Uganda if all donor funds had gone into the type of programs that Uganda implemented when it had control over them. It seems safe to assume that Uganda's program would have had even more impact and certainly at much lower cost.

Another lesson that needs learning concerns the issue of technical expertise. I found the following interesting principle stated in an early book about global AIDS:

The AIDS pandemic is revealing—not for the first time—a fact about development which is more easily stated than taken account of: when it comes to the welfare and survival of Third World and minority communities, the only "experts" are those communities themselves. AIDS prevention can only be effective if it changes people's sexual behaviour. In the Third World, and among ethnic minorities in the North, this is unlikely to happen if AIDS education is perceived to emanate from a predominantly white, relatively privileged, outside establishment. (Sabatier, 1988, p. 121)

That is a useful principle to keep in mind. What a tragedy that these words were not heeded in 1988. But I would go further. We saw that President Museveni and his advisors developed an AIDS prevention model that was suited to the economic and sociocultural realities of Uganda, and that it differed considerably from the model being urged by foreign technical experts. The foreigners urged risk reduction while Museveni did what he could to promote a largely risk avoidance PBC model. Since most of the prevention program was funded by outside donors, and since project activities are earmarked by donors, it is to the credit of Museveni and his early allies (the Ministry of Health, the FBOs, the women's organizations, and the schools) that the PBC model was not pushed aside by the activities the donors wanted. But he had to stand up to donors. An International Labor Organization paper provides some evidence of this in the following section on HIV/AIDS:

President Yoweri Museveni, Uganda, also launched an attack on donors at a Consultative Group meeting in Kampala. He told them he would not stand for them interfering in his country's internal affairs. "This business of 'we will not give you money because you don't dance this way; we will not give you money because you don't dance that way' is squandering the partnership between the donors and the President." (Ramiah, 2003, p. 17)

As one group of researchers in Uganda commented, "Most sexual behaviour interventions to prevent HIV in sub-Saharan Africa are based on external alien models. They are often misunderstood and not trusted by the community" (Whitworth, Muyinda, & Pool, 2000, from abstract). This group went on to design a prevention program in Uganda that took advantage of an existing cultural mechanism, in this case a traditional channel of communication for sex education of adolescent girls. The program led to positive behavior changes that continued after the end of program financial support.

Donors have come to expect that innovative approaches like this last example are more likely to be found in the private sector. This is one of the rationales for donors like USAID channeling most of their AIDS funds through the private sector. Yet it seems that Uganda both pioneered and sustained a great many innovative and high-impact prevention programs through its public sector, mostly through the Ministry of Health. For example, the STI project was funded by a World Bank loan, which meant that the Ugandan government had considerable latitude in deciding how the money was spent as long as it followed the decentralization model required by the Bank. I suspect that decentralization contributed to the cultural and epidemiologic suitability of the Uganda AIDS prevention model perpetuated under this World Bank–supported project. Decisions about how to spend the Bank loan were made to a large extent by district health directors. They were more in touch with what would work and not work at the local level than officials in Kampala, and they were much more in touch than technical experts in Washington or Geneva.

Unlike Uganda, Jamaica did not have government commitment at the highest level. I am not aware that any Jamaican prime minister ever spoke publicly about AIDS, at least by 2000. Jamaica did have a very activist, respected, and competent official in the health ministry, Dr. Peter Figueroa, and this helped a great deal. But this cannot have the same impact as a president or prime minister taking an activist position, such as President Museveni did.

On the other hand, Jamaica developed an effective AIDS prevention program in part because it was able to have more control over its own program after 1996. In addition to the obligatory risk reduction programs, Jamaica also gave some genuine emphasis to PBC, and to implementing these efforts through schools, FBOs, and community-based organizations. There was a lot of face-to-face IEC based on peer education and community leaders. In other words, Jamaica, like Uganda's public sector program funded by WHO and by World Bank loans, was able to decide the kind of interventions that made sense in its own country. We saw even in Thailand that there were interventions aimed at reducing multipartner sex among males in the general population. This seems to have worked, and significant partner reduction by males preceded the mid-1990s decline in national HIV prevalence. Yet most of the promotion and achievement of partner reduction seems to have occurred before there was significant foreign donor support for AIDS prevention in Thailand. Therefore it seems to have been Thai ingenuity, rather than outside expertise, that was largely responsible for at least the PBC part of Thailand's AIDS program, if not for the 100 percent condom policy in brothels as well.

These are uncomfortable conclusions to reach for someone who has been a foreign technical expert in AIDS and broader reproductive health for over twenty years. I don't mean for my tentative conclusions to be taken to an extreme. Technical experts are still needed. But I strongly recommend that we not arrive in the Third World thinking we have all, or even most, of the answers, especially if we are on a mission to change behavior. Instead, we should arrive with a sense of humility and a willingness to learn from our hosts, rather than simply with a determination to teach them, show them the error of their ways, and transfer technology.

Some have argued that we must be extremely cautious in exporting a Ugandan ABC model to other countries, even those of Africa. After all, there is vast cultural diversity in Africa; therefore, each country—indeed each society within each country—needs an approach uniquely adapted to it. Yet these same people say nothing about the United States and other major donors transplanting an intervention to Africa and the world predicated on the premise that if people all over the world will drink Coca Cola, why won't they also use condoms? How culturally sensitive is that? The adaptation of condom social marketing to local sociocultural mileux rarely goes much beyond finding the best commercial marketing channels to exploit. And somehow the socially marketed condoms all end up being promoted in essentially the same way, with the same brand names (Protector, Shield, Trust, etc.), suggesting that there has not been a great deal of social or cultural tailoring of programs. Moreover, abstinence-fidelity behaviors may be rooted in the human survival instinct and therefore universal. When one feels personally at risk of dying, and he or she knows what to do to avoid that risk, it is not surprising that the risk avoidance behavior will often follow, regardless of sociocultural factors.

Another point about being extremely cautious: Where is the risk in expanding a prevention message from condoms and drugs to those plus PBC? How can a broader message be more dangerous than a narrower message when it comes to accommodating varieties and vagaries of human behavior? Specifically, where is the risk in warning about the dangers of having multiple partners in a pandemic driven by having multiple partners? The worst that could happen is that the message would fall on deaf ears. Yet there is considerable risk in *not* promoting PBC. If it turns out that the findings from Uganda and other countries considered here are confirmed, and we have failed to promote the right messages, then it is not too far-fetched to say that millions of lives could have been saved and yet were not.

NOTES

1. Some are already calling this the global ATM machine from which poor countries can draw money.
2. See http://www.boston.com/globe/nation/packages/aids_african/part1.htm.

References

Abdullah, M. (2003, February). HIV/AIDS in Kenya: What went wrong—How we fix it. Paper presented to USAID, Washington DC.

Abma, J. C., & Sonenstein, F. L. (2001). Sexual activity and contraceptive practices among teenagers in the United States, 1988 and 1995. *Vital and Health Statistics, 23* (21), 1–79.

Adetunji, J. (2000). Condom use in marital and nonmarital relationships in Zimbabwe. *International Family Planning Perspectives, 26* (4), 196–200.

ADRA (Adventist Development and Relief Agency). (2002, March). Southern Africa-Indian Ocean Division (SID) of Seventh-day Adventist (SDA) Church Regional Workshop on HIV/AIDS First Phase for Church Administrators. Unpublished paper. Zimbabwe: Harare.

African Medical and Research Foundation/Uganda. (2001, August). *The effects of the Katakwi/ Soroti school health and AIDS prevention project.* Kampala, Uganda: African Medical and Research Foundation (AMREF).

Agha, S. (1999). Consumer intentions to use the female condom in a population to which it has been mass-marketed (Working Paper No. 26). Washington DC: Population Services International, Research Division.

Agha, S. (2002). Declines in casual sex in Lusaka, Zambia: 1996–1999. *AIDS, 16,* 291–293.

Agha, S., & Van Rossem, R. (2002, July). An evaluation to determine whether improvements in risk perception, self-efficacy and normative beliefs regarding abstinence and condom use resulting from a peer sexual health intervention can be sustained over time [Abstract]. *XIV international AIDS conference: Barcelona, July 7–12, 2002: Knowledge and commitment for action.* Barcelona, Spain.

Aggleton, P., & Rivers, K. (1999). Interventions for adolescents. In L. Gibney, R. J. DiClemente, & S. H. Vermund (Eds.), *Preventing HIV in developing countries: Biomedical and behavioral approaches* (pp. 231–255). New York: Kluwer Academic/Plenum Publishers.

Agyei, William K. A., & Epema, Elspeth J. (1992, March). Sexual behavior and contraceptive use among 15–24-year-olds in Uganda. *International Family Planning Perspectives, 18* (1), 7–13.

Ahmed, S., Lutalo, T., Wawer, M., Serwadda, D., & Sewankambo, N. K. (2001). HIV incidence and sexually transmitted disease prevalence associated with condom use: A population study in Rakai, Uganda. *AIDS, 15,* 2171–2179.

Ahmed, S., & Mosley, H. (2003, July 15). ABC, ABCDE, ABCDE . . . Zero HIV/AIDS. Presentation to President's Advisory Council on HIV/AIDS, Washington, DC.

Ainsworth, M., & Semali, I. (1998). Who is most likely to die of AIDS? In M. Ainsworth & A. M. Over (Eds.), *Confronting AIDS: Evidence from the developing world* (pp. 95–109). Washington, DC: World Bank.

Akintola, O. (2002, July). HIV/AIDS risk perception and sexual practices among male commercial drivers in Ibadan, Nigeria [Abstract]. *XIV international AIDS conference: Barcelona, July 7–12, 2002: Knowledge and commitment for action*. Barcelona, Spain.

allAfrica.com. (2002). Zimbabwe: 50pc of New HIV Cases Are People. Available at: allafrica.com/stories/200210030102.html.

Allen, A. (2002, May 27). Sex change. *The New Republic, 226,* 14–15.

Allen, P. L. (2000). *The wages of sin: Sex and disease, past and present*. Chicago: University of Chicago Press.

Altenroxel, L. (2003). Rich, married couples have a high HIV risk. Posted on *Journ-AIDS*, August 7, 2003. Available at: http://www.journ-aids.org/reports/07082003e.htm.

Alwano-Edyegu, M. G., & Marum, E. (1999). *Knowledge is power: Voluntary HIV counseling and testing in Uganda*. Geneva: UNAIDS.

Amarasingham, S., Green, E. C., & Royes, H. (2000). *An evaluation of Jamaica's national AIDS program*. Washington, DC: USAID and TvT Associates.

Ames, F. R. (1974, September 21). Some impressions of family life in Tsolo (Transkei). *South African Medical Journal, 48,* 1961–1964.

Ankrah, E. M. (1993). *Basic country results: Uganda KABP/PR '89*. Louvain-la-Neuve, Belgium: SONECOM.

Ankrah, E. M., Asingwiire, N., & Wangalwa, S. (1991). Sexual behaviours in eastern Uganda. Paper presented at 7th annual AIDS conference, Florence, Italy.

Ankrah, E. M., Wangalwa, S., Abura, A., & Nuwagaba, A. (1990, October). *Ugandan male sexual behaviour*. International conference on AIDS in Africa, Zaire.

Anonymous. (2000). Peers may help reduce teen pregnancy: Programs bring sex education to underserved areas. *Futurist, 34* (1), 10.

Anonymous. (2001). Which success story at ICASSA 2001? Available at: af-aids@healthdev.net. Article extracted from the *SAT News Bulletin, 12*. *SAT News Bulletin* is a publication from the Southern African AIDS Training Programme.

Anonymous. (2002, May 10). *Youngest Crucial to Anti-HIV Efforts: UNAIDS Chief*. New York (Reuters Health).

Ariyaratne, V. (1998). Mobilizing religious leadership for AIDS prevention in Sri Lanka [Abstract]. *12th world AIDS conference: Geneva, June 28–July 3, 1998*. Geneva.

Armstrong, A. K. (1987). Access to health care and family planning in Swaziland: Law and practice. *Studies in Family Planning, 18*, 371–382.

Arya, O. P., & Bennett, F. J. (1974). VD control: a case study of university students in Uganda. *International Journal of Health Education, 27* (1), 53–65.

Asiimwe-Okiror, G. (1995, November). *Brief report on population based survey in Jinja district*. Kampala, Uganda: STD/AIDS Control Programme, Ministry of Health.

Asiimwe-Okiror, Musinguzi, J., Agaba, C., Opio, A., & Madraa, E. (1998, December). *Results of a KABP survey on HIV, AIDS and STDS among commercial sex workers (CSWs) in Kampala, Uganda*. Kampala: STD/AIDS Control Programme, Ministry of Health.

Asiimwe-Okiror, G., Opio, A. A., Musinguzi, J., Madraa, E., Tembo, G., & Carael, M. (1997). Change in sexual behaviour and decline in HIV infection among young pregnant women in urban Uganda. *AIDS, 11*, 1757–1763.

Atwiine, E., Kabarira, C., Kityo, P., Mugyenyi, R., & Nakityo. (2000, July). Prostitution and HIV/AIDS in Uganda: A study of commercial sex workers in Kampala with emphasis on the economic gains vis-à-vis the health risks [Abstract]. *XIII international AIDS conference: Durban, July 9–14, 2000: Break the silence*. Durban, South Africa.

Atwood, J. B. (2001, February 14). Helms's idea could hobble Bush. *The Washington Post*, p. A25.

Auvert, B., Buonamico, G., Lagarde, E., & Williams, B. (2000). Sexual behavior, heterosexual transmission, and the spread of HIV in sub-Saharan Africa: A simulation study. *Computers and Biomedical Research, 33*, 84–96.

Auvert, B., Buvé, A., Ferry, B., Carael, M., Morison, L., Lagarde, E., et al. (2001). Ecological and individual level analysis of risk factors for HIV infection in four urban populations in sub-Saharan Africa with different levels of HIV infection. *AIDS, 15* (Suppl.), S15–S30.

Auvert, B., Buvé, A., Lagarde, E., Kahindo, M., Chege, J., Rutenberg, N., et al. (2001). Male circumcision and HIV infection in four cities in sub-Saharan Africa. *AIDS, 15* (Suppl.), S31–S40.

Auvert, B., Carael, M., Males, S., & Ferry, B. (2002, July). Why is early age at first sex associated with increased HIV infection? A study in four cities of sub-Saharan Africa [Abstract]. *XIV international AIDS conference: Barcelona, July 7–12, 2002: Knowledge and commitment for action*. Barcelona, Spain.

Auvert, B., & Ferry, B. (2002, September). Modeling the spread of HIV infections in four cities of Sub-Saharan Africa. Paper presented at the "ABC" Experts Technical Meeting, USAID, Washington, DC.

Baeten, J. M., Nyange, P. M., Richardson, B. A., Lavreys, L., Chohan, B., Martin, H. L., Jr., Mandaliya, K., Ndiyna-Achola, J. O., Bwayo, J. J., & Kreiss, J. K. (2003). Hormonal contraception and risk of sexually transmitted disease acquisition: results from a prospective study. *American Journal of Obstetrics and Gynecology, 185* (2), 380–385.

Bailey, R. C., Neema, S., & Othieno, R. (1999). Sexual behaviors and other HIV risk factors in circumcised and uncircumcised men in Uganda. *Journal of Acquired Immune Deficiency Syndromes, 22,* 294–301.

Bailey, R. C., Plummer, F., & Moses, S. (2001). Male circumcision and HIV prevention: Current knowledge and future research directions. *Lancet Infectious Diseases, 1,* 223–231.

Barnett, T., & Blaikie, P. (1992). *AIDS in Africa: Its present and future impact.* New York: Guilford Press.

Barton, T. (1997). *Epidemics and behaviours: A review of changes in Ugandan sexual behavior in the early 1990s.* Geneva: UNAIDS.

Barton, T., Thamae, S., & Ntoanyane, M. (1997). *AIDS in Lesotho—A community-based response: A summative evaluation of the CHAL-DCA AIDS Project.* Maseru: Christian Health Association of Lesotho (CHAL) and DanChurchAid.

Barton, T., & Wamai, G. (1994). *Equity and vulnerability: A situation analysis of women, adolescents and children in Uganda.* Kampala: Uganda National Council for Children.

Behavioural sentinel surveillance of CSWs, ICIs, and out-of-school youth. Preliminary findings. (2000, October). Kingston, Jamaica: Market Research Services.

Bennett, A. (2002). Personal communication, January 22.

Bennett, A., & Mills, S. (1996). *Explaining HIV differentials in Asia: The need for a differential response.* Bangkok, Thailand: Family Health International/ Asia Regional Office.

Bernstein, R. S., Sokal, D. C., Seitz, S. T., Auvert, B., Naamara, W., & Stover, J. (1998). Simulating the control of a heterosexual HIV epidemic in a severely affected East African city. *Interfaces, 28,* 101–126.

Bessinger, R., & Akwara, P. (2003). *Trends in sexual and fertility related behavior: Cameroon, Kenya, Uganda, Zambia, and Thailand.* Calverton, MD: ORC Macro, the Measure Project.

Bessinger, R. E., Kasheeka, E. B., Boerma, J. T., Zaba, B., & Kirungi, W. L. (2002, July). Trends in AIDS prevention behaviour in Uganda during the nineties [Abstract]. *XIV international AIDS conference: Barcelona, July 7–12, 2002: Knowledge and commitment for action.* Barcelona, Spain.

Bharath, U., Underwood, C. R., Serlemitsos, E. T., & Hochonda, H. (2002, July). Effects of a media campaign on HIV risk-reduction practices: Findings from the 1999 and 2000 youth surveys in Zambia [Abstract]. *XIV international AIDS conference: Barcelona, July 7–12, 2002: Knowledge and commitment for action.* Barcelona, Spain.

Biener, L., Harris, J. E., & Hamilton, W. (2000). Impact of the Massachusetts tobacco programme: Population based trend analysis. *British Medical Journal, 321,* 351–354.

Blanc, A. K., & Poukouta, P. V. (1997). *Components of unexpected fertility decline in sub-Saharan Africa.* (Demographic and Health Surveys Analytical Reports No. 5). Calverton, Maryland: Macro International.

Bloom, S. S., Banda, C., Songolo, G., Mulendema, S., Cunningham, A. E., & Boerma, J. T. (2000). Looking for change in response to the AIDS epidemic: Trends in AIDS knowledge and sexual behavior in Zambia, 1990 Through 1998. *Journal of Acquired Immune Deficiency Syndromes 25,* 77–85.

Blower, S. M., Aschenbach, A. N., Gershengorn, H. B., & Kahn, J. O. (2001). Predicting the unpredictable: Transmission of drug-resistant HIV. *National Medicine, 7* (9): 1016–1020.

Boerma, J. T., & Mgalla, Z. (2001). *Women and infertility in sub-Saharan Africa.* Amsterdam: Royal Tropical Institute, KIT Publishers.

Bongaarts, J., Reining, P., Way, P., & Conant, F. (1989). The relationship between male circumcision and HIV infection in African populations. *AIDS, 3,* 373–377.

Bonita, F., Stanton, X. L., Kahihuata, S., Fitzgerald, A. M., Neumbo, S., Kanduuombe, G. et al. (1998). Increased protected sex and abstinence among Namibian youth following a HIV risk-reduction intervention: A randomized, longitudinal study. *Aids Online, 12,* 2473–2480.

Brody, S. (1997). *Sex at risk: Lifetime number of partners, frequency of intercourse, adh the low AIDS risk of vaginal intercourse.* Piscataway, NJ: Transaction.

Brown, D. (2001). Study finds drug-resistant HIV in half of infected patients. *The Washington Post,* December 19, p. A2.

Brown, J. E., Ayowa, O. B., & Brown, R. C. (1993). Dry and tight: Sexual practices and potential AIDS risk in Zaire. *Social Science and Medicine, 37,* 989–994.

Brown, T., Sittitrai, W., Vanichseni, S., & Thisyakorn, U. (1994). The recent epidemiology of HIV and AIDS in Thailand. *AIDS, 8* (Suppl. 2), S131–S141.

BUCEN (U.S. Bureau of the Census). (2000). *HIV/AIDS profile: Senegal.* Washington, DC: U.S. Bureau of the Census.

Bui, T. D., Pham, C. K., Pham, T. H., Hoang, L. T., Nguyen, T. V., Vu, T. Q. et al. (2001). Cross-sectional study of sexual behaviour and knowledge about HIV among urban, rural, and minority residents in Viet Nam. *Bulletin of the World Health Organization, 79,* 15–21.

Bukali, F. L., & Mesa, M.I.E. (2002). *HIV/AIDS prevention and care in Mozambique: A socio-cultural approach.* Maputo: UNESCO.

Bulterys, M., Chao, A., Habimana, P., Dushimimana, A., Nawrocki, P., & Saah, A. (1994). Incident HIV-1 infection in a cohort of young women in Butare, Rwanda. *AIDS, 8,* 1585–1591.

Burgess, T. P. (2002a, February 21). Reliable South Africa HIV/AIDS statistics (3). Message posted to the af-aids mailing list, archived at http://www.health dev.net.

Burgess, T. P. (2002b, April 29). One of Feachem's challenges. Message posted to the break-the-silence mailing list, archived at http://www.healthdev.net.

Busulwa, W. R. (1995, July). *Abstinence for AIDS control: A study of adolescents in Jinja district.* Kampala, Uganda: Department of Community Practice, Master of Medicine Dessertation, Makerere University.

Buvé, A. (2002). HIV epidemics in Africa: What explains the variations in HIV prevalence? *IUBMB Life, 53* (4–5), 193–195.

Buvé, A., Carael, M., Hayes, R., Auvert, B., Ferry, B., Robinson, N. et al. (2001). Multicentre study on factors determining differences in rate of spread of HIV in sub-Saharan Africa: Methods and prevalence of HIV infection. *AIDS, 15* (Suppl.), S5–S14.

Buvé, A., Lagarde, E., Carael, M., Rutenberg, N., Ferry, B., Glynn, J. R. et al. (2001, August). Interpreting sexual behaviour data: Validity issues in the multicentre study on factors determining the differential spread of HIV in four African cities. *AIDS, 15* (Suppl. 4), S117–S126.

Byangire, M. B. (2002, July). The advocacy hierarchy for HIV/AIDS prevention and control [Abstract]. *XIV international AIDS conference: Barcelona, July 7–12, 2002: Knowledge and commitment for action*. Barcelona, Spain.

Caldwell, J. C. (1968). The control of family size in tropical Africa. *Demography, 5*, 598–619.

Caldwell, J. C., & Caldwell, P. (2002). Africa: The new family planning frontier. *Studies in Family Planning, 33* (1), 76–86.

Caldwell, J. C., Caldwell, P., & Quiggin, P. (1991). The African sexual system: Reply to Le Blanc et al. *Population and Development Review, 17*, 506–515.

Calvès, A. E. (1999). Condom use and risk perceptions among male and female adolescents in Cameroon: Qualitative evidence from Edéa (Working Paper No. 22). Washingoton, DC: Population Services International, PSI Research Division.

Campolino, A. H., & Adams, I. K. (1992). Involvement of churches in AIDS care and education: The Solidariedade-M.G. experience in Belo Horizonte, Brazil [Abstract]. *VIII international conference on AIDS/III STD world congress, Amsterdam, the Netherlands July 19–24, 1992*. Amsterdam: CONGREX Holland B.V.

Carael, M. (1995). Sexual behavior. In J. Cleland & B. Ferry (Eds.), *Sexual behaviour and AIDS in the developing world* (pp. 77–123). London: Taylor & Francis for the World Health Organization.

Carael, M., Buvé, A., & Awusabo-Asare, K. (1997). The making of HIV epidemics: What are the driving forces? *AIDS, 11* (Suppl. B), S23–S31.

Carael, M., Cleland, J., Deheneffe, J. C., Ferry, B., & Ingham, R. (1995). Sexual behaviour in developing countries: Implications for HIV control. *AIDS, 9*, 1171–1175.

Carael, M., & Holmes, K. (2001). Dynamics of HIV epidemics in sub-Saharan Africa: Introduction. *AIDS, 15* (Suppl. 4), S1–S4.

Carael, M., & Makinwa, B. (2000). AIDS underlines need for action in sub-Saharan Africa. *Global Health and Environment Monitor, 8* (1), 3.

Carey, R. F., Lytle, C. D., & Cyr, W. H. (1999). Implications of laboratory tests of condom integrity. *Sexually Transmitted Diseases, 26* (4), 216–220.

Carter, T. (2003, March 13). Uganda leads by example on AIDS. *Washington Times*, p. A13.

Catania, J. A., Coates, T. J., Stall, R., Turner, H., Peterson, J., Hearst, N., Dolcini, M. M., Hudes, E., Gagnon, J., Wiley, J. et al. (1992). Prevalence of AIDS-related risk factors and condom use in the United States. *Science, 258*, 1101–1106.

Cates, W. (2001). The NIH condom report: The glass is 90% full. *Family Planning Perspectives, 33* (5), 231–233.

Cates, W. (2002). The condom forgiveness factor: The positive spin. *Sexually Transmitted Diseases, 29*, 350–352.

CESDEM. (1996). Encuesta sobre Conocimientos, Creencias, Actitudes y Prácticas acerca del SIDA/ETS con Trabajadores Sexuales en Santo Domingo [Survey of knowledge, beliefs, attitudes and practices about HIV/AIDS among sex workers in Santo Domingo]. Santo Domingo: Proyecto AIDSCAP/USAID.

Chanpong, G. M., Putri, M., Oum, S., An, U. S., & Bunheng, M. (2001). Prevalence of HIV infection in Cambodia: Implications for the future. *International Journal of STD and AIDS, 12,* 413–414.

Charles, M., & Bolye, B. (2002). Excess and access: The continuing controversy regarding HIV and health care in Africa. *The AIDS Reader, 12,* 288–292.

Cheetham, R.W.S., Sibisi, H., & Cheetham, R. J. (1974). Psychiatric problems encountered in urban Zulu adolescents with specific reference to changes in sex education. *Australian and New Zealand Journal of Psychiatry, 8,* 41–48.

Chesney, M. A. (2000). Factors affecting adherence to antiretroviral therapy. *Clinical Infectious Diseases, 30* (Suppl. 2), S171–S176.

Chevannes, B., & Gayle, H. (2000, September). Adolescent and young male sexual and reproductive health study, Jamaica (Report to the Pan American Health Organization). Mona, Jamaica: University of the West Indies.

Chin, J. (2001a). ANNEX 2: The reproductive number (Ro) of HIV infections. In C. Hermann, E. C. Green, J. Chin, M. Taguiwalo, & C. Cortez (Eds.), *Evaluation of the Philippines AIDS Surveillance and Education Project* (pp. 55–56). Philippines: USAID.

Chin, J. (2001b). ANNEX 3. The potential for extensive HIV epidemics in the Asia-Pacific region. In C. Hermann, E. C. Green, J. Chin, M. Taguiwalo, & C. Cortez (Eds.), *Evaluation of the Philippines AIDS Surveillance and Education Project* (pp. 56–58). Philippines: USAID.

Chin, J. (2002). Patterns and measurement of heterosexual risk behaviors. Unpublished manuscript.

Chin, J. (2003). Socio-economic determinants of HIV-risk behaviors. Unpublished paper. Berkeley, California.

Chin, J., Bennett, A., & Mills, S. (1998). Primary determinants of HIV prevalence in Asian-Pacific countries. *AIDS, 12* (Suppl. B), S87–S91.

Chin, J., Bennett, A., & Mills, S. (1999). *HIV prevalence differentials in Asia.* Arlington, Va.: Family Health International (orig. 1995).

Chitwarakorn, A. (2002, December). "National Responses: Factors that make a difference." Department of Communicable Diseases Control, Ministry of Public Health, Thailand. Accelerating the Momentum in the Fight Against HIV/AIDS in South Asia. Geneva, Switzerland.

Clark, S. (2001, March). Non-coital options for sexual expression among young men: Literature review of cross-cultural trends. Paper presented at the annual meeting of the Population Association of America, Washington, DC.

Coates, T., Sangiwa, G., Balmer, D., Furlonge, C., Kamenga, C., & Gregorich, S. (1998). Serodiscordant married couples undergoing couples counseling and testing reduce risk behavior with each other but not with extra-marital partners [Abstract]. *12th world AIDS conference: Geneva, June 28–July 3, 1998.* Geneva.

Cohen, B., & Trussell, J. (Eds.). (1996). *Preventing and mitigating AIDS in sub-Saharan Africa.* Washington, DC: National Academy Press.

Cohen, M. S., & Eron, J. J. (2001, June 27). Sexual HIV transmission and its prevention. Paper in the Continuing Medical Education series. Available at: http://www.medscape.com/viewprogram/704.

Collins, C., Alagiri, P., & Summers, T. (2002). *Abstinence only vs. comprehensive sex education: What are the arguments? What is the evidence?* (Policy Monograph Series). San Francisco: University of California, AIDS Policy Research Center & Center for AIDS Prevention Studies.

Craig, A. P., & Richter-Strydom, L. M. (1983). Unplanned pregnancies among urban Zulu schoolchildren: A summary of the salient results from a preliminary investigation. *Journal of Social Psychology, 121,* 239–246.

Creese, A., Floyd, K., Alban, A., & Guinness, L. (2002). Cost-effectiveness of HIV/AIDS interventions in Africa: A systematic review of the evidence. *Lancet, 359,* 1635–1642.

Croft, T. (2001). Personal communication, May 30.

Crossette, B. (2001, April 30). A wider war on AIDS in Africa and Asia. *The New York Times,* p. A6.

Crossette, B. (2002, June 23). U.N. finds AIDS knowledge still lags in stricken nations. *The New York Times,* p. 6.

Darroch, J. E., & Singh, S. (1999). Why is teenage pregnancy declining? The roles of abstinence, sexual activity and contraceptive use. Occasional Report, No. 1, p. 12. New York: Alan Guttmacher Institute.

Darrow, W. W. (1989). Condom use and use-effectiveness in high-risk populations. *Sexually Transmitted Diseases, 16,* 157–160.

Darrow, W. W. (2001). Latex condoms, human behavior, and public health. *AIDS, 15,* 267–269.

Davidovicha, U., Wita, J. D., Albrechta, N., Geskusa, R., Stroebeb, W., & Coutinhoa, R. (2001). Increase in the share of steady partners as a source of HIV infection: A 17-year study of seroconversion among gay men. *AIDS, 15,* 1303–1308.

DeCock, K. (2001, February). Heterogeneity and public health in the global HIV/AIDS epidemic. In *8th Conference on Retroviruses and Opportunistic Infections.* Chicago, IL: Foundation for Retrovirology and Human Health.

DeLay, P., Stanecki, K., Achibald, C., & Brown, T. (2000). The status and trends of the HIV/AIDS in the world. Preliminary report of a symposium held on July 5–7, 2000 in Durban, South Africa. Available at: http://www.thebody.com/unaids/pdfs/MAP_Stats_2000.pdf

Denison, J. (1996, August). Behavior change—a summary of four major theories: Health belief model, AIDS risk reduction model, stages of change, theory of reasoned action. Arlingon, Va.: Family Health International.

DeYoung, K. (2001, June 19). A deadly stigma in the Caribbean. *The Washington Post,* p. A01.

Diarrah, C. O., & Rielly, C. (2002, July 10). A dose of democracy for Africa's AIDS crisis. *The Boston Globe,* p. A19.

Dieleman, J. P., Jambroes, M., Gyssens, I. C., Sturkenboom, M. C., Stricker, B. H., Mulder, W. M., de Wolf, F., Weverling, G. J., Lange, J. M., Reiss, P., Brinkman, K. (2002). Determinants of recurrent toxicity-driven switches of highly active antiretroviral therapy: The ATHENA cohort. *AIDS, 16,* 737–745.

Diouf, E. D., Paul, S., Leopold, C., & Ibra, N. (2000, July). Religious action at the international level in Africa: The example of international religious alliances against HIV in Africa. Paper presented at the 13th International AIDS Conference, Durban, South Africa.

Dubois-Arber, F., Jeannin, A., Konings, E., & Paccaud, F. (1997). Increased condom use without other major changes in sexual behavior among the majority population in Switzerland. *American Journal of Public Health, 87*, 558–566.

Eaton, L., Flisher, A. J., & Aarø, L. E. (2003.) Unsafe sexual behaviour in South African youth. *Social Science and Medicine 56* (1), 149–165.

Eggleston, E., Leitch, J., & Jackson, J. (2000). Consistency of self-reports of sexual activity among young adolescents in Jamaica. *International Family Planning Perspectives, 26* (2), 79–83.

Elphick, D. (2002, April 13). Memorable patients: Zambia needs basic medicines and HIV education. *British Medical Journal, 324*, 895.

Epstein, H. (2002). Personall communication, March 20.

Etzioni, A. (1996). *The New Golden Rule.* New York: Basic Books, HarperCollins.

Etzioni, A. (2003, March 4). Fight HIV with straight talk. *Christian Science Monitor*, p. 9.

Ezzell, C. (2000, May). Care for a dying continent. *Scientific American, 282*, 96–105.

Family Health International (FHI). (1996). Prevention as policy: How Thailand reduced STD and HIV transmission. *AIDScaptions, 3* (1).

Family Health International (FHI). (2002). Final report for the AIDSCAP program in Thailand: November 1991 to September 1996. Available at: http://www.fhi.org/en/aids/aidscap/aidspubs/special/countryprog/thailand/thaidesc4.html#Evaluation.

Family Health International/UNAIDS. (2001). *Effective strategies in low HIV prevalence countries.* Geneva: UNAIDS.

Farill, E., Romero, M., Ornelas, G., & Urbina, M. (1992, July). Sex education for priests [Abstract]. *VIII international conference on AIDS/III STD world congress, Amsterdam, the Netherlands, July 19–24, 1992.* Amsterdam: CONGREX Holland B.V.

Feinleib, J. A., & Michael, R. T. (1998). Reported changes in sexual behavior in response to AIDS in the United States. *Preventive Medicine, 27* (3), 400–411.

Feldblum, P. J., Kuyoh, M. A., Bwayo, J. J., Feldblum, P. J., Kuyoh, M. A., Bwayo, J. J., Omari, M., Wong, E. L., Tweedy, K. G., & Welsh, M. J. (2001). Female condom introduction and sexually transmitted infection prevalence: Results of a community intervention trial in Kenya. *AIDS, 15*, 1037–1044.

Ferry, B., Carael, M., Buvé, A., Auvert, B., Laourou, M., Kanhonou, L., et al. (2001). Comparison of key parameters of sexual behaviour in four African urban populations with different levels of HIV infection. *AIDS, 15* (Suppl. 4), S41–S50.

Fierstein, H. (2003, July 31). The culture of disease. *The New York Times.* Available at: http://www.nytimes.com/2003/07/31/opinion/31FIER.html?ex=1060641232&ei=1&en=977d2053e66ca196.

Figueroa, J. P., Brathwaite, A. R., Wedderburn, M., Ward, E., Lewis-Bell, K., Amon, J. J. et al. (1998). Is HIV/STD control in Jamaica making a difference? *AIDS, 12* (Suppl. 2), S89–S98.

Fitch, J. T., Stine, C., Hager, W. D., Mann, J., Adam, M. B., & McIlhaney, J. (2002). Condom effectiveness: Factors that influence risk reduction. *Sexually Transmitted Diseases*, 811–817.

Fonck, K. et al. (2001). Healthcare-seeking behavior and sexual behavior of patients with sexually transmitted diseases in Nairobi, Kenya. *Sexually Transmitted Diseases, 28* (7), 367–371.

Fontanet, A. L., Saba, J., Chandelying, V., Sakondhavat, C., Bhiraleus, P., Rugpao, S., Chongsomchai, C., Kiriwat, O., Tovanabutra, S., Dally, L., Lange, J. M., & Rojanapithayakorn, W. (1998). Protection against sexually transmitted diseases by granting sex workers in Thailand the choice of using the male or female condom: Results from a randomized controlled trial. *AIDS, 12*, 1851–1859.

Foster, L. M., Osunwole, S. A., & Wahab, B. W. (1996). Imototo: Indigenous Yoruba sanitation knowledge systems and their implication for Nigerian health policy. In F. Fairfax, B. W. Wahab, L. Egunjobi, & D. M. Warren (Eds.), *Alaafia: Studies of Yoruba concepts of health and well-being in Nigeria* (pp. 26–38). Ames: Iowa State University, Center for Indigenous Knowledge for Agriculture and Rural Development.

Freeman, M., & Motsei, M. (1992). Planning health care in South Africa: Is there a role for traditional healers? *Social Science and Medicine, 34*, 1183–1190.

Frezieres, R. G., Walsh, T. L., Nelson, A. L., Clark, V. A., & Coulson, A. H. (1998). Breakage and acceptability of a polyurethane condom: A randomized, controlled study. *Family Planning Perspectives, 30* (2), 73–78.

Fylkesnes, K., Kasumba, K., Ndhlovu, Z., & Musonda, R. M. (1997). Comparing sentinel surveillance and population-based HIV prevalence rates in Zambia. *AIDS, 11* (Suppl. B), S12–S13.

Fylkesnes, K., Musonda, R. M., Sichone, M., Ndhlovu, Z., Tembo, F., & Monze, M. (2001). Declining HIV prevalence and risk behaviours in Zambia: evidence from surveillance and population-based surveys. *AIDS, 15*, 907–916.

Gamurorwa, A. B., Lettenmaier, C. L., & Lewicky, N. (1997, May). HIV/AIDS prevention: The safer sex campaign for the youth in Uganda. In *Reproductive health and communication at the grassroots: Experiences from Africa and Asia.* Proceedings of the Conference on Reproductive Health and Communication at the Grassroots: Experiences from Africa and Asia, Ethiopian Red Cross Society Training Institute, Addis Ababa, Ethiopia.

Gardner, R., Blackburn, R. D., & Upadhyay, U. D. (1999). *Closing the condom gap.* (Population Reports, Series H). Baltimore: Johns Hopkins University.

Garner, R. (1999). Religion in the AIDS crisis: Irrelevance, adversary or ally? *AIDS Analysis Africa, 10* (2), 4–6.

Garner, R. (2000). Safe sects? Dynamic religion and AIDS in South Africa. *Journal of Modern African Studies, 38* (1), 41–69.

Garnett, G. P., & Rottingen, J. A. (2001). Measuring the risk of HIV transmission. *AIDS, 15*, 641–643.

Gausset, Q. (2001). AIDS and cultural practices in Africa: The case of the Tonga (Zambia). *Social Science and Medicine, 52*, 509–518.

Gebre, Y. (1999). Personal communication, September 14.

Ghys, P. D., Diallo, M. O., Ettiègne-Traoré, V., Kalé, K., Tawil, O., Carael, M. et al. (2002). Increase in condom use and decline in HIV and sexually transmitted diseases among female sex workers in Abidjan, Côte d'Ivoire, 1991–1998. *AIDS, 16*, 251–258.

Gilada, T. I., Gilada, I. S., & Ashar, R. D. (1998, July). AIDS prevention in India through religious festivities and programs [Abstract]. *12th world AIDS conference: Geneva, June 28–July 3, 1998*. Geneva.

Girma, M., & Schietinger, H. (1998, June). Integrating HIV/AIDS prevention, care and support: A rationale (Synergy Discussion Paper No. 1). Washington, DC: TvT Associates.

Glynn, J. R., Buvé, A., Carael, M., Kahindo, M., Macauley, I. B., Musonda, R. M. et al. (2000). Decreased fertility among HIV-1-infected women attending antenatal clinics in three African cities. *Journal of Acquired Immune Deficiency Syndromes, 25*, 345–352.

Glynn, J. R., Buvé, A., Carael, M., Macauleyd, I. B., Kahindoe, M., Musondaf, R. M. et al. (2001). Is long postpartum sexual abstinence a risk factor for HIV? *AIDS, 15*, 1059–1061.

Glynn, J. R., Buvé, A., Carael, M., & Zaba, B. (1999). Adjustment of antenatal clinic HIV surveillance data for HIV-associated differences in fertility [Letter to the editor]. *AIDS, 13*, 1598–1599.

Glynn, J. R., Carael, M., Auvert, B., Kahindo, M., Chege, J., Musonda, R. et al. (2001, August). Why do young women have a much higher prevalence of HIV than young men? A study in Kisumu, Kenya and Ndola, Zambia. *AIDS, 15* (Suppl. 4), S51–S60.

Godwin, P., Bond, K., Fremming, J., & Green, E. C. (1995). *Evaluation of Asia/Near East Bureau regional HIV/AIDS activities*. Arlington, VA: USAID and Health Technical Services.

Goode, E. (2001, August 19). With fears fading, more gays spurn old preventive message. *The New York Times*, p. 1.

Gordon, R. (1989). A critical review of the physics and statistics of condoms and their role in individual versus societal survival of the AIDS epidemic. *Journal of Sex & Marital Therapy, 15* (1), 5–30.

Gorna, R. (1996). *Vamps, virgins and victims: How can women fight AIDS?* London: Cassell.

Gray, R. H., Wawer, M. J., Brookmeyer, R., Sewankambo, N. K., Serwadda, D., Wabwire-Mangen, F. et al. (2001). Probability of HIV-1 transmission per coital act in monogamous, heterosexual, HIV-1-discordant couples in Rakai, Uganda. *Lancet, 357*, 1149–1153.

Gray, R. H., Wawer, M. J., Kiwanuka, N., Serwadda, D., Sewankambo, N. K., & Wabwire-Mangen, F. (2002). Male circumcision and HIV acquisition and transmission: Rakai, Uganda. *AIDS, 16*, 797–812.

Green, E. C. (1987, July). Characterizing the socioeconomic status of consumers in developing nations—New methods from the field in the Dominican Republic. *Occasional Papers: SOMARC, Social Marketing for Change*. Washington, DC: The Futures Group.

Green, E. C. (1988). A consumer intercept study of oral contraceptive users in the Dominican Republic. *Studies in Family Planning, 19* (2), 109–117.

Green, E. C. (1993a). Ethnomedical practices of significance to the spread and prevention of HIV in Southern Africa [Abstract]. *IXth international conference on AIDS in affiliation with the IVth STD World Congress: Berlin, June 6–11, 1993*. London: Wellcome Foundation Ltd.

Green, E. C. (1993b). Uganda trip report. USAID/Uganda and Washington, DC: World Learning, Inc.

Green, E. C. (1994). *AIDS and STDs in Africa: Bridging the gap between traditional healers and modern medicine*. Boulder, CO: Westview Press.

Green, E. C. (1995, March–April). Unpublished field notes, Zambia.

Green, E. C. (1996, November). Analysis and implications of recent market research findings in the Dominican Republic. Arlington, VA: Development Associates and USAID/Dominican Republic.

Green, E. C. (1997). The participation of African traditional healers in AIDS/STD prevention programs. *Tropical Doctor, 27* (Suppl. 1), 56–59.

Green, E. C. (1998, December). Report on the situation of AIDS and the role of IEC in Uganda. Entebbe, Uganda. Washington, DC: The World Bank.

Green, E. C. (1999a). *Indigenous theories of contagious disease*. Walnut Creek, CA: Altamira Press.

Green, E. C. (1999b). The involvement of African traditional healers in the prevention of AIDS and STDs. In R. A. Hahn (Ed.), *Anthropology in public health: Bridging differences in culture and society* (pp. 63–83). Oxford: Oxford University Press.

Green, E. C. (2000a). Calling on the religious community: Faith-based initiatives to help combat the HIV/AIDS pandemic. *Global AIDSLINK, 58,* 4–5.

Green, E. C. (2000b). The Male circumcision and AIDS issue. *Anthropology News, 41* (1), 22.

Green, E. C. (2000c). Male circumcision and HIV infection. *Lancet, 355,* 927.

Green, E. C. (2000d). Traditional healers and AIDS in Uganda. *Journal of Alternative and Complementary Medicine, 6* (1), 1–2.

Green, E. C. (2003). *Faith-based organizations: Contributions to HIV Prevention*. Washington, DC: USAID/Washington and The Synergy Project, TvT Associates.

Green, E. C., & Conde, A. (1988). AIDS and condoms in the Dominican Republic: Evaluation of an AIDS education campaign. In R. Kulstad (Ed.), *AIDS 1988: AAAS Symposium Papers* (pp. 275–288). Washington, DC: American Association for the Advancement of Science Press.

Green, E. C., & Conde, A. (2000). Sexual partner reduction and HIV infection. *Sexually Transmitted Infections, 76* (2), 145.

Green, E. C., & Monger, H. (1989). AIDS and other sexually transmitted diseases in Liberia: Results of a qualitative study. Washington, DC: The Futures Group.

Green, E. C., Nkya, L., & Outwater, A. (2000–2001). Narratives of sex workers in a Tanzanian town. *Global AIDSLINK, 63,* August 2000, October 2000, December 2000, February 2001, April 2001, and May 2001.

Green, E. C., Thornton, R., & Sliep, Y. (2003, March). Traditional healers and the bio-medical health system in South Africa. Summary Report. Washington, DC: Medical Care Development International for the Margaret Sanger Center International, South Africa.

Green, E. C., Zokwe, B., & Dupree, J. D. (1993). Indigenous African healers promote male circumcision for prevention of STDs. *Tropical Doctor, 23,* 182–183.

Green, E. C., Zokwe, B., & Dupree, J. D. (1995). The experience of an AIDS prevention program focused on South African traditional healers. *Social Science and Medicine, 40*, 503–515.

Gregson, S., Nyamukapa, C. A., Garnett, G. P., Mason, P. R., Zhuwau, T., Carael, M. et al. (2002). Sexual mixing patterns and sex-differentials in teenage exposure to HIV infection in rural Zimbabwe. *Lancet, 359*, 1896–1903.

Gregson, S., Zhuwau, T., Anderson, R. M., & Chandiwana, S. K. (1998). Is there evidence for behaviour change in response to AIDS in rural Zimbabwe? *Social Science and Medicine, 46*, 321–330.

Gross, M. (2003). The second wave will drown us. *AJPH 93* (6), 872–882.

Grosskurth, H., Mosha, F., Todd, J., Mwijarubi, E., Klokke, A., Senkoro, K., Mayaud, P., Changalucha, J., Nicoll, A., & Gina, G. (1995). Impact of improved treatment of sexually transmitted diseases on HIV infection in rural Tanzania: Randomized controlled trial. *Lancet, 346*, 530–536.

Grulich, A. E., & Kaldor, J. M. (2002). Evidence of success in HIV prevention in Africa. *Lancet, 360*, 4.

Gruson, L. (1987, August 18). Condoms: Experts fear false sense of security. *The New York Times*, Sec. C, p. 1.

Gunter, M., & Hue, L. (2000, July). Jamaican religious culture and its role in acceleration of HIV/AIDS and stigmatization of PLWAs [Abstract]. *XIII international AIDS conference, Durban, July 9–14, 2000: Break the silence.* Durban, South Africa.

Gupta, N., & Mahy, M. (2001). *Sexual initiation among adolescent women and men: Trends and differentials in sub-Saharan Africa.* Calverton, MD: Macro International, Demographic and Health Research Division.

Guyer, J. I. (1994). Lineal identities and laternal networks: The logic of polyandrous motherhood. In C. Bledsoe & G. Pison (Eds.), *Nuptiality in sub-Saharan Africa: Contemporary anthropological and demographic perspectives* (pp. 231–252). Oxford, UK: Clarendon Press.

Gysels, M., Pool, R., & Bwanika, K. (2001). Truck drivers, middlemen and commercial sex workers: AIDS and the mediation of sex in south west Uganda. *AIDS Care, 13* (3), 373–385.

Gysels, M., & Whitworth, J. (2001, September 26). Driving home the message— HIV prevention among African truck drivers. Available at: http://www.id21.org.

Hachonda, H. M., Serlemitsos, R. T., Mwaba, C., & Bharath, U. (2000, July). Youth leadership in mass media to bring about behavior change among their peers [Abstract]. *XIII international AIDS conference, Durban, July 9–14, 2000: Break the silence.* Durban, South Africa.

Halperin, D. T. (1999a). Dry sex practices and HIV infection in the Dominican Republic and Haiti. *Sexually Transmitted Infections, 75* (6), 445–446.

Halperin, D. T. (1999b) Heterosexual anal sex practices in Latin America and the U.S. *AIDS Patient Care, 13* (12), 717–730.

Halperin, D. T., & Allen, A. (2000). Is poverty the root cause of African AIDS? *AIDS Analysis Africa, 11* (4), 15.

Halperin, D. T., & Bailey, R. C. (1999). Male circumcision and HIV infection: 10 years and counting. *Lancet, 354*, 1813–1815.

Halperin, D. T., de Moya, A., Pérez-Then, E. (in preparation). Between patterns I and II: A stabilized, apparently bisexual AIDS epidemic in the Dominican Republic. Manuscript in preparation.

Hanenberg, R. S, Rojanapithayakorn, W., Kunasol, P., & Sokal, D. C. (1994). Impact of Thailand's HIV-control programme as indicated by the decline of sexually transmitted diseases. *Lancet, 344*, 243–245.

Hearst, N. (2003). Personal communication, January 23,

Hearst, N., & Chen, S. (2003a). Condoms for AIDS prevention in the developing world: A review of the scientific literature. Geneva: UNAIDS.

Hearst, N., & Chen, S. (2003b). Condom promotion for AIDS prevention in the developing world: Is it working? Presentation to President's Advisory Council on HIV/AIDS, Washington, DC, August 8.

Hellman, H. (2001). *Great feuds in medicine.* New York: Wiley.

Henry, K. (1998). New guidelines on monitoring HIV risk behavior. *Global AIDSLINK, 53*, 12–13.

Herman, B. (2002, April 22). Food and Drug Administration, Personal communication.

Hitchcock, P., & Fransen, L. (1999). Preventing HIV infection: Lessons from Mwanza and Rakai. *Lancet, 353*, 513–515.

Hodgins, S. (2003, June 10). USAID/Zambia, Personal communication.

Homsy, J., Katabira, E., Kabatesi, D., Mubiru, F., Kwamya, L., Tusaba, C. et al. (1999). Evaluating herbal medicine for the management of Herpes zoster in human immunodeficiency virus-infected patients in Kampala, Uganda. *Journal of Alternative and Complementary Medicine, 5*, 553–565.

Hooper, E. (1999). *The river: A journey to the source of HIV and AIDS.* Boston: Little, Brown.

Hope Enterprises. (2000, October). National KABP survey on HIV/AIDS in Jamaica: Preliminary findings. Kingston, Jamaica: Hope Enterprises.

Hospers, H. J., & Kok, G. (1995). Determinants of safe and risk-taking sexual behaviour among gay men: A review. *AIDS Education and Prevention, 7*, 74–96.

Hulley, S. B., Cummings, S. R., Browner, W. S., Grady, D., Hearst, N., & Newman, T. B. (2001). *Designing clinical research: An epidemiologic approach.* 2d ed. Philadelphia: Lippincott, Williams & Wilkins.

Hygea/FHI. (1998). Behavioral surveillance survey Senegal: 1997 and 1998. Dakar: Institut Supérieur Africain pour le Développement de l'Entreprise (ISADE) and the Cabinet d'Etudes et de Recherche (HYGEA).

Hygea/FHI. (2001). *Enquete de Surveillance du Comportement ESC 2001.* Senegal Ministry of Health and Prevention.

Imani, M. R. (1998). Findings from the "Straight Talk" radio program listeners survey (Contract No. 623-0133-C-00-4027-00 DISH Project, USAID). Unpublished report.

Iwere, N., Ojidoh, J. C., & Okide, N. (2000, July). Engaging religious communities in breaking the silence on HIV/AIDS [Abstract]. *XIII international AIDS conference, Durban, July 9–14, 2000: Break the silence.* Durban, South Africa.

Jeannin, A., Konings, E., Dubois-Arber, F., Landert, C., & Van Melle, G. (1998). Validity and reliability in reporting sexual partners and condom use in a Swiss population survey. *European Journal of Epidemiology, 14* (2), 139–146.

Jemmott, J. B., & Fry, D. (2002). The abstinence strategy for reducing sexual risk behavior. In A. O'Leary (Ed.), *Beyond condoms: Alternative approaches to HIV prevention* (pp. 109–137). New York: Kluwer Academic.

Jones, R., & Wasserheit, J. (1991). Introduction to the biology and natural history of sexually transmitted diseases. In J. N. Wasserheit, S. Aral, & K. Holmes (Eds.), *Research issues in human behavior and sexually transmitted diseases in the AIDS era* (p.25). Washington, DC: American Society for Microbiology.

Jones, S. G. (2002, June). From pill fatigue to pill counts: Medication adherence in HIV/AIDS. *Lighting the future of HIV/AIDS nursing: 14th annual conference of the association of nurses in AIDS care.* Retrieved November 11–14, 2001. Available at: http://www.medscape.com/viewarticle/412901.

Kagimu, M., Marum, E., Wabwire-Mangen, F., Nakyanjo, N., Walakira, Y., & Hogle, J. (1998). Evaluation of the effectiveness of AIDS health education interventions in the Muslim community in Uganda. *AIDS Education & Prevention, 10* (3), 215–228.

Kaijage, F. J. (1989). The AIDS crisis in the Kagera region, Tanzania, from an historical perspective. In J.Z.J. Killewo, G. K. Lwihula, A. Sandstrom, & L. Dahlgren (Eds.), *Behavioural and epidemiological aspects of AIDS research in Tanzania: Proceedings from a workshop held in Dar es Salaam, Tanzania, December 6–8, 1989.* Stockholm, Sweden: SAREC.

Kaiser Daily HIV/AIDS Report. (2001, November). HIV "virgin" myth suspected behind rapes of children in South Africa. Retrieved April 9, 2002. Available at: af-aids@healthdev.net.

Kagimba, J. (2003, July 19). Office of the President of Uganda, Personal communication.

Kaleeba, N., Namulondo, J., Kalinki, D., & Williams, G. (2000). *Open secret: People facing up to HIV and AIDS in Uganda* (Strategies for Hope Series no. 15). London: ActionAIDS.

Kamali, A., Nakamanya, S., Mitchell, K., & Whitworth, J.A.G. (2001). Community-based HIV/AIDS education in rural Uganda: Which channel is most effective? *Health Education Research, 16* (4), 411–423.

Kamya, R. M., Ssali, A., Busulwa, R., Grant, B., & Hearst, N. (1993). Condom use and marketing issues in an urban village of Kampala, Uganda [Abstract]. HIV/AIDS surveillance data base: Marrakech conference update: *VIIIth International Conference on AIDS in Africa/VIIIth African Conference on STDs, Marrakech, Morocco, December 12–16, 1993.* Washington, DC: Center for International Research, U.S. Bureau of the Census.

Kanki, P. J. (2002, April). Understanding and prevention of the HIV/AIDS epidemic in West Africa. Paper presented to Takemi Fellows, Harvard University, Cambridge, MA.

Kanyesigye, E., Kinsman, J., Kengeya-Kayondo, J., Kamulegeya, I., Nakiyingi, J., & Whitworth, J. A. (1998, July). A standardized community based sexual behaviour intervention in southwest Uganda: Progress in the first year [Abstract]. *12th world AIDS conference: Geneva, June 28–July 3, 1998.* Geneva.

Kanyunyuzi-Asaba, J. F., & Mwesigye, R. K. (1998, July). Audio-visual communication as an intervention in preventing HIV spread: Experience from Uganda [Abstract]. *12th world AIDS conference: Geneva, June 28–July 3, 1998.* Geneva.

Kapiga, S. (2002). Personal communication, February 15.

Karim, A. Q. (2001). Barriers to preventing human immunodeficiency virus in women: Experiences from KwaZulu-Natal, South Africa. *Journal of the American Medical Women's Association, 56* (4), 193–196.

Kasirye, S., Sentumbwe, S. S., & Nakkazi, N. D. (1998). Evaluation of HIV/AIDS prevention program among the students, youth and adolescents at Makerere University in Uganda. *Int-Conf-AIDS, 12,* 1133.

Kelly, R., Kiwanuka, N., Wawer, M. J., Serwadda, D., Sewankambo, N. K., Wabwire-Mangen, F. et al. (1999). Age of male circumcision and risk of prevalent HIV infection in rural Uganda. *AIDS, 13,* 399–405.

Kepka, D. (2000, July). Utilizing the performing arts to engender behavior change for young residents of an inner-city Jamaican community [Abstract]. *XIII international AIDS conference, Durban, July 9–14, 2000: Break the silence.* Durban, South Africa.

Kies, C. W. (1987). Family planning in rural Kwazulu: Transition from traditional to contemporary practices. *Southern African Journal of Demography, 1* (1), 16–19.

Kilian, A. H., Gregson, S., Ndyanabangi, B., Walusaga, K., Kipp, W., Sahlmuller, G. et al. (1999). Reductions in risk behaviour provide the most consistent explanation for declining HIV-1 prevalence in Uganda. *AIDS, 13,* 391–398.

Kilmarx, P. H., Supawitkul, S., Wankrairoj, M., Uthaivoravit, W., Limpakarnjanarat, K., Saisorn, S. et al. (2000). Explosive spread and effective control of human immunodeficiency virus in northernmost Thailand: The epidemic in Chiang Rai province, 1988–99. *AIDS, 14,* 2731–2740.

King, R. (2000). *Collaboration with traditional healers in HIV/AIDS prevention and care in sub-Saharan Africa: A literature review.* Geneva: UNAIDS.

Kipp, W., Kabagambe, G., & Konde-Lule, J. (2001). Low impact of a community-wide HIV testing and counseling program on sexual behavior in rural Uganda. *AIDS Education and Prevention, 13* (3), 279–289.

Kiragu, K. (2001, Fall). Youth and HIV/AIDS: Can we avoid catastrophe? (Population Reports, Series L, No. 12, Bloomberg School of Public Health, Population Information Program). Baltimore: Johns Hopkins University.

Kirby, D. (2003, April 24). Changing youth behaviors: Findings from U.S. and developing country research and their implications for A, B and C. Presentation to USAID, conference on HIV prevention for young people in developing countries. U.S. Agency for International Development (USAID) Office of HIV/AIDS, the Institute for Youth Development, and FHI/YouthNet Project. Washington, DC.

Kirungi, F. (2001, June). Uganda beating back AIDS. *Africa Recovery, 15* (1–2), 26.

Kirungi, W. L., Musinguzi, J. B., Opio, A., & Madraa, E. (2002, July). Trends in HIV prevalence and sexual behaviour (1990–2000) in Uganda [Abstract]. *XIV international AIDS conference: Barcelona, July 7–12, 2002: Knowledge and commitment for action.* Barcelona, Spain.

Kissling, F. (2003, March 5). Bush cripples his AIDS initiative. Available at: af-aids@healthdev.net.

Kiyonga, C. (2001, October 13). Keynote address by H. E. Yoweri Kaguta Museveni, president of the Republic of Uganda. Presented by chairman of the working group to establish the global AIDS and health fund. Africa Prize For Leadership. Available at: http://www.thp.org/prize/01/ceremony/museveni.htm.

Knodel, J., & Pramualratana, A. (1996). Prospects for increased condom use in marital unions in Thailand. *International Family Planning Perspectives 22* (3): 97–102.

Konde-Lule, J. K. (1993). The social and demographic impact of AIDS in a rural Ugandan community: Results of a 5 year follow-up study, 1987–1992. Paper presented at the Population Association of Uganda Annual Conference, Kampala, Uganda.

Konde-Lule, J. K., Berkley, S., & Downing, R. (1989). Knowledge, attitudes and practices concerning AIDS in Ugandans. *AIDS, 3*, 513–518.

Konde-Lule, J. K., Musagara, M., & Musgrave, S. (1993). Focus group interviews about AIDS in Rakai District of Uganda. *Social Science and Medicine, 37*, 679–684.

Kunda, A. (2001, January 2). Zambia's churches win fight against anti-AIDS ads. *Christianity Today*. Available at: http://www.christianitytoday.com/ct/2001/102/56.0.html.

Kretzschmar, M., & Morris, M. (1996). Measures of concurrency in networks and the spread of infectious disease. *Mathematical Biosciences, 133*, 165–195.

Kwesigabo, G. (2001). *Trends of HIV infection in the Kagera region of Tanzania 1987–2000*. Umea, Sweden: Umea University.

Kwesigabo, G., Killewo, J., Godoy, C., Urassa, W., Mbena, E., Mhalu, F. et al. (1998). Decline in the prevalence of HIV-1 infection in young women in the Kagera region of Tanzania. *Journal of Acquired Immune Deficiency Syndromes and Human Retrovirology, 17* (3), 262–268.

Kwesigabo, G., Killewo, J. Z., Urassa, W., Mbena, E., Mhalu, F., Lugalla, J. L. et al. (2000). Monitoring of HIV-1 infection prevalence and trends in the majority population using pregnant women as a sentinel population: 9 years experience from the Kagera region of Tanzania. *Journal of Acquired Immune Deficiency Syndromes 23* (5), 410–417.

Ladame, M. (1998). The First International Colloquium on AIDS and Religion. GTZ AIDS NETWORK. May (2), 18.

Laga, M., Schwartlander, B., Pisani, E., Sow, P. S., & Carael, M. (2001). To stem HIV in Africa prevent transmission to young women. *AIDS, 15*, 931–934.

Lagarde, E., Carael, M., Glynn, J. R., Kanhonou, L., Abega, S. C., Kahindo, M. et al. (2001). Educational level is associated with condom use within non-spousal partnerships in four cities of sub-Saharan Africa. *AIDS, 5*, 1399–1408.

Lagarde, E., Enel, C., Seck, K., Gueye-Ndiaye, A., Piau, J. P., Pison, G. et al. (1999). Religion and protective behaviours towards AIDS in rural Senegal. *AIDS, 13*, 1397–1405.

Lagarde, E., Pison, G., & Enel, C. (1997). Improvement in AIDS knowledge, perceptions and risk behaviours over a short period in a rural community of Senegal. *International Journal of STD & AIDS, 8*, 681–687.

Lauman, E. O. (1994). *The social organization of sexuality: Sexual practices in the United States.* Chicago: University of Chicago Press.

Lazzarini, Z. (1998, June). Human Rights and HIV / AIDS (Discussion Paper no. 2 on HIV / AIDS Care and Support). Washington, DC: The Synergy Project.

Leakey, L.S.B. (1931). The Kikuyu problem of the initiation of girls. *Journal of the Royal Anthropological Institute of Great Britain and Ireland, 61,* 277–285.

Leclerc-Madlala, S. (2002, October 4). South Africa: Prevention means more than condoms. *Daily Mail and Guardian,* p. 19.

Leonard, L., Ndiaye, I., Kapadia, A., Eisen, G., Diop, O., Mboup, S. et al. (2000). HIV prevention among male clients of female sex workers in Kaolack, Senegal: Results of a peer education program. *AIDS Education & Prevention, 12* (1), 21–37.

Lewicky, N., Kiragu, K., Young, S., & Barth, S. (1998). Delivery of improved services for health project Uganda: Evaluation of the safer sex or AIDS communication campaign. Unpublished manuscript, Johns Hopkins School of Public Health, Center for Communication Programs, Baltimore, MD.

Liebmann-Smith, J. (2001). Preteenage relationship with an older partner may lead to early first sex. *Family Planning Perspectives, 33* (3), 134.

Ling, J. C., Franklin, B., Lindsteadt, J., & Gearon, S. (1992). Social marketing: Its place in public health. *Annual Review of Public Health, 13,* 341–362.

Lom, M. M. (2001). Senegal's recipe for success. Early mobilization and political commitment keep HIV infections low. *Africa Recovery, 15* (1–2), 24–25, 29.

Longfield, K., Agha, S., Kusanthan, T., Klein, M., & Berman, J. (2001, December). Non-use of condoms: What role do supply, demand, & acceptance play in the condom gap? Paper presented at the International Conference on AIDS & STDs in Africa, Ouagadougou, Burkina Faso.

Low-Beer, D. (in press). Uganda and the challenge of AIDS. In A. Whiteside & N. K. Poku (Eds.), *Political Economy of AIDS in Africa.*

Low-Beer, D. (2002, November 30). HIV-1 incidence and prevalence trends in Uganda [Letter]. *Lancet, 360* (9347): 1788.

Low-Beer, D., & Stoneburner, R. (2002, July). Evidence of distinctive communication channels related to population level behaviour changes and HIV prevalence declines in Uganda [Abstract]. *XIV international AIDS conference: Barcelona, July 7–12, 2002: Knowledge and commitment for action.* Barcelona, Spain.

Low-Beer, D., Stoneburner, R., Barnett, T., & Whiteside, A. (2000, July). Knowledge diffusion and personalizing risk: Key indicators of behaviour change in Uganda compared to South Africa [Abstract]. *XIII international AIDS conference, Durban, July 9–14, 2000: Break the silence.* Durban, South Africa.

Lule, E. (2003, April 24). Personal communication.

Lutalo, T., Kidugavu, M., Wawer, M. J., Serwadda, D., Zabin, L. S., & Gray, R. H. (2000). Trends and determinants of contraceptive use in Rakai District, Uganda, 1995–98. *Studies in Family Planning, 31* (3), 217–227.

Lyons, M. (1996, January 20). *Summative evaluation: AIDS prevention and control project.* Kampala: USAID/Uganda.

MacFarlane, C. (1999). Reproductive health survey: Final report 1997, Jamaica. Kingston, Jamaica: National Family Planning Board.

Macintyre, K., Brown, L., & Sosler, S. (2001). It's not what you know, but who you knew: Examining the relationship between behavior change and AIDS mortality in Africa. *AIDS Education and Prevention, 13* (2), 160–174.

Macro International. (1995). *Uganda demographic and health survey 1995.* Calverton, MD: ORC Macro.

Macro International. (2000). *Senegal demographic and health survey 1999.* Calverton, MD: ORC Macro.

Macro International. (2001, December). *Uganda demographic and health survey 2000–2001.* Calverton, MD: ORC Macro.

Macro International. (2002). *República Dominicana Encuesta demográfica y de Salud 2002 Informe Preliminar Sobre VIH/SIDA.* Calverton, MD: Macro International/DHS+ Program.

Macro International, CESDEM, PROFAMILIA, & ONAPLAN. (1997). *República Dominicana: Encuesta demográfica y de Salud, 1996.* ENDESA-96 [Dominican Republic: Demographic and Health Survey]. Informe Preliminar. Santo Domingo.

Magnani, R. J., Karim, A. M., Weiss, L., Bond, K., Lemba, M., & Morgan, G. (2002). Reproductive health risk and protective factors among youth in Lusaka, Zambia. *Journal of Adolescent Health, 30* (1), 76–86.

Mahathir, M. (2002). President, Malaysian AIDS Council to a list-serve. *RE: Malaysia—HIV no longer to be feared.* Available at: http://archives. healthdev.net/sea-aids/msg00293.html.

Mahmud, H., Kabir, M. A., Mian, M. A., & Ali, M. M. (1998, July). HIV/AIDS prevention and control through creation of awareness by motivating and mobilizing religious leaders [Abstract]. *12th world AIDS conference: Geneva, June 28–July 3, 1998.* Geneva.

Mahy, M., & Gupta, N. (2002). Trends and differentials in adolescent reproductive behavior in sub-Saharan Africa (DHS Analytical Studies no. 3). Calverton, MD: Macro International, Measure DHS Project.

Mann, J. M., Nzilambi, N., Piot, P., Bosenge, N., Kalala, M., Francis, H., Colebunders, R. C., Azila, P. K., Curran, J. W., & Quinn, T. C. (1988). HIV infection and associated risk factors in female prostitutes in Kinshasa, Zaire. *AIDS, 2* (4), 249–254.

Mann, J. R., Stine, C. C., & Vessey, J. (2002). The role of disease-specific infectivity and number of disease exposures on long-term effectiveness of the latex condom. *Sexually Transmitted Diseases, 29,* 344–349.

MAP International. (1997, November). Religious-based initiatives. Arlington, VA: AIDSCAP/Family Health International.

Marck, J. (1997). Aspects of male circumcision in sub-equatorial African culture history. *Health Transition Review, 7* (Suppl.), 337–360.

Marin, B. V., Coyle, K. K., Gómez, C. A., Carvajal, S. C., & Kirby, D. B. (2000). Older boyfriends and girlfriends increase risk of sexual initiation in young adolescents. *Journal of Adolescent Health, 27,* 409–418.

Marum, E. (2002, September). USAID–Uganda ABC experience. Paper presented at the "ABC" Experts Technical Meeting, USAID, Washington, DC.

Marum, E., & Madraa, E. (2000, July). The role of donors in empowering an effective national response to AIDS: The Uganda example. Paper presented at the *XIIIth International AIDS Conference,* Durban, South Africa.

Marum. E. (1993). Personal communication, March 18.

Maund, L., Bennoun, R. M., & Chaimalee, P. W. (1998, July). The role of Buddhist monks and communities in HIV/AIDS prevention and care [Abstract]. *12th world AIDS conference: Geneva, June 28–July 3, 1998*. Geneva.

Mbizvo, M. T., Ray, S., Bassett, M., McFarland, K. W., Machekano, R., & Katzenstein, D. (1994) Condom use and the risk of HIV infection: Who is being protected? *Central African Journal of Medicine, 40* (11), 294–299.

Meda, N., Ndoye, I., M'Boup, S., Wade, A., Ndiaye, S., Niang, C. et al. (2000). Low and stable HIV infection rates in Senegal: Natural course of the epidemic or evidence for success of prevention? *AIDS, 14*, 1276–1277.

Meekers, D. (1999). Patterns of use of the female condom in urban Zimbabwe (Working Paper no. 28). Washington, DC: Population Services International, Research Division.

Mekonen, E., & Mekonen, A. (1999). Breakage and slippage of condoms among users in north Gondar Province, Ethiopia. *East African Medical Journal, 76*, 481–483.

Merson, M. (1993, May 28). Slowing the spread of HIV: Agenda for the 1990s. *Science, 260*, 266–268.

Messersmith, L. J., Kane, T. T., Odebiyi, A. I., & Adewuyi, A. A. (2000). Who's at risk? Men's STD experience and condom use in southwest Nigeria. *Journal of the Association of Nurses in AIDS Care, 11* (4), 46–54.

Mill, J. E., & Anarfib, J. K. (2002). HIV risk environment for Ghanaian women: Challenges to prevention. *Social Science and Medicine, 54* (3), 325–337.

Mills, S., Benjarattanaporn, P., Bennett, A., Na Pattalung, R., Sundhagul, D., Trongsawad, P., Gregorich, S. E., Hearst, N., & Mandel, J. S. (1997). HIV risk behavioral surveillance in Bangkok, Thailand: Sexual behavior trends among eight population groups. *AIDS, 11* (Suppl. 1), S43–S51.

Ministry of Health/Uganda AIDS Commission. (1997, December). *National strategic framework for HIV/AIDS activities in Uganda 1998–2002*. Entebbe, Uganda: Ministry of Health.

Ministry of Health/Uganda AIDS Commission. (2000–2001). Unpublished reports, tables, raw data from population surveys, STD/AIDS Control Programme.

Monitoring the AIDS Pandemic Network Symposium. (2000, July). *The status and trends of the HIV/AIDS in the world*. Durban, South Africa.

Moodie, R., Katahoire, A., Kaharuza, F., Balikowa, D. O., Busuulwa, J., & Barton, T. (1991, July–December). An evaluation study of Uganda AIDS control programme's information education and communication activities. Uganda Ministry of Health AIDS Control Programme, and WHO, Global Programme on AIDS.

Morris, M., & Kretzschmar, M. (1997). Concurrent partnerships and the spread of HIV. *AIDS, 11*, 641–648.

Morris, M., Wawer, M. J., Makumbi, F., Zavisca, J. R., & Sewankambo, N. (2000). Condom acceptance is higher among travelers in Uganda. *AIDS, 14*, 733–741.

Moses, S., Bailey, R. C., & Ronald, A. R. (1998). Male circumcision: assessment of health risks and benefits." *Sexually Transmitted Infections, 74*, 368–373.

Moses, S., Plummer, F. A., Bradley, J. E., Ndinya-Achola, J. O., Nagelkerke, N.J.D., & Ronald, A. R. (1994). The association between lack of male circumcision and risk for HIV infection: A review of the epidemiological data. *Sexually Transmitted Infections, 21,* 201–210.

Mostad, S. B., Overbaugh, J., DeVange, D. M., Welch, M. J., Chohan, B., Mandaliya, K., Nyange, P., Martin, H. L. Jr., Ndinya-Achola, J., Bwayo, J. J., & Kreiss, J. K. (1997). Hormonal contraception, vitamin A deficiency, and other risk factors for shedding of HIV-1 infected cells from the cervix and vagina. *Lancet, 350,* 922–927.

Msamanga, G. I., Urassa, E., Spiegelman, D., Hertzmark, E., Kapiga, S. H., Hunter, D. J. et al. (1996). Socioeconomic status and prevalence of HIV infection among pregnant women in Dar es Salaam, Tanzania. *Int Conf AIDS, 11* (1), 345.

Mukoyogo, M. C., & Williams, G. (1991, June). *AIDS orphans: A community perspective from Tanzania* (Strategies for Hope no. 5). London: ACTIONAID.

Murphy, E. (2003, February). Gender and ABCs. Paper presented at USAID Expert's Meeting on AIDS and ABC, Washington, DC.

Musara, T. M. (1991). Interview with a traditional healer. In M. A. Mercer & S. Scott (Eds.), *Tradition and transition: NGOs respond to AIDS in Africa.* Baltimore: Johns Hopkins University School of Public Health and Hygiene.

Museveni, Y. K. (2000). *What is Africa's problem?* Minneapolis: University of Minnesota Press.

Musinguzi, J. G., Asiimwe-Okiror, A., Madraa, E., Nsubuga, P., Talamoi, L. O., Byabamazima, C., & Kaweesa, D. (1997, October). Results of population-based KABP survey on HIV/AIDS and STDs in Kotido district, northeastern Uganda. Entebbe, Uganda: STD/AIDS Control Programme, Ministry of Health.

Nakiyingi, J., Ruberantwari, A., Kamali, A., & Mbulaiteye, S. M. (2000, July). Falling HIV incidence: One decade of follow up of a rural cohort in south-west Uganda [Abstract]. *XIII international AIDS conference, Durban, July 9–14, 2000: Break the silence.* Durban, South Africa.

Nantulya, V. (2002, February). HIV/AIDS prevention: Policy and program context of Uganda's success story. Paper presented to USAID, Washington, DC.

N'Diaye, S., Ayad, M., & Gaye, A. (1994). *Enquête démographique et de Santé au Sénégal (EDS-II), 1994* [Demographic and Health Survey]. Calverton, MD: Macro International.

N'Diaye, S., Ayad, M., & Gaye, A. (1997). Enquête démographique et de Santé au Sénégal (EDS-III), 1997 [Demographic and Health Survey]. Calverton, MD: Macro International.

Ng, H. (2000, Winter). AIDS in Africa: A regional overview. *Harvard AIDS Review,* 2–5.

Ng'weshemi, J. Z., Boerma, J. T., Pool, R., Barongo, L., Senkoro, K., Maswe, M. et al. (1996). Changes in male sexual behaviour in response to the AIDS epidemic: Evidence from a cohort study in urban Tanzania. *AIDS, 10,* 1415–1420.

NIH: National Institute of Allergy and Infectious Diseases, Workshop Summary. (2001, July 20). *Scientific evidence on condom effectiveness for sexually transmitted disease (STD) prevention.*

Norman, L. R., & Gebre, Y. (2002, July). HIV-related sexual behaviours among students at a Caribbean university [Abstract]. *XIV international AIDS conference: Barcelona, July 7–12, 2002: Knowledge and commitment for action.* Barcelona, Spain.

Ntozi, J., Ahimbisibwe, F., Mulindwa, I. K., Ayiga, N., & Odwee, J. (2001, August). Has HIV/AIDS epidemic changed sexual behaviour of high risk groups in Uganda? Paper presented at the Conference of the International Union for Scientific Study of Population, Salvador, Brazil.

Nyblade, J., Menken, M., Wawer, N., Sewankambo, D., Serwadda, R., Gray, F. et al. (2000, July). HIV risk behavior change subsequent to participation in voluntary counseling and testing in rural Rakai, Uganda [Abstract]. *XIII international AIDS conference, Durban, July 9–14, 2000: Break the silence.* Durban, South Africa.

Nzioka C., (1996). Lay perceptions of risk of HIV infection and the social construction of safer sex: Some experiences from Kenya. *AIDS Care, 8* (5), 565–579.

O'Connor, M. L. (2001). Men who have many sexual partners before marriage are more likely to engage in extramarital intercourse. *International Family Planning Perspectives, 27* (1), 48–49.

O'Farrell, N. (2001). Enhanced efficiency of female-to-male HIV transmission in core groups in developing countries. *Sexually Transmitted Diseases, 28* (2), 84–91.

Okware, S. (2003, July 21). Uganda Ministry of Health. Personal communication.

Okware, S., Opio, A., Musinguzi, J., & Waibale, P. (2001). Fighting HIV/AIDS: Is success possible? *Bulletin of the World Health Organization, 79,* 1113–1120.

Olowo-Freers, B.P.A., & Barton, T. G. (1992). *In pursuit of fulfillment: Studies of cultural diversity and sexual behaviour in Uganda.* Kisubi, Uganda: Marianum Press (UNICEF).

OMSA. (1997, July). Evaluation of Triquilar commercial (Report). Santo Domingo: PROFAMILIA and Development Associates.

OMSA. (1997, July). Final report: Pre-test of protector commercial and sexual behavior inquiry (Report). Santo Domingo: PROFAMILIA and Development Associates.

OMSA. (2000, November). Cambios en al comportamento sexual por el SIDA [Change in sexual behavior due to AIDS]. Santo Domingo: OMSA, SA.

ORC Macro. (2003). *Zambia demographic and health survey 2001–2.* Calverton, MD: Macro International.

O'Reilly, K. R. (1986). Sexual behaviour, perceptions of infertility and family planning in sub-Saharan Africa. *African Journal of Sexually Transmitted Diseases, 2* (2), 47–49, 80.

Orroth, K. K., Korenromp, E. L., White, R. G., Gavyole, A., Sewankambo, N. K., Wawer, M. J. et al. (2002, July). Differences between the Mwanza, Rakai and Masaka populations: A reanalysis of trial data [Abstract]. *XIV international AIDS conference: Barcelona, July 7–12, 2002: Knowledge and commitment for action.* Barcelona, Spain.

Ostrow, D. E., Fox, K. J., Chmiel, J. S., Silvestre, A., Visscher, B. R., Vanable, P. A., Jacobson, L. P., & Strathdee, S. A. (2002, March 29). Attitudes towards highly active antiretroviral therapy are associated with sexual risk taking among HIV-infected and uninfected homosexual men. *AIDS, 16* (5), 775–780.

Outwater, A., Nkya, L., Lwihula, G., O'Connor, P., Leshabari, M., Nguma, J. et al. (2000). Patterns of partnership and condom use in a population of CSWs in Morogoro, Tanzania. *Journal of the Association of Nurses in AIDS Care, 11* (4), 46–54.

Over, M., & Piot, P. (1993). HIV infection and sexually transmitted disease. In D. T. Jamison, W. H. Mosely, A. R. Mensham, & J. L. Bobadilla (Eds.), *Disease control priorities in developing countries.* Oxford, UK: Oxford University Press.

Packard, R. M., & Epstein, P. (1991). Epidemiologists, social scientists, and the structure of medical research on AIDS in Africa. *Social Science and Medicine, 33* (7), 771–783.

Painter, T. M. (2001). Voluntary counseling and testing for couples: A high-leverage intervention for HIV/AIDS prevention in sub-Saharan Africa. *Social Science and Medicine, 53,* 1397–1411.

Palmer, A. (2002). Reaching youth worldwide: The Johns Hopkins Center for Communication Programs, 1995–2000 (Working Paper no. 6, Population Communication Services). Baltimore: Johns Hopkins University.

Parker, R. (2002). The global HIV/AIDS pandemic, structural inequalities, and the politics of international health. *American Journal of Public Health, 92* (3), 343–346.

Parkhurst, J. O. (2001, September). Myths of success: The use and misuse of Ugandan HIV data. Paper presented at the Sixth UKFIET Oxford International Conference For Education and Development, Oxford, United Kingdom.

Pattalung, R. N., & Bennett, A. (1990). Private sector initiative: AIDS prevention in Thailand. Unpublished manuscript.

Perez-Peña, R. (2003, August 9). Study finds many ignore warnings on sex practices. *The New York Times.* Available at: http://www.nytimes.com/2003/08/09/nyregion/09SEX.html?ex=1061457769&ei=1&en=2f80afb1 2bdb48fe.

Phoolcharoen, W. (1998). HIV/AIDS prevention in Thailand: Success and challenges. *Science, 280* (5371), 1873–1874.

Phoolcharoen, W., Ungchusak, K., Sittitrai, W., & Brown, T. (1998). Thailand: Lessons from a strong national response to HIV/AIDS. *AIDS, 12* (Suppl. B), S123–S135.

Pielemeier, J., de George, S., Fluty, H., O'Loughlin, W., Odhiambo D., & Wagner, K. (1996, June). Process evaluation of the AIDS technical support project (ATSP). Washington, DC: USAID, Division of HIV/AIDS.

Piliero, P. J., & Purdy, B. (2001). Nevirapine-induced hepatitis: A case series and review of the literature. *AIDS Reader, 11* (7), 379–382.

Piot, P. (1994). Differences between African and western patterns of heterosexual transmission. In A. Nicolai (Ed.), *HIV epidemiology: Models and methods* (pp. 77–82). New York: Raven Press.

Pisani, E. (1999, June). Acting early to prevent AIDS: The case of Senegal (UNAIDS/99.34E, Best Practice Collection). Geneva, Switzerland: Joint United Nations Programme for HIV/AIDS.

Pisani, E., Brown, T., Saidel, T., Rehle, T., & Carael, M. (1998, May). Meeting the behavioural data collection needs of national HIV/AIDS and STD programmes. Arglinton, VA: Family Health International.

Pool, R., Maswe, M., Boerma, J. T., & Nnko, S. (1996). The price of promiscuity: Why urban males in Tanzania are changing their sexual behavior. *Health Transition Review, 6,* 203–221.

Popp, D., & Fisher, J. D. (2002). First, do no harm: A call for emphasizing adherence and HIV prevention interventions in active antiretroviral therapy programs in the developing world. *AIDS, 16,* 676–678.

Porapakkham, Y., Pramarnpol, S., Athibhoddhi, S., & Bernhard, R. (1996). The evolution of HIV/AIDS policy in Thailand: 1984–94. USAID and FHI/AIDSCAP project.

Qu, S., Liu, W., Choi, K. H. et al. (2002). The potential for rapid sexual transmission of HIV in China: Sexually transmitted diseases and condom failure highly prevalent among female sex workers. *AIDS and Behavior, 6* (3), 267–275.

Quinn, T. C., Gray, R., Sewankambo, N. et al. (2000, July). Therapeutic reductions of HIV viral load to prevent HIV transmission: Data from HIV discordant couples, Rakai, Uganda [Abstract]. *XIII international AIDS conference, Durban, July 9–14, 2000: Break the silence.* Durban, South Africa.

Quinn, T. C., Wawer, M. J., Sewankambo, N., Serwadda, D., Li, C., Wabwire-Mangen, F. et al. (2000). Viral load and heterosexual transmission of human immunodeficiency virus type 1. *New England Journal of Medicine, 342,* 921–929.

Ramiah, I. (2003, March 31). The HIV/AIDS epidemic and poverty reduction strategy papers: A case for greater integration of HIV/AIDS issues in PRSPs and policy options for the International Labour Office. HIV/AIDS and the World of Work. Geneva: International Labour Office.

Ranjit, N., Bankole, A., Darroch, J. E., & Singh, S. (2001). Contraceptive failure in the first two years of use: Differences across socioeconomic subgroups. *Perspectives on Sexual and Reproductive Health, 33* (1), 19–27.

Reid, E., & Bailey, M. (1992). Young women: Silence, susceptibility and the HIV epidemic. *UNDP Issues Paper No. 12.* Available at: http://www.undp.org/hiv/publications/issues/english/issue12e.htm.

Reuters. (2001, May 23). High rate of severe liver toxicity associated with antiretroviral therapy. Posted on Medscape.com and CBSHealthwatch. Atlanta (Reuters Health).

Reuters. (2002, October 10). Probe widens into stolen African HIV drugs—Glaxo. Reuters NewMedia. Available at: http://www.aegis.com/news/re/2002/RE021016.html.

Richens, J., Imrie, J., & Copas, A. (2000). Condoms and seat belts: The parallels and the lessons. *Lancet, 29,* 400.

Richens, J., Imrie, J., & Weiss, H. (2003). Sex and death: Why does HIV continue to spread when so many people know about the risks? *Journal of Royal Statistical Society Association, 166,* 207–215.

Rimal, R. N. (2001). Perceived risk and self-efficacy as motivators: Understanding individuals' long-term use of health information. *Journal of Communication, 51* (4), 633–654.

Robinson, N. J., Mulder, D. W., Auvert, B., & Hayes, R. J. (1995). Modeling the impact of alternative HIV intervention strategies in rural Uganda. *AIDS, 9,* 1263–1270.

Roesin, R. (1998, July). Islamic response to HIV/AIDS impact in Indonesia [Abstract]. *12th world AIDS conference: Geneva, June 28–July 3, 1998.* Geneva.

Rogers, E. M. (1962). *Diffusion of innovations.* New York: The Free Press.

Rogers, E. M., & Shoemaker, F. F. (1971). *Communications of innovations.* New York: The Free Press.

Rojanapithayakorn, W., & Hanenberg, R. (1996). The 100% condom program in Thailand. *AIDS, 10* (1), 1–7.

Root-Bernstein, R. (1998). *Rethinking AIDS.* New York: Macmillan.

Rosenberg, J. (2001). Condoms reduce women's risk of herpes infection, but do not protect men. *International Family Planning Perspectives, 27* (4), 213–214.

Rosenberg, J. (2002). In Zimbabwe, sexual relationships with older men put young women at high risk of HIV infection. *International Family Planning Infections, 28* (4), 230–231.

Rossi, E. E., Raharisoa, M. B., Ny, A., & Ralison, A. (2002, July). Increasing condom use through community mobilization and social marketing in Madagascar [Abstract]. *XIV international AIDS conference: Barcelona, July 7–12, 2002: Knowledge and commitment for action.* Barcelona, Spain.

Rotello, G. (1998). *Sexual ecology.* New York: Dutton.

Rotello, G. (2003, August 15). Personal communication.

Runganga, A., Pitts, M., & McMaster, J. (1992). The use of herbal and other agents to enhance sexual experience. *Social Science and Medicine, 35,* 1037–1042.

Ruteikara, S. L., Byamugisha, G. B., Miiro, H., Wabwire, D., James, T. M., & Marum, E. (1996, July). Religious beliefs and dogmas on population issues and HIV and AIDS prevention [Abstract]. *XI international conference on AIDS: Vancouver, July 7–12, 1996.* Vancouver, B.C.

Ruteikara, S. L., Nassanga-Miiro, H., Byamugisha, G., James, T. M., & Church Human Services AIDS Prevention Programme (CHUSA) Project. (1995, July). Follow-up Evaluation Report. Church Human Services, the Church of the Province of Uganda, World Learning.

Rutenberg, N., Kehus-Alons, C., Brown, L., Macintyre, K., Dallimore, A., & Kaufman, C. (2001, March). Transitions to adulthood in the context of AIDS in South Africa: Report of wave I. Washington, DC: The Population Council, Horizons Project.

Rwomushana, J. (2000, July). Breaking the silence around traditional medicine for HIV/AIDS prevention and care [Abstract]. *XIII international AIDS conference, Durban, July 9–14, 2000: Break the silence.* Durban, South Africa.

Sabatier, R. (1988). *Blaming others: Prejudice, race, and worldwide AIDS.* London: Panos Institute.

Samson, M., Libert, F., Doranz, B. J., Rucker, J., Liesnard, C., Farber, C. M., Saragosti, S., Lapoumeroulie, C., Cognaux, J., Forceille, C., Muyldermans, G., Verhofstede, C., Burtonboy, G., Georges, M., Imai, T., Rana, S., Yi, Y., Smyth, R. J., Collman, R. G., Doms, R. W., Vassart, G., & Parmentier, M. (1996). Resistance to HIV-1 infection in caucasian individuals bearing mutant alleles of the CCR-5 chemokine receptor gene. *Nature, 382*, 722–725.

Sanderson, W. (2001). The mixed blessing of anti-retroviral therapy. *AIDS Analysis Africa, 12* (1), 12–13.

Saracco, A., Musicco, M., Nicolosi, A., Angarano, G., Arici, C., Gavazzeni, G., Costigliola, P., Gafa, S., Gervasoni, C., Luzzati, R. et al. (1993). Man-to-woman sexual transmission of HIV: Longitudinal study of 343 steady partners of infected men. *Journal of Acquired Immune Deficiency Syndrome, 6*, 497–502.

Schietinger, H., & Sanei, L. (1998, June). Systems for delivering HIV/AIDS care and support (HTS Discussion Paper no. 8). Washington, DC: TvT Associates.

Schoepf, B. G. (2001). International AIDS research in anthropology: Taking a critical perspective on the crisis. *Annual Review of Anthropology, 30*, 335–361.

Schoofs, M. (1997, April 15). The law of desire. *The Village Voice*.

Schopper, D. (1992). Design of a population-based AIDS control program in Northern Uganda. Unpublished Ph.D. diss., Harvard University, Cambridge, MA.

Schreiner, R. (2002, March 4). Letter to the editor: Abstinence won't sell. *USA Today*, p. 11A.

Sekirevu, D. M., & Lukenge, D. L. (1998, July). People living with HIV/AIDS reaching out to schools [Abstract]. *12th world AIDS conference: Geneva, June 28–July 3, 1998*. Geneva.

Serenata, C. M. (2002, October 7). Women reusing female condom, despite risks. Message posted on af-aids@healthdev.net.

Serwadda, D., Gray, R. H., Wawer, M. J., Sewankambo, N. K., Li, C., & Konde-Lule, J. (1996). HIV-1 incidence and prevalence among pregnant women in a population-based rural cohort, Rakai district, Uganda [Abstract]. *XI international conference on AIDS: Vancouver, July 7–12, 1996*. Vancouver, BC.

Sharma, R. (2001). Condom use seems to be reducing number of new HIV/AIDS cases. *British Medical Journal, 323*, 417.

Shelton, J., & Johnston, B. (2001). Condom gap in Africa: Evidence from donor agencies and key informants. *British Medical Journal, 323*, 139.

Shillinger, K. (1999, October 10). AIDS and the African. *Boston Globe Online*, p. A1.

Shoumatoff, A.(1988). *African madness*. New York: Alfred Knopf.

Shuey, D. A, Babishangire, B. B., Omiat, S., & Bagarukayo, H. (1999). Increased sexual abstinence among in-school adolescents as a result of school health education in Soroti district, Uganda. *Health Education Research, 14*, 411–419.

Simmons, A. M. (2001, March 9). In AIDS-ravaged Africa, Senegal is a beacon of hope. *Los Angeles Times*, p. A1.

Simon, G., Zhuwau, T., Anderson, R. M., & Chandiwana, S. K. (1998). Is there evidence for behaviour change in response to AIDS in rural Zimbabwe? *Social Science and Medicine, 46*, 321–330.

Singh, S., Darroch, J. E., & Bankole, A. (2002). *The role of behavior change in the decline in HIV prevalence in Uganda*. New York: Guttmacher Institute.

Singh, S., Wulf, D., Samara, R., & Cuca, Y. P. (2000). Gender differences in the timing of first intercourse: Data from 14 countries. *International Family Planning Perspectives, 26* (1), 21–28, 43.

Sittitrai, W. (2001). *HIV prevention needs and success: A tale of three countries*. Geneva: UNAIDS.

Sliep, Y. (2003, September 3). Transcripts of interviews conducted under Dr. Yvonne. Part of Green, Thornton, and Sliep 2003.

Smith, A. M., Jolley, D., Hocking, J., Benton, K., & Gerofi, J. (1998). Does penis size influence condom slippage and breakage? *International Journal of STD & AIDS, 9*, 444–447.

Smith, J., Nalagoda, F., Wawer, M. J., Serwadda, D., Sewankambo, N., Konde-Lule, J. T. et al. (1999). Education attainment as a predictor of HIV risk in rural Uganda: Results from a population-based survey. *International Journal of STD & AIDS, 10*, 452–459.

Soper, D. C., Shoupe, D., Shangold, G. A., Shangold, M. M., Gutmann, J., & Mercer, L. (1993). Prevention of vaginal trichomoniasis by compliant use of the female condom. *Sexually Transmitted Diseases, 20* (3), 137–139.

Soto-Ramirez, L. E., Renjifo, B., McLane, M. F., Marlink, R., Hara, C., Sutthent, R. et al. (1996). HIV-1 Langerhans' cell tropism associated with heterosexual transmission of HIV. *Science, 271*, 1291–1293.

Ssemwogerere, P. (2002, April 11). Personal communication.

Ssengonzi, R., Morris, M., Sewankambo, N., Serwadda, D., Wawer, W., & Konde-Lule, J. (1996). Socio-economic status and sexual networks in a high HIV prevalence population in rural Uganda [Abstract]. *XI international conference on AIDS: Vancouver, July 7–12, 1996*. Vancouver, B.C.

STD/ACP. (1998). *Surveillance Report March 1998*. Entebbe, Uganda: Ministry of Health, Epidemiology and Surveillance Unit.

Steen, R. (2001). Eradicating chancroid. *Bulletin of the World Health Organization, 79*, 818–826.

Steyn, A. F., & Rip, C. M. (1968). The changing urban Bantu family. *Journal of Marriage and the Family, 30* (3), 499–517.

Stillwagon, E. (2002). HIV/AIDS in Africa: Fertile terrain. *Journal of Development Studies 38* (6), 1–22.

St. Louis, M. E., & Holmes, K. K. (1999). Conceptual framework for STD/HIV prevention and control. In M.K.K. Holmes, P. F. Sparling, & P. A. Mardh (Eds.), *Sexually transmitted diseases* (3d ed.). New York: McGraw-Hill.

Stolberg, S. G. (2003, February 2). The White House gets religion on AIDS in Africa. Available at: http://www.nytimes.com/2003/02/02/weekinre view/02STOL.html?ex=1045212267&ei=1&en=61bfca898fea7807.

Stone, V. E., Catania, J. A., & Binson, D. (1999). Measuring change in sexual behavior: Concordance between survey measures. *Journal of Sex Research, 36* (1), 102–108.

Stoneburner, R. L. (2000, July). Analyses of HIV trend and behavioral data in Uganda, Kenya, and Zambia: Prevalence declines in Uganda relate more to reduction in sex partners than condom use [Abstract]. *XIII international AIDS conference, Durban, July 9–14, 2000: Break the silence*. Durban, South Africa.

Stoneburner, R. L., Asiimwe-Okiror, G., Musinguzi, J., Opio, A., Biryahwaho, B., Byabamazima, C. et al. (1996). Declines in HIV prevalence in Ugandan pregnant women and its relationship to HIV incidence and risk reduction [Abstract]. *XI international conference on AIDS: Vancouver, July 7–12, 1996*. Vancouver, B.C.

Stoneburner, R. L., & Carballo, M. (1997). An assessment of emerging patterns of HIV incidence in Uganda and other East African countries. Geneva: International Centre for Migration and Health and FHI/AIDSCAP.

Stoneburner, R. L., Carballo, M., Bernstein, R., & Saidel, T. (1998). Simulation of HIV incidence dynamics in the Rakai cohort. *AIDS, 12*, 226–228.

Stoneburner, R. L., & Low-Beer, D. (2000, July). Is condom use or decrease in sexual partners behind HIV declines in Uganda? Paper presented at the *13th International AIDS Conference*, Durban, South Africa.

Stoneburner, R. L., & Low-Beer, D. (2002a). Epidemiological elements associated with HIV declines and behavior change in Uganda: Yet another look at the evidence. Paper presented at the "ABC" Experts Technical Meeting, USAID, Washington, DC.

Stoneburner, R. L., Low-Beer, D., & Green, E. (in preparation). Population level HIV declines and behavioral risk avoidance in Uganda: Evidence for a largely successful (and economical) public health prevention program—but why doesn't it sell?

Stoneburner, R. L., Low-Beer, D., Tembo, G., Mertens, T. E., & Asiimwe-Okiror, G. (1996). HIV incidence dynamics in East Africa deduced from surveillance data. *American Journal of Epidemiology, 144*, 682–695.

Stover, J. (2002, February). The effects of behavior change on trends in HIV incidence in Kenya and Uganda. Paper presented to USAID, Washington, DC.

Strathdee, S. A. et al. (2002). Safer sex fatigue: Confidence in HIV treatment lead to risky sex behavior. *AIDS, 16*, 775–780.

Sweat, M., & Dennison, J. (1995). Reducing HIV incidence in developing countries with structural and environmental interventions. *AIDS, 9* (Suppl. A), S251–S257.

Sy, F. S., Lacson, R., Theocharis, T., Osteria, T., Jimenez, P., Vincent, M. et al. (1996, July). Correlates of sexual abstinence among urban university students in the Philippines [Abstract]. *XI international conference on AIDS: Vancouver, July 7–12, 1996*. Vancouver, B.C.

Taha, T. E., Canner, J. K., Chiphangwi, J. D., Dallabetta, G. A., Yang, L. P., Mtimavalye, L. A., & Miotti, P. G. (1996). Reported condom use is not associated with incidence of sexually transmitted diseases in Malawi. *AIDS 10*, 207–212.

Talbot, D. (1990, January). Condom conundrum. *Mother Jones*, pp. 39–47.

Tangwa, G. B. (2002). The HIV/AIDS pandemic, African traditional values and the search for a vaccine in Africa. *Journal of Medicine & Philosophy, 27*, 217–230.

Tarantola, D., & Schwartlander, B. (1997). HIV/AIDS epidemics in sub-Saharan Africa: Dynamism, diversity and discrete declines? *AIDS, 11* (Suppl. B), S5–S21.

Thesenvitz, J. (2000, February). *Fear appeals for tobacco controls*. Ontario: Council for a Tobacco Free Ontario, the Program Training and Consultation Centre, and the Health Communication Unit.

Thornton, R. (2003). Personal communication, July 18.

Thornton, R. (2003, February). Flows of "sexual substance" and representation of the body in South Africa. Unpublished manuscript. Johannesburg: Department of Anthropology, University of the Witwatersrand.

Torres, J. (2000, September 9). Condom crazy. From the online magazine: *World on the Web.* http://www.worldmag.com/world/issue/09-09-00/cover_3.asp.

Trussell, J., & Kowal, D. (1998). The essentials of contraception. In R. A. Hatcher, J. Trussell, & F. Stewart (Eds.), *Contraceptive technology* (17th ed.). New York: Ardent Media.

Turner, R. (1993, June). Young Ugandans know condoms prevent STDs, but disagree on whether use shows respect for partner. *International Family Planning Perspectives, 19* (2), 7–76.

Uganda AIDS Commission. (2001). *The national strategic framework for HIV/AIDS activities in Uganda (2000/1–2005/6).* Kampala.

Uganda AIDS program gets results. (Lutheran World Federation efforts to reduce AIDS transmission). (1998). *The Christian Century, 115* (33), 1139.

Uganda Ministry of Health. (1997). Unpublished reports, tables, raw data from population-pased surveys, STD/AIDS Control PRogramme.

Uganda Ministry of Health. (1998). STD/AIDS control programme. Population survey: English questionnaire. Kampala: Ministry of Health.

Uganda Ministry of Health. (1998). Surveillance report March 1998. Kampala: Ministry of Health.

Uganda Ministry of Health. (2001a). Surveillance report June 2001. Kampala: Ministry of Health.

Uganda Ministry of Health. (2001b), Unpublished reports, tables, raw data from population-based KABP surveys, STD/AIDS Control Programme. 2000, 2001.

UNAIDS. (1998a). *Global report on the HIV/AIDS epidemic.* Geneva: UNAIDS.

UNAIDS. (1998b). *A measure of success in Uganda: The value in monitoring both HIV prevalence and sexual behaviour.* Geneva, UNAIDS.

UNAIDS. (1998c). *Relationships of HIV and STD declines in Thailand to behavioural change: A synthesis of existing studies.* Geneva: UNAIDS.

UNAIDS. (1999a). *Acting early to prevent AIDS: The case of Senegal.* Geneva: UNAIDS.

UNAIDS. (1999b). *Sexual behaviour change for HIV: Where have theories taken us?* Geneva: UNAIDS.

UNAIDS. (1999c). *Summary booklet of best practices.* Geneva: UNAIDS.

UNAIDS. (1999d). *Trends in HIV incidence and prevalence: Natural course of the epidemic or results of behavioural change?* Geneva: UNAIDS.

UNAIDS. (2000a). *Collaboration with traditional healers in HIV/AIDS prevention and care in sub-Saharan Africa: A literature review.* Geneva: UNAIDS.

UNAIDS. (2000b). *Report on the global HIV/AIDS epidemic.* Geneva: UNAIDS.

UNAIDS. (2001). *Report of the secretary general to the special session of the general assembly on HIV/AIDS.* Geneva: UNAIDS.

UNAIDS/Kenya. (2000). *Kenya: Epidemiological fact sheet on HIV/AIDS and sexually transmitted diseases.* Geneva: UNAIDS.

UNAIDS/Senegal. (2000). *Senegal: Epidemiological fact sheet on HIV/AIDS and sexually transmitted diseases.* Geneva: UNAIDS.

UNAIDS/Thailand. (2002). *Thailand epidemiological fact sheet on HIV/AIDS and sexually transmitted infections* (2002 Update). Geneva: UNAIDS.

UNAIDS/Uganda. (2000). *Uganda: Epidemiological fact sheet on HIV/AIDS and sexually transmitted diseases.* Geneva: UNAIDS.

UNAIDS/Zambia. (2000). *Zambia: Epidemiological fact sheet on HIV/AIDS and sexually transmitted diseases.* Geneva: UNAIDS.

UNAIDS/MAP. (2000, July). *Report of the Durban Monitoring the AIDS Pandemic (MAP) Network Symposium.* Available at the UNAIDS Web site, http://www.UNAIDS.org.

UNAIDS/WHO. (2002). *AIDS epidemic update December 2002.* Geneva: Joint United Nations Programme on HIV/AIDS (UNAIDS) World Health Organization (WHO).

Underwood, C., Hachonda, H., Serlemitsos, E., & Bharath, U. (2001, November). Impact of the HEART campaign: Findings from the youth surveys 1999 and 2000. Lusaka, Zambia: Zambia Integrated Health Programme and Johns Hopkins Center for Communication Programs.

Underwood, C. R., Serlemitsos, E. T., Bharath, U., & Hachonda, H. M. (2002). Effects of a media campaign on HIV risk-reduction practices: Findings from the 1999 and 2000 youth surveys in Zambia.

UNFPA. 2003. *State of the world population: People, poverty and possibilities*, chap. 6: HIV/AIDS and Poverty, pp. 42–44.

Ungphakorn, J., & Sittitrai, W. (1994). The Thai response to the HIV/AIDS epidemic. *AIDS, 8* (Suppl. 2), S155–S163.

United Nations. (2002). *HIV/AIDS awareness and behavior.* New York: United Nations.

Urdaneta, C. (2003, September). Best practices: What do we know about prevention programs that work? *AIDSLink, 81.*

USAID. (2000, March). *Handbook of indicators for HIV/AIDS/STI programs.* Washington, DC: USAID.

USAID/Uganda. (1996). *USAID/Uganda support for AIDS prevention activities with the Ugandan Military.* Kampala: USAID.

USAID/Uganda. (2000). *USAID/Uganda support for AIDS prevention activities with the National Resistance Army, Uganda.* Kampala: USAID.

U.S. Census Bureau. (1998). *Recent HIV seroprevalence levels by country: January 1998.* Washington, DC.

U.S. Census Bureau. (2000). *HIV/AIDS Surveillance Data Base.* Available on CD.

Valenti, W. M. (2002). Managing HIV care: A global perspective. *The AIDS Reader, 12* (8), 328–331.

Vandemoortele, J. (2000, December 1). The "education vaccine" against HIV. *Current Issues In Comparative Education, 3*, (1).

Van de Wijgert, J. H. (1997). The effect of douching, wiping and inserting herbs inside the vagina on the vaginal and cervical mucosa, on the vaginal flora, and on the transmission of human immunodeficiency virus and other sexually transmitted diseases in women in Zimbabwe. Unpublished Ph.D. diss., University of California at Berkeley.

Van Griensven, G. J., de Vroome, E. M., Tielman, R. A., Coutinho, R. A. (1988). Failure rate of condoms during anogenital intercourse in homosexual men. *Genitourinary Medicine, 64* (5), 344–346.

Van Lith, L. M., Hachonda, H., & Underwood, C. 2002. Abstinence—Zambian youth are asking for it. Abstract code: ThPeF8115. *Presentation at AIDS 2002 Barcelona: XIV international AIDS conference. July 7–12, 2002.*

Van Rossem, R., Meekers, D., & Zkinyemi, Z. (2001). Consistent condom use with different types of partners: Evidence from two Nigerian surveys. *AIDS Education and Prevention, 13* (3), 252–267.

Varga, C. (2001). Coping with HIV/AIDS in Durban's commercial sex industry. *AIDS Care, 13* (3), 351–365.

Vavrus, F. (2000). The contributions of cultural theory to the study of AIDS and education. *Current Issues in Comparative Education 3* (1). Available at: www.tc.columbia.edu/cice.

Velimirovic, B. (1984). Traditional medicine is not primary health care: A polemic. *Curare, 7* (1), 61–79.

Veloso, V. G., Pilotto, J. H., Azambuja, R., do Valle, F. F., Perez, M., Grinsztein, B. et al. (1998). High prevalence of HIV infection in low income pregnant women in Rio de Janeiro-Brazil [Abstract]. *12th world AIDS conference: Geneva, June 28–July 3, 1998.* Geneva.

Voelker, R. (2001). HIV/AIDS in the Caribbean: Big problems among small. *Journal of the American Medical Association, 285,* 2961–2963.

Vos, T. (1988). Attitudes to sex and sexual behaviour in rural Matabeleland, Zimbabwe. *Population Today, 16* (2), 5.

Wald, A., Langenberg, A. G., Link, K., Izu, A. E., Ashley, R., Warren, T., Tyring, S., Douglas, J. M. Jr., & Corey, L. (2001). Effect of condoms on reducing the transmission of herpes simplex virus type 2 from men to women. *Journal of the American Medical Association, 285,* 3100–3106.

Wawer, M. J., Sewankambo, N. K., Serwadda, D., Quinn, T. C., Paxton, L. A., Kiwanuka, N., Wabwire-Mangen, F., Li, C., Lutalo, T., Nalugoda, F., Gaydos, C. A., Moulton, L. H., Meehan, M. O., Ahmed, S., & Gray, R. H. (1999). Control of sexually transmitted diseases for AIDS prevention in Uganda. *Lancet, 353,* 525–535.

Wedderburn, M., Amon, J., & Figueroa, P. (1998). Knowledge, attitudes, beliefs and practices (KABP) about HIV/AIDS among youth aged 12–14 in Jamaica. *AIDS, 12,* 191.

Weller, S., & Davis, K. (2002). Condom effectiveness in reducing heterosexual HIV transmission. *Cochrane Library.* Available at: http://www.update-software.com/abstracts/ab003255.htm.

Welsh, M. J., Puello, E., Meade, M., Kome, S., & Nutley, T. (2001). Evidence of diffusion from a targeted HIV/AIDS intervention in the Dominican Republic. *Journal of Biosocial Science, 33* (1), 107–119.

Weniger, B., & Brown, T. (1996). The march of AIDS through Asia. *New England Journal of Medicine, 335,* 343–345.

Westinghouse Health Systems. (1985). Encusesta nacional de prevalencia de anticonceptivos: Hombres. Informe de resultados, 1984–85 [National Contraceptive Prevalence Survey: Results for Men]. Columbia, MD: Westinghouse Health Systems.

White, R., Cleland, J., & Carael, M. (2000). Links between premarital sexual behavior and extramarital intercourse: Multi-site analysis. *AIDS, 14,* 2323–2331.

White, R. G., Orroth, K. K., Korenromp, E. L., Bakker, R., Wambura, M., Sewankambo, N. K., et al. (2002). Can population differences in Mwanza, Rakai and Masaka explain the contrasting outcomes of the intervention trials? A modelling study [Abstract]. *XIV international AIDS conference: Barcelona, July 7–12, 2002: Knowledge and commitment for action*. Barcelona, Spain.

Whitworth, J., Muyinda, H., & Pool, R. (2000). Harnessing traditional sex education institutions: The senga model in Uganda [Abstract]. *XIII international AIDS conference, Durban, July 9–14, 2000: Break the silence*. Durban, South Africa.

Wierzba, T. F., & Tumushabe, J. (1994). *Rakai AIDS Information Network Baseline Survey*. APCP. Washington, DC: Worled Learning, Inc.

Wilson, D. (2002, September). Epidemiological overview. Paper presented at the "ABC" Experts Technical Meeting, USAID, Washington, DC.

Witte, K. (1992, December). Putting the fear back into fear appeals: The extended parallel process model. *Communication Monographs, 59*. Available at: http://www.msu.edu/~wittek/fearback.htm.

Witte, K. (1998). Fear as motivator, fear as inhibitor: Using the EPPM to explain fear appeal successes and failures. In P. A. Andersen and L. K. Guerrero (Eds.), *The Handbook of Communication and Emotion* (pp. 423–450). New York: Academic Press.

Witte, K., & Allen, M. (2000). A meta-analysis of fear appeals: Implications for effective public health campaigns. *Health Education & Behavior, 27* (5): 608–632.

Witte, K., Girma, B., & Girgre, A. (in press). Addressing the underlying mechanisms to HIV/AIDS preventive behaviors in Ethiopia. *International Quarterly of Community Health Education, 21* (2).

Wolitski, R., MacGowan, R., Higgins, D., & Jorgensen, C. (1997). The effects of HIV counseling and testing on risk-related practices and help-seeking behavior. *AIDS Education and Prevention, 9* (Suppl. B), 52–67.

World Bank. (1997). *Confronting AIDS: Public priorities in a global epidemic*. New York: Oxford University Press.

World Bank. (1999, January). Uganda: The sexually transmitted infections project: Findings (World Bank Publication no. 127). Washington, DC.

Yamey, G. (2001). San Francisco's HIV infection rate doubles. *British Medical Journal, 322*, 260.

Zaba, B. W., Carpenter, L. M., Boerma, J. T., Gregson, S., Nakiyingi, J., & Urassa, M. (2000). Adjusting ante-natal clinic data for improved estimates of HIV prevalence among women in sub-Saharan Africa. *AIDS, 14*, 2741–2750.

Zaba, B. W., & Gregson, S. (1998). Measuring the impact of HIV on fertility in Africa. *AIDS, 12* (Suppl. 1), S41–S50.

Zaba, B. W., Boerma, J. T., Pisani, E., & Baptiste, N. (2002, March). Estimation of levels and trends in age of first sex from surveys using survival analysis (Measure/Evaluation Working Paper). Calverton, MD: Macro International.

Zenilman, J. M., Weisman, C. S., Rompalo, A. M., Ellish, N., Upchurch, D. M., Hook E. W. et al. (1995). Condom use to prevent incident STDs: The validity of self-reported condom use. *Sexually Transmitted Diseases, 22*, 15–21.

Zvinavashe, G., & Rusakaniko, M. (2000) The reported quality of condom use by young adult Zimbabwean males at higher learning centres in Harare. *Central African Journal of Medicine, 46* (6), 158–161.

Index

'i' indicates an illustration; 't' indicates a table; 'n' indicates a note.

ABOUT THE AUTHOR

Edward C. Green is a member of the President's Advisory Committee on HIV/AIDS. He is a medical anthropologist and Senior Research Scientist at the Harvard Center for Population and Development Studies, part of Harvard University's School of Public Health.